Titles of related int

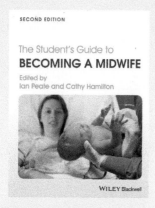

ISBN: 978-1-118-41093-6
"The Student's Guide to Becoming a Midwife is an excellent all-round book to accompany any midwifery student throughout their training … I would recommend it to students in direct entry and shortened programmes of study as well as any practitioners returning to practice or wishing to update their study skills." (British Journal of Midwifery)

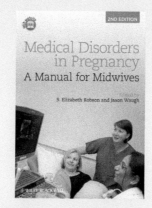

ISBN: 978-1-4443-3748-8
Praise for the 1st edition:
"This book is a must have for any midwife, particularly those working in the community, clinics and in high-risk areas… This book is an extremely useful reference tool." (MIDIRS Midwifery Digest)

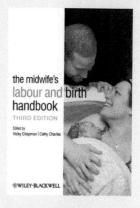

ISBN: 978-0-470-65513-9
Praise for previous editions:
"An excellent resource for both student midwives and qualified staff alike." (Alison James, Midwifery Lecturer, Plymouth University)

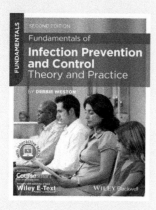

ISBN : 978-1-118-30665-9
"This book would also serve as an excellent quick reference to any healthcare practitioner exploring issues related to everyday practice in infection control and prevention." (Journal of Perioperative Practice)

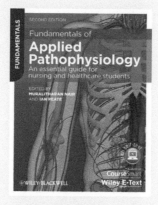

ISBN : 978-0-470-67062-0
Reviews from 1st edition:
"An exceptional book looking at the anatomy and physiology of the human body which would be an invaluable addition to any nursing students' studies … It was a pleasure to read and will be a valuable resource for my studies." (1st year student nurse, Glyndwr University)

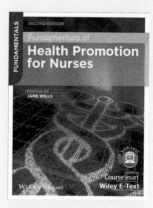

ISBN: 978-1-118-51577-8
Reviews from 1st edition:
"This is a really useful text. Health promotion, an essential aspect of the nurse's role, has not previously been given sufficient prominence. The chapters are written by notable authors and despite their diversity, there is continuity to it, giving it an overall coherence and sense of whole. This is a thoroughly useful text." (Nursing Times)

This title is also available as an e-book. For more details, please see
www.wiley.com/buy/9781118528020
or scan this QR code:

Fundamentals of

Midwifery

A Textbook for Students

EDITED BY

LOUISE LEWIS RGN, RM, BSc(Hons), MSc, PGCE

Lecturer in Midwifery
Faculty of Health and Social Care
University of Hull
Hull, United Kingdom

WILEY Blackwell

This edition first published 2015 © 2015 by John Wiley & Sons, Ltd

Registered Office
John Wiley & Sons Ltd, The Atrium, Southern Gate, Chichester, West Sussex, PO19 8SQ, UK

Editorial Offices
350 Main Street, Malden, MA 02148-5020, USA
9600 Garsington Road, Oxford, OX4 2DQ, UK
The Atrium, Southern Gate, Chichester, West Sussex, PO19 8SQ, UK

For details of our global editorial offices, for customer services, and for information about how to apply for permission to reuse the copyright material in this book please see our website at www.wiley.com/wiley-blackwell.

The rights of Louise Lewis to be identified as the author of the editorial material in this work has been asserted in accordance with the UK Copyright, Designs and Patents Act 1988.

Library of Congress Cataloging-in-Publication Data

Fundamentals of midwifery : a textbook for students / edited by Louise Lewis.
    p. ; cm.
Includes bibliographical references and index.
ISBN 978-1-118-52802-0 (pbk.)
I. Lewis, Louise (Midwife)
[DNLM: 1. Midwifery–methods–Great Britain. WQ 160]
RG525
618.2–dc23

                                   2014032475

A catalogue record for this book is available from the British Library.

Cover image: Shutterstock © Monkey Business Images

Set in 10/12 pt MyriadPro by Toppan Best-set Premedia Limited
Printed and bound by CPI Group (UK) Ltd, Croydon, CR0 4YY

C001022_120922

Contents

Contents

Contents

About the series

Wiley's *Fundamentals* series are a wide-ranging selection of textbooks written to support preregistration nursing, midwifery and other healthcare students throughout their programme of study. Packed full of useful features such as learning objectives, activities to test knowledge and understanding, and clinical scenarios, the titles are also highly illustrated and fully supported by interactive MCQs. Each one includes access to a **Wiley E-Text: powered by VitalSource** – an interactive digital version of the book including downloadable text and images, with highlighting and note-taking facilities. Accessible on your laptop, mobile phone or tablet device, the *Fundamentals* series are *the* most flexible, supportive textbooks available for nursing, midwifery and other healthcare students today.

Contributors

Lynda Bateman RM, Adv.Dip, BSc (Hons), MA, PGCE, FHEA
Lecturer in Midwifery
Faculty of Health and Social Care
University of Hull
Hull, United Kingdom

Mary Beadle SRN, RM, ADM, Cert Ed, BA, MA
Lecturer in Midwifery
Faculty of Health and Social Care
University of Hull
Hull, United Kingdom

Nicky Clark RGN, RM, ADM, Cert Ed, MA
Lead Midwife in Education
Deputy Head of Department, Maternal and Child Health
Faculty of Health and Social Care
University of Hull
Hull, United Kingdom

Julie Flint SRN, RM, BSc (Hons), MSc, PGCE
Lecturer in Midwifery
Supervisor of Midwives
Faculty of Health and Social Care
University of Hull
Hull, United Kingdom

Andrea Hilton BPharm, MSc, PhD, MRPharms, PGCHE, FHEA
Pharmacist and Lecturer in Health Professional Studies
Faculty of Health and Social Care
University of Hull
Hull, United Kingdom

Julie Jomeen RGN, RM, MA, PhD
Professor of Midwifery
Head of Department, Maternal and Child Health
Acting Head of Department, Psychological Health and Wellbeing
Faculty of Health and Social Care
University of Hull
Hull, United Kingdom

Catriona Jones RM, BSc (Hons), MSc, PGCE
Lecturer in Midwifery and Research Associate
Faculty of Health and Social Care
University of Hull
Hull, United Kingdom

Lisa Lachanudis RGN, RM, BSc (Hons), PGCE
Community Midwife
Women and Children's Hospital
Hull and East Yorkshire Hospitals NHS Trust
Hull, United Kingdom

Carol Lambert RM, PG Dip, BSc (Hons), PhD
Lecturer in Midwifery
School of Health Sciences
City University
London, United Kingdom

Louise Lewis RGN, RM, BSc (Hons), MSc, PGCE
Lecturer in Midwifery
Faculty of Health and Social Care
University of Hull
Hull, United Kingdom

Jane Marsh RM, BSc (Hons), MSc, MBAcC
Acupuncturist, Owner of Hull and East Yorkshire Community Acupuncture
Cottingham, United Kingdom

Liz Mason SRN, RM, BA (Hons), Dip App SS, IBCLC
Former Infant Feeding Coordinator
Lactation Consultant and Frenotomy Practitioner
Women and Children's Hospital
Hull and East Yorkshire Hospitals NHS Trust
Hull, United Kingdom

Olanma Ogbuehi RM, PG Dip, BSc (Hons), MSc, PGCE
Lecturer in Midwifery
Faculty of Health and Social Care
University of Hull
Hull, United Kingdom

xiv

Carol Paeglis RN, RM, ADM, BSc (Hons), MA
Former Supervisor of Midwives and Local
Supervising Authority Midwifery Officer
Yorkshire and the Humber, United Kingdom

Jacqui Powell RGN, RM, BSc (Hons)
Clinical Governance Midwife
Health Education Midwife and Supervisor of
Midwives
Women and Children's Hospital
Hull and East Yorkshire Hospitals NHS Trust
Hull, United Kingdom

Fiona Robinson RGN, RM, BSc (Hons)
Healthy Lifestyle Midwife
Women and Children's Hospital
Hull and East Yorkshire Hospitals NHS Trust
Hull, United Kingdom

Liz Smith SRN, SCM, Dip HE, MSc, MA, PGCE(A)
Lecturer in Midwifery and Health Professional
Studies
Faculty of Health and Social Care
University of Hull
Hull, United Kingdom

Sue Townend SRN, RM, BSc (Hons), MSc
Consultant Midwife and Supervisor of Midwives
Calderdale and Huddersfield NHS Foundation
Trust
West Yorkshire, United Kingdom

Brenda Waite SRN, RM, Dip HE, BSc (Hons)
Advanced Midwifery Practitioner and Labour
Ward Co-ordinator
Diana Princess of Wales Hospital
Grimsby, United Kingdom

Sarah Wise RGN, RM, BSc (Hons), MSc
Consultant Midwife, Teenage Pregnancy and
Sexual Health and Supervisor of Midwives
Diana Princess of Wales Hospital
Grimsby, United Kingdom

Foreword

The world of midwifery is changing, whilst much stays the same: the importance of the relationship with women and the need for autonomous professional practise by midwives able to provide sensitive effective care, based on a foundation of scientific understanding; the world we work in is changing. Life and the world of midwifery practice grows more complicated, the knowledge base is expanding, but above all, during a renaissance of midwifery and the development of new ways of practice, of rigorous innovative research, we are reforming what it is to be a midwife, what it means to be a midwife, what our purpose is.

The aim of a healthy mother and baby while necessary is no longer enough. Just as important is a positive experience, preparation for mothering and parenting, caring for women with dignity and respect for their autonomy, supporting the growth of love and family integrity. These form part of a more complex aim that reflects the fundamental contribution of midwifery to the start of life and the new family. And in reflection of these more complicated aims, the fundamentals of midwifery require more complex, more nuanced and rich understanding, knowledge and approaches as a basis.

Today's midwifery students require practical and academic, interpersonal, social and intellectual skills. The many students I have met during my Presidency are articulate, passionate, compassionate and skilled. They are highly motivated and in many ways very demanding of themselves and others in pursuit of excellent midwifery. The 'Fundamentals of Midwifery' will provide students with an excellent resource to lay a foundation to practice. I anticipate that qualified midwives will love it and find it helpful too. The authors of the chapters, experts in their field, and with practical as well as academic experience, lay here a solid rigorous foundation.

Student midwives who are inheriting a renaissance of thinking, understanding and awareness of the nature of modern day midwifery will be tasked with spreading the renaissance into reform. They will form a new world order in midwifery and will help create a new world for women, babies and families. These fundamentals for midwifery will support the reform to a better world of midwifery.

The fundamentals in these pages will be a must read for every student of midwifery, and for many others too.

Professor Lesley Page
President of The Royal College of Midwives,
Visiting Professor, King's College London and Adjunct Professor,
University of Technology Sydney

Preface

The aim of this book is to provide foundational and essential, evidence-based knowledge for midwifery practice. Theoretical and practical perspectives are used to discuss the provision of safe, high-quality professional care to women, babies and their families. Standards for pre-registration midwifery education (NMC 2009) insist student midwives need to be prepared to demonstrate competence and sound knowledge to practise safely and effectively so that, at the point of registration they can assume full responsibility and accountability to undertake the role and responsibilities of a midwife. This book brings together knowledge from a collection of clinical experts and experienced academics to support student's leaning and prepare them for the challenges faced in contemporary midwifery healthcare. There is a good balance between theory and its application to practice using numerous illustrations figures, tables, and interactive text to provide clear insight into the fundamentals of midwifery practice. Each chapter's content is preceded by learning outcomes and an introduction with key points, conclusion, glossary and an extensive reference list at the end. The book is interspersed with student-friendly teaching methods throughout, including: clinical considerations, activities and further reading to encourage in-depth learning, reflection and critical discussion.

This book provides contemporary knowledge, with application to practical skills to develop students professionally, clinically and academically enhancing the learning process. This book will enable the student to explore the midwife's roles and responsibilities and the involvement of the interprofessional team within the wider healthcare setting, providing the foundations for effective evidence-based practice. The book promotes essential skill acquisition and knowledge for students to practise under the supervision of qualified midwives.

The book is aimed at pre-registration student midwives undertaking the Bachelor of Science and Postgraduate Diploma Midwifery Programmes. It is relevant to practising midwives and health and social care provider organisations and educational institutions. The book will also be applicable globally, not just in the United Kingdom, but the wider European market and developing countries, because the fundamentals of midwifery education are recognisable worldwide.

Louise Lewis

Acknowledgements

I would sincerely like to thank all the authors that have contributed their specialised knowledge, clinical expertise and time to the growth and quality of this book. The commitment and dedication from all the authors to ensure the book consistently provides current evidence-based knowledge and illustrative, interactive content has been instrumental to the development of the book. Without the continued support and experienced input from my colleagues both at the University of Hull and in clinical practice, the book would not have been possible.

A special thanks to Jack Green who has drawn some of the artworks for the book and many thanks to Pauline Alexander.

I would like to thank everyone who has given kind permission to use their photographs to illustrate the content.

I would also like to thank Lesley Page for writing the foreword for this book and the Wiley Blackwell team.

Last, but not least, thank you to my partner Jay and family who have encouraged and supported me in being able to sacrifice my time with them.

L.L.

How to use your textbook

Features contained within your textbook

Learning outcome boxes give a summary of the topics covered in a chapter.

Learning outcomes

By the end of this chapter the reader will be able to:

* understand how midwifery has evolved as a profession
* examine how midwifery as a profession is regulated in the united kingdom
* identify the support processes available to student midwives undertaking a pre-registration midwifery programme
* be cognisant of the demands working within the midwifery profession
* identify factors that can facilitate successful course completion.

Clinical consideration boxes give inside information on a topic.

Clinical consideration

Remember that listening is an important skill in communication. Never forget that the woman is more in tune with herself than anyone else is, and her voice must be heard, her views respected and her contribution acknowledged and valued. This can be particularly challenging where women are hesitant or reluctant to participate in decision-making.

Key point boxes highlight points to remember.

Key points

* Midwifery regulation is extensive and rigorous.
* Essential characteristics for student midwives and midwives are deemed paramount to cope with the demands of the profession.
* Clinical practice, supervision of midwifery and education are closely aligned.
* Student support is varied and readily available.

Glossary boxes provide definitions of important terms.

Glossary of terms

CHRE   Centre for Healthcare Regulatory Excellence
CMB   Central Midwives Board
CQC   Care Quality Commission
DBS   Disclosure and Barring Service
EEA   European Economic Area
EI   Emotional intelligence
EMA   European Midwives Association
EU   European Union
ICM   International Confederation of Midwives
ITP   Intention to practise
IQ   Intelligence Quotient
LME   Lead Midwife for Education
LSA   Local Supervising Authority
MINT   Midwives in Teaching
NHS   National Health Service
NMC   Nursing and Midwifery Council
PLF   Practice Learning Facilitator
PIN   Personal Identification Number
PREP   Post-registration ongoing education and practice
PSA   Professional Standards Authority
RCM   Royal College of Midwives
SOM   Supervisor of Midwives
UK   United Kingdom
UKCC   United Kingdom Central Council
VLE   Visual learning environment

Activities and further reading boxes help consolidate learning. These can also be found on the book's companion website (www. wileyfundamentalseries.com/ midwifery) so that you can easily click through to the useful websites referenced in these boxes.

Activity 1.1

Ask yourself why you wanted to become a midwife. It will be useful to revisit this as you progress on your programme. At difficult times within your programme these statements can be very helpful.

Your textbook is full of **photographs, illustrations and tables**.

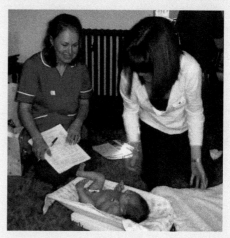

Figure 8.2   Community midwife visiting a woman at home in the postnatal period.

Crosswords and **'Find out more'** exercises help you test yourself after each chapter.

Find out more

1. For more information on the history of midwifery read:
   - Cowell, B., Wainwright, D. (1981) *'Behind the Blue Door: The History of the Royal College of Midwives 1881–1981'.* London: Balliere Tindall.
   - Leap, N., Hunter, B. (1993) *The Midwife's Tale: An oral history from handywoman to professional midwife.* London: Scarlet Press.

2. Read the article below and consider how you can prepare yourself and maximise the many invaluable learning experiences you will encounter during your programme and indeed as a midwife.
   - Healey, J., Spence, M. (2007) *Surviving Your Placement in Health and Social Care A Student Handbook.* Open University Press.

3. Read the article below and think if you can see yourself in any of the student midwives comments? Does this give any advice around how to keep your motivation in the real world of maternity care?
   - Carolan, M., Kruger, G. (2011) Understanding midwifery studies: Commencing students' views. *Midwifery* 27, pp. 642–647.

4. Read the article
   - Snow, S. (2010) Mutual newness mothers experiences of student midwives. *British Journal of Midwifery* 18(1), pp. 38–41
     a. Think about how you can and do foster an effective relationship with the woman.
     b. How can you ensure that you reflect this in your assessment documents?

The anytime, anywhere textbook

Wiley E-Text

For the first time, your textbook comes with free access to a **Wiley E-Text: Powered by VitalSource**version – a digital, interactive version of this textbook which you own as soon as you download it.

Your **Wiley E-Text** allows you to:

Search: Save time by finding terms and topics instantly in your book, your notes, even your whole library (once you've downloaded more textbooks)

Note and Highlight: Colour code, highlight and make digital notes right in the text so you can find them quickly and easily

Organize: Keep books, notes and class materials organized in folders inside the application

Share: Exchange notes and highlights with friends, classmates and study groups

Upgrade: Your textbook can be transferred when you need to change or upgrade computers

Link: Link directly from the page of your interactive textbook to all of the material contained on the companion website

The **Wiley E-Text** version will also allow you to copy and paste any photograph or illustration into assignments, presentations and your own notes.

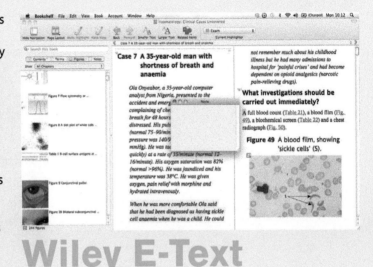

To access your Wiley E-Text:

- Find the redemption code on the inside front cover of this book and carefully scratch away the top coating of the label. Visit **www.vitalsource.com/software/bookshelf/downloads** to download the Bookshelf application to your computer, laptop, tablet or mobile device.
- If you have purchased this title as an e-book, access to your **Wiley E-Text** is available with proof of purchase within 90 days. Visit **http://support.wiley.com** to request a redemption code via the 'Live Chat' or 'Ask A Question' tabs.
- Open the Bookshelf application on your computer and register for an account.
- Follow the registration process and enter your redemption code to download your digital book.
- For full access instructions, visit **www.wileyfundamentalseries.com/midwifery**.

The VitalSource Bookshelf can now be used to view your Wiley E-Text on iOS, Android and Kindle Fire!

- **For iOS:** Visit the app store to download the VitalSource Bookshelf: http://bit.ly/17ib3XS
- **For Android:** Visit the Google Play Market to download the VitalSource Bookshelf: http://bit.ly/ZMEGvo
- **For Kindle Fire, Kindle Fire 2 or Kindle Fire HD:** Simply install the VitalSource Bookshelf onto your Fire (see how at http://bit.ly/11BVFn9). You can now sign in with the email address and password you used when you created your VitalSource Bookshelf Account

Full E-Text support for mobile devices is available at: http://support.vitalsource.com

CourseSmart

CourseSmart gives you instant access (via computer or mobile device) to this Wiley-Blackwell e-book and its extra electronic functionality, at 40% off the recommended retail print price. See all the benefits at **www.coursesmart.com/students**.

Instructors … receive your own digital desk copies!

CourseSmart also offers instructors an immediate, efficient, and environmentally-friendly way to review this textbook for your course.

For more information visit **www.coursesmart.com/instructors**.

With **CourseSmart**, you can create lecture notes quickly with copy and paste, and share pages and notes with your students. Access your **CourseSmart** digital textbook from your computer or mobile device instantly for evaluation, class preparation, and as a teaching tool in the classroom.

Simply sign in at **http://instructors.coursesmart.com/bookshelf** to download your Bookshelf and get started. To request your desk copy, hit 'Request Online Copy' on your search results or book product page.

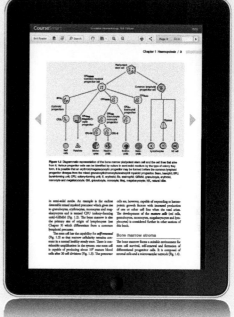

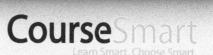

Learn Smart. Choose Smart.

We hope you enjoy using your new textbook. Good luck with your studies!

About the companion website

Don't forget to visit the companion website for this book:

www.wileyfundamentalseries.com/midwifery

There you will find valuable material designed to enhance your learning, including:

* Interactive multiple-choice questions
* Interactive true/false questions
* Case studies to test your knowledge
* Glossary of key terms

Scan this QR code to visit the companion website:

Chapter 1

To be a midwife

Nicky Clark
University of Hull, Hull, UK

Carol Paeglis
Former Supervisor of Midwives and Local Supervising Authority Midwifery Officer, Yorkshire and the Humber, UK

Learning outcomes

By the end of this chapter the reader will be able to:

- understand how midwifery has evolved as a profession
- examine how midwifery as a profession is regulated in the united kingdom
- identify the support processes available to student midwives undertaking a pre-registration midwifery programme
- be cognisant of the demands working within the midwifery profession
- identify factors that can facilitate successful course completion.

Introduction

Midwifery is a dynamic profession that is responsive to change. In recent years, the social, economic and technological forces have altered the context of midwifery significantly. The scale of healthcare provision has changed greatly; philosophies and values have been adjusted and the restructuring of healthcare provision has been dramatic. Public expectation regarding involvement in care and opportunities for informed choice has increased; consequently women and their babies expect more than ever before to be partners in the care process.

Midwives provide high-quality professional care to women and their families, acting autonomously, accountably and responsibly within their sphere of practice. This chapter aims to explore the development of midwifery and its professional regulation with the subsequent evolution of the role and responsibilities of a midwife. The quality of midwifery education and the supervision of midwifery will also be examined.

Fundamentals of Midwifery: A Textbook for Students, First Edition. Edited by Louise Lewis.
© 2015 John Wiley & Sons, Ltd. Published 2015 by John Wiley & Sons, Ltd.
Companion website: www.wileyfundamentalseries.com/midwifery

Activity 1.1

Ask yourself why you wanted to become a midwife. It will be useful to revisit this as you progress on your programme. At difficult times within your programme these statements can be very helpful.

To be a midwife is to understand the role and responsibilities of being a midwife. The midwifery profession is recognised globally and is defined by the International Confederation of Midwives (ICM) (2011) as:

> …A midwife is a person who has successfully completed a midwifery education programme that is duly recognized in the country where it is located and that is based on the ICM Essential Competencies for Basic Midwifery Practice and the framework of the ICM Global Standards for Midwifery Education; who has acquired the requisite qualifications to be registered and/ or legally licensed to practice midwifery and use the title 'midwife'; and who demonstrates competency in the practice of midwifery…

This definition is complex; therefore the professional status and regulation of midwifery nationally and internationally will now be clarified.

The professional status and regulation of midwifery

Historically the professional status of midwifery in England and Wales began with The Midwives Act 1902. This enabled the state enrolment of midwives and established the Central Midwives Board (CMB) for England and Wales. The Midwives Institute was established in the 1880s and was instrumental in the application of the Midwives Act. The Midwives Institute became known as the Royal College of Midwives (RCM) in 1941. All practising midwives were enrolled with the CMB by 1910. A Midwives Act was not passed in Scotland until 1915, which built on the experience of the CMB for England and Wales when setting up the CMB for Scotland.

The CMB produced an annual Roll of Midwives, which was a list of qualified midwives, indicating which were practising. The CMB was independent from nursing, although many midwives were nurses. In 1983 the United Kingdom Central Council for Nursing, Midwifery and Health Visiting (UKCC) replaced the General Nursing Council (Nursing) and the CMB (Midwifery), which brought the nursing, and midwifery records together for the first time. The Nursing Midwifery Council (NMC) was established under the Nursing and Midwifery Order 2001 ('the order') (SI:2002/253) and came into being on 1 April 2002, abolishing the UKCC and its four National Boards.

Midwifery, as a profession is recognised globally, although there are wide variations in education and scope of practice between the different continents. Currently, in the United Kingdom, the NMC is the nursing and midwifery regulator for England, Wales, Scotland, Northern Ireland and the Islands. The aims of the NMC are outlined in Box 1.1.

The NMC

The NMC are governed by legislation approved by the Houses of Parliament and this is detailed in what is known as the Statutory Instruments (SIs). SIs allow an Act of Parliament to be brought

Box 1.1   Aims of the NMC

- Exist to safeguard the health and wellbeing of the public.
- Set standards of education, training, conduct and performance so that nurses and midwives can deliver high quality healthcare consistently throughout their careers.
- Ensure that nurses and midwives keep their skills and knowledge up to date and uphold the professional standards.
- Have clear and transparent processes to investigate nurses and midwives who fall short of the standards.

into force or altered. The Statutory Instrument 2002 No. 253 is The Nursing and Midwifery Order 2001, and replaced the Nurses, Midwives and Health Visitors Act 1997.

The main objective of the NMC in exercising its functions under The Order is to safeguard the health and wellbeing of persons using or needing the services of registrants. The principal functions of the Council are to establish from time to time standards of education, training, conduct and performance for nurses and midwives and to ensure the maintenance of those standards.

Part VIII of the Nursing and Midwifery Order is specific to Midwifery and is concerned with:

- The Midwifery Committee.
- Rules as to midwifery practice.
- Local supervision of midwives.

Since 1 December 2012, following the Health and Social Care Act (2012) the NMC has been regulated by the Professional Standards Authority for Health and Social Care (PSA). The PSA replaced the Council for Healthcare Regulatory Excellence (CHRE). The PSA's function is to ensure that the NMC and other healthcare regulators promote the best interests of patients and the public and ensure consistency across the professions (Yearley and Dawson-Goodey 2014).

European Union

The UK became part of the European community in 1973, and after the Maastricht Treaty was signed in 1992, the European Union (EU) was formed. As a member state of the EU, all EU legislation must be enforced and UK law must adhere to the EU framework and refer to the European Court of Justice. The NMC maintains close partnerships with colleagues and decision makers in Europe to ensure they can influence EU legislation in the interests of patients and the public in the UK.

There are three main institutions involved in EU legislation:

- The European Parliament, which represents the EU's citizens and is directly elected by them.
- The Council of the European Union, which represents the governments of the individual member countries. The Presidency of the Council is shared by the member states on a rotating basis.
- The European Commission, which represents the interests of the Union as a whole.

Together, these three institutions produce the new policies and laws that apply throughout the EU. In principle, the Commission proposes new laws, and the Parliament and Council adopt them. The Commission and the member countries then implement them, and the Commission ensures that the laws are properly applied and implemented.

EU directives

The purpose of the EU is to facilitate the freedom of movement of people, goods and services. In the case of seven professions who have to be registered to practice (doctors, nurses, dentists, midwives, veterinarians, opticians and architects); specific sectarian directives were developed as the EU recognised that the purpose of the registration is first and foremost the protection of the public. To ensure the protection of the public throughout the EU, directives were developed so that a minimum standard of education and practice could be identified. Midwifery education and practice are determined by the Directive 2005/36/EC of the European Parliament and of the Council (2005). This Directive has just been amended on 20 November 2013 to ensure greater efficiency and transparency with the recognition of professional qualifications and has placed value on the use of a European Professional Card (Directive 2013/55/EU, 2013).

The NMC set standards for education and practice and give guidance to professionals. The latest standards for pre-registration midwifery education (NMC 2009) are guided by the international definition of a midwife and the requirements of the European Union Directive Recognition of Professional Qualifications 2005/36/EC Article 40 (training of midwives) and amendments to the EU Directive as stated above. These directives stipulate the experience that students must demonstrate before registering as a qualified midwife and are listed in Box 1.2.

All member states that adopt this directive must ensure that midwives are at least entitled to take up and pursue the following activities listed in Box 1.3.

The NMC insist that education programmes prepare students to practise safely and effectively so that, on registration, they can assume full responsibility and accountability to undertake the

Box 1.2 The European Union Article 40 (training of midwives) of Directive 2005/36/EU

- Advising of pregnant women, involving at least 100 antenatal examinations.
- Supervision and care of at least 40 women in labour. (The student should personally carry out at least 40 deliveries; where this number cannot be reached owing to the lack of available women in labour, it may be reduced to a minimum of 30, provided that the student participates actively in 20 further deliveries.)
- Active participation with breech deliveries. (Where this is not possible because of lack of breech deliveries, practice may be in a simulated situation.)
- Performance of episiotomy and initiation into suturing. Initiation shall include theoretical instruction and clinical practice. The practice of suturing includes suturing of the wound following an episiotomy and a simple perineal laceration. (This may be in a simulated situation if absolutely necessary.)
- Supervision and care of 40 women at risk in pregnancy, or labour or postnatal period.
- Supervision and care (including examination) of at least 100 postnatal women and healthy newborn infants.
- Observation and care of the newborn requiring special care including those born pre-term, post-term, underweight or ill.
- Care of women with pathological conditions in the fields of gynaecology and obstetrics.
- Initiation into care in the field of medicine and surgery. Initiation shall include theoretical instruction and clinical practice.

(NMC 2009)

Box 1.3   Article 42 of Directive 2005/36/EU

- To provide sound family planning information and advice.
- To diagnose pregnancies and monitor normal pregnancies; to carry out examinations necessary for the monitoring of the development of normal pregnancies.
- To prescribe or advise on the examinations necessary for the earliest possible diagnosis of pregnancies at risk.
- To provide a programme of parenthood preparation and a complete preparation for childbirth including advice on hygiene and nutrition
- To care for and assist the mother during labour and to monitor the condition of the fetus in utero by the appropriate clinical and technical means.
- To conduct spontaneous deliveries including where required an episiotomy and, in urgent cases, a breech delivery.
- To recognise the warning signs of abnormality in the mother or infant which necessitate referral to a doctor and to assist the latter where appropriate; to take the necessary emergency measures in the doctor's absence, in particular the manual removal of the placenta, possibly followed by a manual examination of the uterus.
- To examine and care for the newborn infant; to take all initiatives which are necessary in case of need and to carry out where necessary immediate resuscitation.
- To care for and monitor the progress of the mother in the postnatal period and to give all necessary advice to the mother on infant care to enable her to ensure the optimum progress of the newborn infant.
- To carry out treatment prescribed by a doctor.
- To maintain all necessary records.

(NMC 2009)

activities of a midwife as directed by the EU Directive. To meet this in the UK, the NMC expect students, at the end of their midwifery programme to demonstrate competence in the following tasks, listed in Box 1.4:

Box 1.4   Students must demonstrate competence in:

- Sound, evidence-based knowledge of facilitating the physiology of childbirth and the newborn, and be competent in applying this in practice.
- A knowledge of psychological, social, emotional and spiritual factors that may positively or adversely influence normal physiology, and be competent in applying this in practice.
- Appropriate interpersonal skills (as identified in the Essential Skills Cluster – Communication) to support women and their families.
- Skills in managing obstetric and neonatal emergencies, underpinned by appropriate knowledge.

(Continued)

- Being autonomous practitioners and lead carers to women experiencing normal childbirth and being able to support women throughout their pregnancy, labour, birth and postnatal period, in all settings including midwife-led units, birthing centres and the home.
- Being able to undertake critical decision-making to support appropriate referral of either the woman or baby to other health professionals or agencies when there is recognition of normal processes being adversely affected and compromised.

(NMC 2009)

The International Confederation of Midwives

In view of the Global Midwifery agenda, the International Confederation of Midwives (ICM) is active and current. The use of global standards, competencies, tools and guidelines ensures that midwives in all countries have effective education, regulation and strong associations. The ICM has developed various interrelated ICM Core Documents, which guide Midwives Associations and their Governments to review and improve on the education and regulation of midwives and midwifery, and enable countries to review their midwifery curricula for the production and retention of a quality midwifery workforce.

The ICM supports, represents and works to strengthen professional associations of midwives throughout the world. There are currently 108 national Midwives Associations, representing 95 countries across every continent. This includes the Royal College of Midwives in the UK, which is the UK's only professional organisation and trade union led by midwives for midwives. The ICM is organised into four regions: Africa, the Americas, Asia Pacific and Europe. Together these associations represent more than 300,000 midwives globally. Its first recorded meeting was in 1919 in Belgium after World War I.

ICM Scope of Practice

…The midwife is recognised as a responsible and accountable professional who works in partnership with women to give the necessary support, care and advice during pregnancy, labour and the postpartum period, to conduct births on the midwife's own responsibility and to provide care for the newborn and the infant. This care includes preventative measures, the promotion of normal birth, the detection of complications in mother and child, the accessing of medical care or other appropriate assistance and the carrying out of emergency measures.

The midwife has an important task in health counselling and education, not only for the woman, but also within the family and the community. This work should involve antenatal education and preparation for parenthood and may extend to women's health, sexual or reproductive health and child care.

A midwife may practise in any setting including the home, community, hospitals, clinics or health units…

(Revised and adopted by ICM Council June 15, 2011. Due for review 2017)

Key midwifery concepts

(See Box 1.5.)

The European Midwives Association (EMA) is a non-profit and non-governmental organisation of midwives, representing midwifery organisations and associations from the member states of the European Union (EU), members of the Council of Europe, the European Economic Area (EEA) and EU applicant countries.

Box 1.5   Key midwifery concepts that define the unique role of midwives

- Partnership with women to promote self-care and the health of mothers, infants, and families.
- Respect for human dignity and for women as persons with full human rights.
- Advocacy for women so that their voices are heard.
- Cultural sensitivity, including working with women and healthcare providers to overcome those cultural practices that harm women and babies.
- A focus on health promotion and disease prevention that views pregnancy as a normal life event.

Activity 1.2

After thinking about why you wanted to become a midwife, identify how this links to the role, responsibilities and regulation of the midwife.

Interpersonal skills and attributes

Preparedness to learn, accept, and not judge, to give advice and support are key characteristics of all healthcare professionals today. Emotional maturity to facilitate trust, respect and confidence from the women and families being cared for is also crucial. Maturity does not mean age. It is now recognised that to be a midwife requires in-depth tacit knowledge, competence and confidence to undertake the activities of a midwife, which are, as evidenced laid down in statute. In recognition of this, all midwifery programmes are now at a minimum level of degree. However, midwifery, although demanding and requiring a diverse knowledge base also needs compassion, caring and commitment. These are harder to measure.

Emotional intelligence (EI) as a concept has been researched extensively within other professions, but not within midwifery. It has been a major topic of debate since its appearance in the psychological literature in 1990 (Salovey and Mayer 1990). The interest in EI seems to stem from the view that despite seemingly average intelligence, some individuals appear to do well in life, whereas others with a seemingly high intelligence quotient (IQ), struggle with life challenges (Goldenberg et al. 2006). EI is defined as:

> …the capacity to reason about emotions to enhance thinking. It includes the ability to accurately perceive emotions, to access and generate emotions so as to assist thought, to understand emotions and emotional knowledge, and to reflectively regulate emotions as to promote emotional and intellectual growth…
>
> (Mayer et al. 2004, p. 197)

Patterson and Bagley (2011) believe that raising the profile of EI will increase effectiveness and capacity in midwives to manage the constant change and challenges facing the profession. To be emotionally intelligent appears to evidence higher coping strategies, successful problem solving, higher academic achievement, improved interpersonal relationships and the ability to feel less anxious and to be more resilient (Kun et al. 2012). Attributes deemed desirable within a highly emotive and challenging profession such as midwifery.

These attributes are arguably as individual as the women with whom midwives provide care. How your own emotions and those of others are managed, combined with empathy and communication skills, without provoking conflict in a practice situation that is becoming increasingly challenging, are important components that must be considered in midwifery practice. However, these are profound concepts; therefore the challenge to identify, measure and apply meaning to them, in an attempt to facilitate appropriate recruitment and retention to a profession that is currently at the height of media attention and scrutiny is one that must now be faced.

Healthcare education has evolved beyond recognition since the NHS was formed. With the move into Higher Education in the early 1990s for all midwifery education, the emphasis on academic achievement is consistently in the spotlight. With the decision for all pre-registration midwifery programmes to be at degree level by 2009 (NMC 2009) academic entry and degree classifications are now seen as key to a university's success. Academic achievement is naturally aligned with IQ; however midwifery is more naturally aligned with care and compassion. Therefore it is reasonable to assume that a successful midwife today should possess a high IQ, should aim for academic success, and have the personality to care for and cope with the demands of the nature of midwifery practice. However, as the literature disputes the association between EI and IQ (Cherniss et al, 2006; Davis 2012; Faguy 2012), recruitment and retention strategies have limited evidence on which to be based.

Performance in practice is largely observable and constitutes a minimum of 50% of the midwifery programme; it must be undertaken in clinical practice. The reliability of the practice assessments undertaken by clinical midwives has been scrutinised since their introduction by the NMC and continues to be open to criticism of subjectivity, unreliability and inequity.

Working within the NHS is a unique experience, and many studies have considered socialisation to the culture of midwifery and the NHS as both a barrier and a coping mechanism for those working within it. Even those with experience as healthcare support workers have reported experiencing a culture and reality shock (Brennan and McSherry 2007). Socialisation can lead to a loss of idealism and identification of negative aspects of care, which can decrease the ability to cope (Mackintosh 2006). Organisational socialisation, where interpersonal relationships are to be maintained, together with adaptation to the ward rules and culture, can create frustration and stress (Feng and Tsai 2012). However, resilience and mental toughness (Clough and Strycharczyk 2012), can foster clinical reasoning and critical decision-making abilities, which are vital in this profession. Midwives must have the ability to question and challenge practices and make difficult decisions based on available evidence and the preferences of women in their care (Parsons and Griffiths 2007).

There is currently a great deal in the press about the kind of skills and attitudes healthcare professionals need to have. This is related to the recent Francis Report (2010) and the Care Quality Commission (CQC) (2013) report into maternity services at Barrow in Furness. This has led to the Department of Health (DH) strategy to set out the requirement for care and compassion around those who are in the caring profession (DH 2012).

Further reading activity

Read: The vision for midwifery care within the Department of Health strategy.
[Available online] http://www.england.nhs.uk/wp-content/uploads/2012/12/6c-midwifery.pdf

Activity 1.3

Think about how you can be caring and compassionate at all times and what aspects of the caring environment could challenge this?

Effective communication is crucial. Midwives work in a multidisciplinary environment and therefore must be able to consistently communicate accurately and clearly with women, their families and to other professionals. Being able to communicate effectively both verbally, and in writing to ensure that all care provided is safe, is essential. The NMC (2009) standards reflect this requirement and assessment aims to reduce and challenge barriers.

Professional expectations

As soon as a person commences a professional programme that on completion will allow entry onto the NMC register, then their behaviour is under scrutiny. This behaviour is set out in NMC documents, which are periodically updated. The code of practice and the NMC guide for students sets out clearly what is classed as acceptable and unacceptable behaviour.

Further reading activity

Read: The Code (NMC 2008a) and student guidance on professional conduct (NMC 2011a) and think about what aspects of your behaviour you might need to change in order to meet these codes.

One of these aspects of behaviour may be the use of social networking sites. Practitioners and students must not put anything on these sites that they would not be happy for the entire world to see. This has implications in relation to the confidentiality of patients and other health-care workers, as well as to appropriate language and comments (Jones and Hayter 2013). The transition to a student midwife can be a challenging one and it is useful to revisit the code and student guidance, as well as discussing this with midwifery lecturers and midwives.

Life as a student midwife

Further reading activity

Read: Lisa McTavish's article about her experiences as a student midwife and think about what lessons you can learn from her story and write your own story.

McTavish, L. (2010) 'A student midwives' experience in the 21st century' *British Journal of Midwifery* 18 (1), pp. 43–47.

Student midwives often face challenging times on their demanding midwifery programmes. This is good preparation for post-registration practice: some 'mental resilience' is needed for students and midwives alike. This is currently more challenging due to the latest changes to the NHS structure which are underway and the financial situation within the NHS. This means that students and midwives need to develop coping strategies in order to manage the working environment, whilst still giving good quality care.

Further reading activity

For more information on the latest changes in the NHS, read: The New NHS 2013. [Available online] http://www.nhs.uk/NHSEngland/thenhs/about/Pages/nhsstructure.aspx

As midwifery education is very intimate in its delivery and practice, 'people' skills are paramount. This is where, arguably, the emotionally intelligent element plays a significant role in course progression. Generally, mentor/student relationships are acknowledged as compatible or not; adjustments can easily be made if required. The important thing is to recognise if there is a problem and address it. This requires a confident, self-compassionate and resilient individual and highlights that appropriate student recruitment is vital.

There is undisputed evidence to suggest that healthcare practitioners cope better than others with the challenge of the demands placed upon them, and there are also those who actively flourish and thrive. Resilience has been defined as:

> …The inner strength, competence, optimism, flexibility and the ability to cope effectively when faced with adversity…
>
> (Wagnild 2009, p. 105)

Control is crudely, a cognitive ability, which requires knowledge and skill. It is seen as important when coping within the workplace and cited as a major cause of burnout if lost. Resilience has a core philosophy, which makes individuals take responsibility for their own success or failure, and it is a measure of self-worth (self-compassion). It focuses on emotional flexibility, responsiveness, strengths and resilience. Compassion has been defined as:

> …Being open to and moved by the suffering of others, so that one desires to ease their suffering. It also involves offering others' patience, kindness and non-judgmental understanding, recognising that all humans are imperfect and make mistakes…
>
> (Neff 2003, p. 224)

Buddhist belief regards the self and others as interdependent; therefore to be compassionate to others is not possible without compassion for the self (Baer 2010).

University students must be adult learners who must develop and enhance their own learning skills. Student midwives therefore should identify their needs; self-assess and be able to seek help and support proactively. Seeking help retrospectively, following poor performance in assessments, indicates earlier missed opportunities. There are many people within the university and the clinical practice areas who can help and support students; it is the student's role to seek them out when necessary.

The programme

The midwifery degree is a degree of two awards: first, the professional award, Midwifery, which is regulated by the NMC, and must adhere to all the NMC documentation, standards and guidance. The second award is the academic award of a degree, which is regulated and monitored by the university where it is being studied.

With the professional recognition of becoming a midwife, having evidenced all the requirements and competences to be admitted to the professional register and achieve the University's
academic standard to be awarded a degree, comes an increase in workload and commitment.
Despite being forewarned of this, this creates a major struggle for some student midwives.

There are two lengths of programme. One is 156 weeks in length, or 3 years (NMC 2009); the
other is where the student is already registered with the NMC as a nurse level 1 (adult). The
length of this programme is not less than 78 weeks full time. Both student groups are *pre-
registration* midwifery students, who will be competent to practise, at the point of registration.
The theoretical content is driven by the Standards (NMC 2009); the clinical practice is driven by
local provision and the EU Directive. The university processes generate the structure, assessment, teaching style and resources. All universities that provide pre-registration midwifery must
appoint a Lead Midwife for Education (LME).

> …*The lead midwife for education is an expert in midwifery education and has the knowledge
> and skills to develop policy, as well as to advise others on all matters relating to midwifery educa-
> tion. She should liaise directly with commissioning and purchasing agencies for midwifery edu-
> cation, as well as being involved in any decisions regarding midwifery education…*
>
> (NMC 2009, p. 8)

Midwifery lecturers are practising midwives who hold a recognised teaching qualification.
Universities who run pre-registration midwifery programmes employ them. Midwifery programmes usually exist within University Faculties or Departments encompassing Health, Social
Care, or Medicine and Allied Health. The number of midwifery lecturers within each university
was traditionally determined by student numbers and worked on a ratio of 1:10; however this
is variable across the country and does impact on the quality of the teaching resource. Midwifery lecturers are all practising midwives; they must maintain their competence and confidence as a midwife, notify their intention to practise annually and remain up-to-date with
mandatory training and education. Midwifery lecturers, in addition to teacher training, should
hold or be working towards a higher degree or doctorate. In meeting these requirements, midwifery lecturers are able to apply contemporary practice to the classroom. This is to address the
theory/practice divide which can occur if practice taught away from the clinical area is not
consistent with practice that is taught/observed within the clinical area.

The students' theory elements are assessed generally in the university by the midwifery lecturers employed by that university. Midwives in the clinical areas who are employed by the local
Trusts assess midwifery practice. Assessment of practice must be graded and must contribute
to the award of the degree as per the Standards (NMC 2009). Therefore, as it is the university
who awards the degree, it is exceptional if university staff are not solely responsible for the
assessment of that award. This has and does cause difficulties when seeking university approval,
which must be granted by the university to offer and support pre-registration midwifery programmes. To address this anomaly, the university seeks reassurance that equity and parity of all
assessments are assured.

Midwives who assess student midwives must be sign-off mentors. The role of the sign-off mentor
is to make judgments about whether a student has achieved the required standards of proficiency
for safe and effective practice for entry to the NMC register. The LME confirms to the approved
education institution assessment board that both the theoretical and practice elements have been
achieved on completion of the programme (NMC 2008b).

The midwife with whom the student will be working mainly provides placement support. The
NMC stipulate that a minimum of 40% of the time is spent working with a sign-off midwifery

mentor, who is an experienced midwife and has undergone additional training to be able to assess the students' practice. Additional support is available by a Supervisor of Midwives who is available 24 hours every day, and a Practice Learning Facilitator (PLF). A PLF is a person who is generally jointly employed by the Trust and the university where students undertake their programme. The PLFs are visible within the clinical areas, and are a point of contact should issues arise; they work alongside a link lecturer. The link lecturer is usually a member of the midwifery teaching team at the university; along with the PLFs they provide ongoing education and training to clinical staff on curriculum issues and student assessment.

A minimum of 50% of the programme must be spent in the clinical area: clinical systems of care will vary between Trusts and some students find that they prefer one system to another. The advantage of the team approach is consistency of mentor and continuity of carer for those accessing that service. The advantage of the non-integrated approach is working with different mentors and adjusting to different placement areas. All midwives, despite the same common goal and mission as depicted in the Midwives Rules and Standards (NMC 2012) work slightly differently. This is the autonomous element of the midwives' role. All students have different learning styles and all educators and mentors have different teaching styles. Therefore some students and mentors/teachers work better together than others. However experiences can be unpredictable and there are times of stress in all systems.

Different students have different learning styles whether in academic or clinical learning; therefore some teaching methods will appeal to some and not others. All curricula should evidence different styles in an attempt to meet the needs of all. All learners can be helped by knowing their own learning styles.

Activity 1.4   Learning styles

The websites below will assist you in identifying your learning style and also examine the learning situations which suite you best. If you have done one of these assessments before, it can still be worth doing this again as these can change over time.

[Available online] http://www.brainboxx.co.uk/A2_LEARNSTYLES/pages/learningstyles.htm and http://www.vark-learn.com/english/page.asp?p=questionnaire

The statutory supervision of midwives

Supervision of midwives was introduced over 110 years ago as a purely inspectorial function to lower maternal mortality rates and to protect mothers and babies from unsafe midwifery practice. It is enshrined in law and has evolved to support the protection of mothers and babies by promoting excellence in midwifery care, through the leadership roles of Supervisors of Midwives. This is achieved by every midwife in the UK having a named Supervisor of Midwives, whether they practise clinically, or in education, or in a research post or whether they practise in the NHS, or are privately employed. Supervisors of Midwives work within a framework of supervision outlined by their Local Supervising Authority (LSA) Midwifery Officer who appoints them to practise within that LSA area. They have a caseload of midwife 'supervisees' and have a responsibility to ensure their supervisees' eligibility to practise by undertaking an annual supervisory review to identify and discuss how best to address any developmental needs. On the basis of that review and on any other relevant information, the supervisor then submits the midwife's annual Intention to Practise (ITP) to the NMC which is displayed to the public on the NMC register.

Clinical consideration

Intrapartum stillbirths are a central indicator of patient safety and quality of care, but despite this stillbirth rates have changed little in the English National Health Service over the past two decades. Increasing evidence indicates that fetal growth restriction is currently missed in most pregnancies in the NHS, and that better antenatal detection needs to become a cornerstone and key indicator of safety and effectiveness in maternity care. This has, therefore, been an LSA priority over recent years with the LSA and supervisors disseminating best practice evidence to midwives within local conferences, presentations, newsletters and during annual supervisory reviews. Preventing poor practice has occurred by the LSA producing a best practice competency assessment tool for fundal height measurement, which supervisors have worked through with midwives to ensure that midwives consistently and competently measure and respond to fetal growth in the same way. Intervening in unacceptable practice has occurred by LSA reviews where clusters of stillbirths have been noted. Reviews have led to some changes to generic practice within Trusts, e.g. the implementation of customised growth charts. Other reviews have led to additional supervisory input to aid the development of individual midwives' practice where required.

All maternity services are required to ensure the availability of 24-hour access to support and advice from a Supervisor of Midwives for midwives and service users. Supervisors practise in a team within maternity services; hold regular supervisors' meetings to determine their local work priorities; are involved in the maternity services' clinical governance systems, for example, audit meetings and risk management meetings; and ensure that their supervisory framework encompasses involvement with their local universities in the recruitment to and progress of student midwives through their midwifery education programmes. Evidence from the diaries of newly qualified midwives (MINT research commissioned by the NMC 2010) indicates that where the role of a Supervisor of Midwives for student midwives occurs it enhances students' understanding of supervision.

The example in Box 1.6 demonstrates how supervisors work to promote excellence in midwifery care, prevent poor midwifery practice and intervene in unacceptable practice.

A Supervisor of Midwives is now commonly assigned to every student midwife undergoing a pre-registration midwifery programme. The student midwife can contact the Supervisor of Midwives, in confidence, at any time to voice concerns or to debrief following an upsetting or difficult situation in the clinical area.

Raising and escalating concerns

Raising and escalating concerns is a fundamental responsibility of all healthcare workers, and the NMC have published guidance on this (NMC 2013). If students or practitioners are worried generally about an issue, wrongdoing or risk which may affect or is affecting others in the workplace or in their care, they should raise a point of concern. This is not an easy thing to do, which is why students are advised where to access support at the start of the programme. These include their personal supervisors, university lecturers, midwifery mentors and Supervisor of Midwives.

Quality assurance

The quality measure of midwife lecturer to student ratio at the university demonstrates the resource commitment from the university to that provision, where 1:10 is seen as best practice.

Clinically, the birth rate to midwife ratio should also be considered, with the additional quality measures of Care Quality Commission reports, Professional Standards for Health and Social Care, Maternity Liaison Committee, LSA audits, all of which are readily available to the public. Evidence suggests that if the team of teachers includes a Supervisor of Midwives, it can enhance communication between the universities and their clinical placement areas and provide an additional level of support to newly qualified midwives during their transition period from that of student midwife.

Midwifery educationalists are often invited members of LSA working groups and receive routine communication, for example newsletters from the LSA, which are disseminated to student midwives. This ensures close links between education and supervision, with resultant benefits to education, supervision and to the LSA. Any forums that bring education, practice, Supervisors of Midwives and the LSA together are in line with Maternity Matters (Department of Health 2007) and research advocating closing the theory–practice gap.

Universities value student evaluations and seek student representation on committees at programme, departmental, faculty and university levels. Student evaluations of modules, placements, programmes and the university are sought and acted upon. The National Student Survey is undertaken annually; all students are invited to complete this in their final year of study. The results are available to the public, and are valued as a serious quality measure of student satisfaction.

Student support

Personal supervision is an element found in all pre-registration midwifery education programmes, and is generally undertaken by a member of the midwifery teaching team. University processes tend to determine the format this takes. The personal supervisor role can play a significant part in a student's progress whilst on the midwifery programme. It allows a relationship to be developed between the personal supervisor and the student, with mutual respect, honesty and confidentiality being crucial components. Ideally the student and personal supervisor meet early after the programme commences agreeing the subsequent frequency and format for further contact. As with the mentor–student relationship, a rapport between the two parties must be established in order to maximize the benefit; therefore the option of changing should always be available. Changing mentors clinically, or personal supervisors in the university, is not a failure, but merely recognition of different learning styles and personality traits.

Student support services are also a feature of Higher Education Institutions, but these vary. The student union is an example. Student midwives/nurses may find it more challenging to participate in student unions and campus life for various reasons (see Figure 1.1). They are still eligible to receive student union support and to participate in any student ballots. It is important to also access various study support services available to all students, including library services, study skills advice and information and communication technologies (ICT). These are all essential to learning and continuing education post-registration. Additionally, most universities will have confidential counselling services, which can be accessed by students; at times these may help to cope with the conflicting demands and stresses which may accompany student life.

Health screening

Health screening has consistently been a feature of all healthcare programmes, with all student midwives requiring health clearance prior to the course commencement and to declare annually their good health and good character (NMC 2009), whilst on the programme and prior to

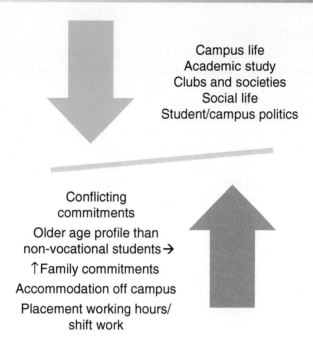

Campus life
Academic study
Clubs and societies
Social life
Student/campus politics

Conflicting
commitments

Older age profile than
non-vocational students→

↑Family commitments

Accommodation off campus

Placement working hours/
shift work

Figure 1.1 Conflicting commitments faced by midwifery students.

their admittance to the NMC professional registers. Students with long-term health issues must be passed as fit to undertake the programme from the occupational health department. Students whilst on clinical placement can also access the Trust occupational health department should the need arise. Students and midwives must take responsibility for their own health, and are required to have all vaccinations recommended by the Department of Health to protect themselves and the people in their care. These include rubella, measles and seasonal influenza. All midwifery students prior to commencing the programme are tested for blood-borne viruses due to the risk of exposure prone procedures.

Criminal record

All students and midwives upon appointment have to undergo a Disclosure and Barring Service (DBS) investigation. Should this return with a positive record, a meeting would be convened between the applicant, an admissions representative and a Trust representative to discuss this in more depth. This meeting would be to determine the gravity of the record, and to determine whether this would preclude the applicant from being successful with this application. Generally, decisions are dependent upon the nature of the offence, circumstances surrounding the offence and the time elapsed since it was committed. All applicants are routinely asked at interview if they have anything to declare; therefore the opportunity is afforded to discuss this frankly and honestly. Should any offence, subsequently disclosed on the DBS not be declared at this point, it is generally viewed unfavourably. It is worthy of note that all offences will be disclosed with an enhanced DBS enquiry, even speeding offences and offences committed as a juvenile. Any subsequent offence, warning, reprimand or caution received whilst on the programme, or as a midwife must be notified to the university (if applicable) or the NMC and may initiate a Fitness to Practise investigation (NMC 2011a).

Life as a midwife

Upon successful course completion, the LME has to be satisfied of the student's good health and character, and that they have completed all the required statutory elements. The LME then notifies the NMC of the student's successful completion and that he/she is satisfied that all requirements have been fulfilled. The successful student is allocated an NMC Personal Identification Number (PIN) and her/his name appears on Part 2 of the professional register. At this point the candidate has become a registered midwife and is licensed to practise midwifery in the UK and other regions of the world, where this is recognised.

Midwives practising in the UK utilise statutory supervision for support and professional development. Annual LSA audit visits to maternity services indicate the substantial psychological, clinical and professional support that Supervisors of Midwives provide to midwives during their careers. Midwives undertake Post-Registration ongoing Education and Practice (PREP) (NMC 2011b) requirements and mandatory training, which is to be superseded by the Revalidation process in 2015. Additionally there are different career routes to consider.

Activity 1.5   What kind of midwife do you want to be?

Think about a midwife you admire and that you feel is a good role model. Undertake a SWOT analysis (Strengths, Weaknesses, Opportunities, and Threats) to identify challenges and support frameworks for you to achieve your goals.

Career routes

To remain firmly rooted in clinical practice is the most popular career choice, with many opportunities to advance experience and scope of practice. These include: intravenous cannulation skills; examination of the newborn; ultrasound techniques; labour ward co-ordinator; Supervisor of Midwives and sign-off midwifery mentor. Some midwives become advanced practitioners and/or consultant midwives by specialising in certain areas, for example, ultrasound, family planning, teenage pregnancy, domestic violence and healthy lifestyles. There is the option of undertaking further academic study by undertaking a master's degree, or a doctorate. These provide the opportunity to undertake research positions. Midwifery management is a vital element to any maternity provision, which again can be a career choice. Some midwives become midwife educators, working within higher education or in a statutory capacity. This list is not exhaustive, but indicative of the pathways available upon qualification as a registered midwife.

Key points

- Midwifery regulation is extensive and rigorous.
- Essential characteristics for student midwives and midwives are deemed paramount to cope with the demands of the profession.
- Clinical practice, supervision of midwifery and education are closely aligned.
- Student support is varied and readily available.

Conclusion

What it means to be a midwife, how you become a midwife and how to remain a midwife is entrenched in EU legislation, and professional standards. The professional status of a midwife is protected, the regulation complex and internationally compliant, the quality and academic rigour of pre-registration midwifery programmes is assured and career choices diverse. Statutory supervision is a major strength of the midwifery profession. The pre-registration midwifery programme is challenging, as is the current climate of maternity service provision. The support systems in place are robust, and are there to be accessed. Completion of the programme and successful retention of high calibre recruits to the profession is pivotal to maintaining the high quality provision women and their families deserve.

This chapter has aimed to provide clarity to the evolvement of midwifery, and how student midwives are recruited and supported to become a confident, competent, compassionate, accountable and autonomous practitioner in the world of midwifery. The following chapters outline the roles and responsibilities of a midwife.

End of chapter activities
Crossword

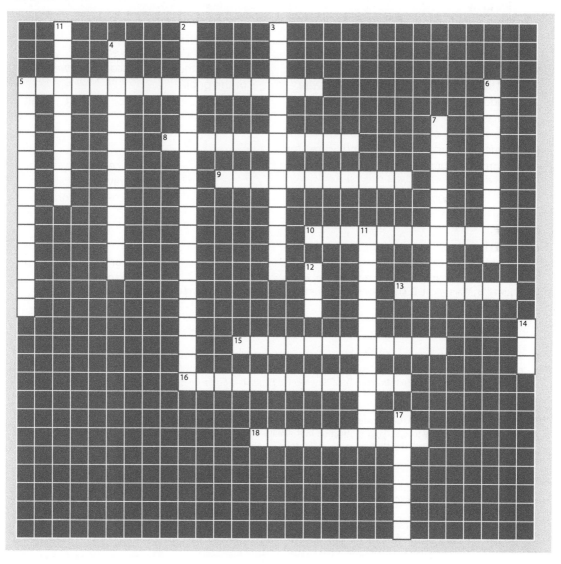

Across

5. Midwives must have the ability to do this.
8. What all care should be.
9. What a midwife and student midwife should have with a woman and her partner.
10. What a midwife needs to be as described by the ICM.
13. A key midwifery concept.
15. What a midwife must be able to do.
16. It can be a barrier and a coping mechanism.
18. Being open to and moved by the suffering of others, so that one desires to ease their suffering.

Down

1. Inner strength, competence, optimism and flexibility.
2. What a midwife or student midwife must have 24 hour access to.
3. An essential characteristic of a midwife.
4. An essential skill which a mentor will demonstrate and teach to a student midwife.
5. Students need to demonstrate competence in this.
6. The number of postnatal women which students must supervise and care for during their programme.
7. A minimum standard for the education and practice of midwives.
11. Something which is paramount in midwifery education.
12. An expert in midwifery education.
14. Exist to safeguard the health and wellbeing of the public.
17. A key characteristic of all health professionals.

Find out more

1. For more information on the history of midwifery read:
   - Cowell, B., Wainwright, D. (1981) *'Behind the Blue Door: The History of the Royal College of Midwives 1881–1981'.* London: Balliere Tindall.
   - Leap, N., Hunter, B. (1993) *The Midwife's Tale: An oral history from handywoman to professional midwife.* London: Scarlet Press.

2. Read the article below and consider how you can prepare yourself and maximise the many invaluable learning experiences you will encounter during your programme and indeed as a midwife.
   - Healey, J., Spence, M. (2007) *Surviving Your Placement in Health and Social Care A Student Handbook.* Open University Press.

3. Read the article below and think if you can see yourself in any of the student midwives comments? Does this give any advice around how to keep your motivation in the real world of maternity care?
   - Carolan, M., Kruger, G. (2011) Understanding midwifery studies: Commencing students' views. *Midwifery* 27, pp. 642–647.

4. Read the article
   - Snow, S. (2010) Mutual newness mothers experiences of student midwives. *British Journal of Midwifery* 18(1), pp. 38–41
     a. Think about how you can and do foster an effective relationship with the woman.
     b. How can you ensure that you reflect this in your assessment documents?

5. For more information visit:
   http://www.europeanmidwives.eu/eu
   http://www.internationalmidwives.org/
   http://www.nmc-uk.org/
   http://www.rcm.org.uk/
   https://www.rcn.org.uk/
   http://www.6cs.england.nhs.uk/pg/dashboard
   http://www.nhs.uk/NHSEngland/thenhs/about/Pages/nhsstructure.aspx
   http://www.england.nhs.uk/wp-content/uploads/2012/12/6c-midwifery.pdf
   http://www.legislation.gov.uk/uksi/2008/1485/pdfs/uksi_20081485_en.pdf
   http://www.brainboxx.co.uk/A2_LEARNSTYLES/pages/learningstyles.htm
   http://www.vark-learn.com/english/page.asp?p=questionnaire

Glossary of terms

CHRE Centre for Healthcare Regulatory Excellence
CMB Central Midwives Board
CQC Care Quality Commission
DBS Disclosure and Barring Service
DH Department of Health
EEA European Economic Area
EI Emotional intelligence
EMA European Midwives Association
EU European Union
ICM International Confederation of Midwives
ITP Intention to practise
IQ Intelligence Quotient
LME Lead Midwife for Education
LSA Local Supervising Authority
MINT Midwives in Teaching
NHS National Health Service
NMC Nursing and Midwifery Council
PLF Practice Learning Facilitator
PIN Personal Identification Number
PREP Post-registration ongoing education and practice
PSA Professional Standards Authority
RCM Royal College of Midwives
SOM Supervisor of Midwives
UK United Kingdom
UKCC United Kingdom Central Council
VLE Visual learning environment

References

Baer, R. (2010) Self-compassion as a mechanism of change in mindfulness and acceptance-based treatments. In: *Assessing Mindfulness and Acceptance Processes in Clients: Illuminating the Processes of Change.* Oakland, CA: New Harbinger Publications.

Brennan, G., McSherry, R. (2007) Exploring the transition and professional socialization from healthcare assistants to student nurses. *Nurse Education in Practice* 7, pp. 206–214.

Care Quality Commission Inspection Report (2013) Furness General Hospital, Barrow in Furness.

Cherniss, C., Extein, M., Goleman, D., Weissberg, R.P. (2006) Emotional intelligence: what does the research really indicate? *Educational Psychologist* 41 (4), pp. 239–245.

Clough, P., Strycharczyk, D. (2012) *Developing Mental Toughness: Improving Performances, Well-Being and Positive Behaviour in Others.* Kogan Page: London.

Davis, S.K., Humphrey, N. (2012) Emotional Intelligence as a moderator of stressor-mental heath relations in adolescence: Evidence for specificity. *Personality and Individual Differences* 52, pp. 100–105.

Department of Health (2007) Maternity Matters Choice, access and continuity of care in a safe service. London: DH [online] Available: http://webarchive.nationalarchives.gov.uk/20130107105354/http://www.dh.gov.uk/prod_consum_dh/groups/dh_digitalassets/@dh/@en/documents/digitalasset/dh_074199.pdf

Department of Health: NHS England (2012) *Compassion in Practice: Vision and Strategy: An Approach in Midwifery Care.* London: DH.

Directive 2005/36/EC of the European Parliament and of the Council of 7 September 200 on the recognition of professional qualifications. *Official Journal of the European Union* 2005: L.255, pp. 22–142.

Directive 2013/55/EU of the European Parliament and of the Council of 20 November 2013 amending Directive 2005/35/EU on the recognition of professional qualifications. *Official Journal of the European Union* 2013: L.354/321.

Faguy, K. (2012) Emotional intelligence in health care. *Radiologic Technology* 83 (3), pp. 237–253.

Feng, R.F., Tsai, Y.F. (2012) Socialisation of new graduate nurses to practicing nurses. *Journal of Clinical Nursing* 21, pp. 2064–2071.

Francis Report (2010) Independent Inquiry into care provided by Mid Staffordshire NHS Foundation Trust January 2005–March 2009, HMSO.

Goldenberg, I., Matheson, K., Mantler, J. (2006) The assessment of emotional intelligence: A comparison of performance-based and self-Report methodologies. *Journal of Personality Assessment* 86 (1), pp. 33–45.

International Confederation of Midwives (2011) International Definition of the Midwife [online] Available: http://www.internationalmidwives.org

Jones, C., Hayter, M. (2013) Editorial: Social media use by nurses and midwives: 'a recipe for disaster' or 'a force for good'. *Journal of Clinical Nursing* 22, pp. 1495–1496.

Kun, B., Urban, R., Paksi, B., Csobor, L.V., Olah, A., Demetrovics, Z. (2012) Psychometric characteristics of the emotional quotient inventory, youth version, short form, in Hungarian high school students. *Psychological Assessment* 24 (2), pp. 518–523.

Mackintosh, C. (2006) The socialization of pre-registration student nurses: A longitudinal qualitative descriptive study. *International Journal of Nursing Studies* 43, pp. 953–962.

Mayer, J.D., Salovey, P., Caruso, D.R. (2004) Emotional intelligence: theory, findings and implications. *Psychological inquiry* 15 (3), pp. 197–215.

McTavish, L. (2010) A student midwives' experience in the 21st century. *British Journal of Midwifery* 18 (1), pp. 43–47.

Neff, K.D. (2003) The development and validation of a scale to measure self-compassion. *Self and Identity* 2, pp. 223–250.

Nursing and Midwifery Council (2008a) *The code: Standards of conduct, performance and ethics for nurses and midwives.* London: NMC.

Nursing and Midwifery Council (2008b) *Standards to support learning and assessment in practice* London: NMC.

Nursing and Midwifery Council (2009) *Standards for Pre-registration midwifery education.* London: NMC.

Nursing and Midwifery Council (2010) *Midwives in Teaching The MINT Project* [online] Available: http://www.nmc-uk.org/Documents/Midwifery-Reports/MINT-annexe5.1.pdf

Nursing and Midwifery Council (2011a) *Guidance on professional conduct for nursing and midwifery students.* London: NMC.

Nursing and Midwifery Council (2011b) *The Prep Handbook*. London: NMC.

Nursing and Midwifery Council (2012) *Midwives Rules and Standards*. London: NMC.

Nursing and Midwifery Council (2013) *Raising and escalating concerns: guidance for Nurses and Midwives*. London: NMC.

Parsons, M., Griffiths, R. (2007) The effect of professional socialization on midwives practice. *Women and Birth* 20, pp. 31–34.

Patterson, D., Begley, A. (2011) An exploration of the importance of emotional intelligence in midwifery. *Evidence Based Midwifery* 9 (2), pp. 53–60.

Salovey, P., Mayer, J.D. (1990) Emotional Intelligence. *Imagination, Cognition and Personality* 9, pp. 185–211.

The New NHS [online] Available http://www.nhs.uk/NHSEngland/thenhs/about/Pages/nhsstructure.aspx

The Nursing and Midwifery order (2001) 2002 No. 253 [online] Available http://www.legislation.gov.uk/uksi/2002/253/pdfs/uksi_20020253_en.pdf

Wagnild, G. (2009) A review of the resilience scale. *Journal of Nursing Measurement* 17 (2), pp. 105–113.

Yearley, C., Dawson-Goodey, E. (2014) Regulating the midwifery profession. In: Peate, I., Hamilton, C. (eds) *The Student's Guide to Becoming a Midwife*. Chichester: Wiley Blackwell.

Chapter 2

Team working

Mary Beadle
University of Hull, Hull, UK

Sue Townend
Calderdale and Huddersfield NHS Foundation Trust, West Yorkshire, UK

Learning outcomes

By the end of this chapter the reader will be able to:

* recognise, respect and value the role that women and their partners have within the team
* define the terms 'team', 'management' and 'leadership'
* discuss the possible differences between a manager and a leader
* describe what makes an effective team
* identify the characteristics of a team player
* reflect on own team working skills
* discuss the challenges of collaboration
* examine the importance of handovers.

Introduction

Before embarking on this chapter, it is important to make the distinction that when discussing teamwork in maternity care, the woman must be acknowledged as a key team member.

The National Health Service (NHS) Constitution (Department of Health (DH) 2013a) states quite clearly that the patient must be at the heart of everything that the NHS does. This is further supported by the report of the Mid Staffordshire NHS Foundation Trust Public Inquiry (Francis 2013, p. 4) which states that the NHS must *foster a common culture shared by all in the service of putting the patient first*. Therefore everyone who works within the NHS and social care must find a way to do this, in a way that is acceptable to the patient. Within midwifery the voice of the woman's partner and where they sit within the team is also an important consideration. The Nursing and Midwifery Council (NMC) (2009) are explicit in their identification that all midwives must be able to work in partnership with women to facilitate and encourage team working, whether this be intraprofessional, interprofessional or interagency. Effective communication and team working is the cornerstone to best practice. This chapter will examine the dynamics

Fundamentals of Midwifery: A Textbook for Students, First Edition. Edited by Louise Lewis.
© 2015 John Wiley & Sons, Ltd. Published 2015 by John Wiley & Sons, Ltd.
Companion website: www.wileyfundamentalseries.com/midwifery

of teams, the role of leadership and characteristics of team leaders and members. The purpose and features of effective communication with be explored including the value of accurate record keeping in accordance with professional standards.

Woman-centred care

The woman should be seen as the key to all care decisions, and is essential for good quality care. One way to illustrate this is to see the woman as the owner of a boat, 'Emancipation'; they decide who is allowed onto the boat and who is responsible for steering the boat. Who is needed on the boat depends on the condition of the sea and the weather forecast, and the potential challenges of the journey. If the sea is calm and the forecast is good, then the woman will only need the midwife and her partner on board. If the seas become rough then she may need other members to join the crew, including doctors and anaesthetists. If the forecast demonstrates risk then doctors may be already on board. The type of boat, the crew and journey will depend on what the woman wants based on her previous experiences. An inexperienced woman may want more crew on board, and further support, whereas an experienced woman may feel more comfortable with less crew. The crucial element is that the woman is in charge, based on her knowledge and experience and that it is her decision on the type of journey she wants. What everyone plans is a safe journey which is plain sailing and to reach their destination in good health, having had a successful trip. Figure 2.1 illustrates a woman on her journey with different crew members on board.

Effective team working

There is a general consensus that the ability to work effectively as part of a team is a key transferable skill and is something that is seen as an essential attribute for all employers. There has

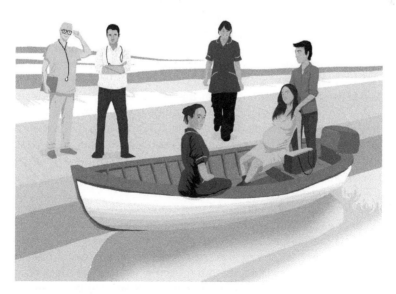

Figure 2.1   The woman as the owner of a boat with different crew members to support her journey. Source: Reproduced with permission from J. Green.

been a strong drive towards this within the NHS in the United Kingdom and worldwide, particularly around interprofessional working (NMC 2009). This is often articulated in terms of what happens if teams do not work well together, therefore setting a negative tone to team working. The consequences of poor team working are well documented within many reports (Francis 2013; Healthcare Commission 2006; Mencap 2009). Lessons can be learned from these reports, but it is also important to reinforce what key characteristics are needed for good team working, as well as the benefits to the worker of being a good team player. It is important not to get bogged down in terminology; however, it is important to be clear what is being discussed, to facilitate the practice of working as part of a team.

What is a team?

Newson (2006, p. 541) defines a team as:

> …A small number of people with complementary knowledge and skills who are committed to a common purpose…

This is the definition that will be used throughout this chapter, although, there are multiple other definitions and an identification of the difficulties in defining the term (Bleakley 2013).

Activity 2.1

Take a few minutes to think about what a team is, and the types of teams that you have belonged to.

There are team-working theories, which attempt to identify roles and responsibilities within teams (Belbin 2000; 2010; Bayliss 2009; Day 2013). These can be helpful when exploring how teams work and what roles individuals within a team take on. They can however be limiting, in that it is not always possible to ascribe a relevant descriptor to a person within the team. This is particularly the case when identifying the role of the woman and their partner who should be part of any healthcare team. This could be seen as a fundamental flaw in using frameworks, which are not specifically designed for use within the healthcare setting. There is a great deal of literature around the role of the woman and her partner within the decision-making process (DH 2007) and therefore it is essential that they are seen as part of the team. Care cannot be women-centred if she is not recognised as part of the team. However, there are many examples of where the patient is not so identified (Tingle 2012). Women themselves may not see their role within the team, relying on the health professionals to either make decisions for them or to recommend a course of action. There are women who have little or no experience of making their own decisions and therefore may find the need to make a choice unsettling and overwhelming. This will be discussed later in this chapter.

Every team needs to have an attainable goal to work towards, with clear identification and understanding of each member's role and responsibilities in meeting the desired goal. There also needs to be a mechanism for evaluating the team's success in achieving the goal.

Within maternity services the goal is for a healthy and successful birth outcome for both mother and baby. Difficulties can arise in the team when there is a lack of consensus on how to reach this goal. Issues can arise around team members' role boundaries, blurring of those boundaries and a lack of understanding in the team of each other's roles. This can be as a result of conflict in the risk assessment versus normality debate, changes of leadership of the team and poor communication between team members including the woman. Such tensions are evident in many healthcare settings around the world, with issues of unequal partnerships (McIntyre et al. 2012), and conflict between professional groups around whether to submit or collaborate with each other (Fujita et al. 2012).

Activity 2.2

Think about how you would find out about the different roles and responsibilities of a team you are member of. You might find the article identified below gives you some ideas.

Wright, A., Hawkes, G., Baker, B., Lindqvist, S. (2012) Reflections and unprompted observations by healthcare students of an interprofessional shadowing visit. *Journal of Interprofessional Care* 26, pp. 305–311.

Leadership

Armstrong (2012, p. 30) defines leadership as:

> …*A process of social influence, concerned with the traits and styles and behaviours of individuals that causes others to follow them…*

The Professional Standards Authority (2012, p. 1) has identified the importance of leadership within the NHS by challenging people to take responsibility for their own actions, to challenge the behaviour of others and to recognise and resolve conflict. These standards are based around seven core values: 'responsibility, honesty, openness, respect, professionalism, leadership and integrity'. It could be argued that except for the leadership value these are essential characteristics of everyone who works within the NHS.

Carnell (2013) also highlights essential qualities for leadership in the NHS as being: shared values, not to be or become cynical, build bridges, be resilient, support new ideas, communicate clearly and honestly, manage upwards, manage time carefully, say sorry and thank you and build a team that will challenge you. All these have to be built around a system that has many constraints and at a time of great change and financial adversity.

There are theories around different types of leadership and which best meet the needs of the NHS. These theories tend to focus on the skills a person needs to have in particular situations (Doody and Doody 2012; Day 2013), often focusing on key skills such as: motivation, flexibility, managing change, communication and being a good role model. Wong and Laschnger (2012) identify how important it is that leaders and managers facilitate staff to gain knowledge and skills, opportunities to 'learn and grow' and support staff with appropriate resources. They see this as a way to develop a positive working and learning environment, which will improve and enhance both staff and patient experiences.

Management

Armstrong (2012, pp. 24 & 30) defines management as:

> …*the process of 'making things happen', and 'getting things done through exercising leadership'. He sees management as 'the act of getting people together to accomplish desired goals…*

There is confusion within many institutions around the differences between a manager and a leader; this may be because these terms are often used interchangeably in many arenas. In practice, there is a manager for each area who ensures that the work is done and that policies and procedures are followed. They deal with operational issues such as staffing and the day-to-day running of the practice area. These managers may have leadership qualities, in that they can inspire staff, but this is not necessarily seen as essential for their role. Pinnock (2012) highlights the role of managers in developing an effective environment for safe care. He identifies the importance of the managers in making the link between the Trusts and the staff. He argues that ward managers should be clearly identified as leaders.

There can be difficulties in relation to management of teams in that practitioners are often organised in multiple teams. Within these different teams there may be different managers for different team members. Bucknall and Forbes (2009) identify that this can lead to role boundary issues and conflict. Managers are often easily identified within a framework, but leaders are less clearly identified unless they have a specific title. Practitioners may choose who they see as a leader, and this may be someone they do not work with directly, but who they admire and aspire to be more like. These issues can be further complicated with the use of other terms, such as: co-ordinators, team leaders, consultant midwives, Supervisor of Midwives and preceptors. The key issue is not to get bogged down in terminology, but to seek out and identify leaders (who may also be managers) to inspire and challenge us.

Activity 2.3

Think of a person who has inspired you. What was it about that person that made you feel the way you did? Would you call this person a leader? Have you recognised this in some of the women in your care?

The importance of having a good working environment is well documented with working in 'a positive working environment' identified as a right for staff (DH 2013a, p. 13). Each individual has their own idea of what this is, often based on experiences of positive and negative working environments. There is a general consensus that the environment within health services influences the quality of care offered and the job satisfaction and motivation of staff (DH 2013a; Glasper 2010; Hutchinson et al. 2010; NICE 2009). The report by the National Advisory Group on Safety of Patients in England (2013, p. 8) identifies:

> …good people can fail to meet patient's needs when their working conditions do not provide them with the conditions for success…

One of the recommendations of the report is that leaders take action when they identify poor team working, giving specific examples of the change in practices that are needed to build the leaders that are needed in today's NHS.

Activity 2.4

Read: page 17 of the report: National Advisory Group on the Safety of Patients in England (2013) [available online] https://www.gov.uk/government/uploads/system/uploads/attachment_data/file/226703/Berwick_Report.pdf

Reflect on how the changes could impact on you, midwives and women. Then read page 44, which is a letter to all staff that work in the NHS and think about what this message means to you.

Ortega et al. (2012) demonstrates how important a learning environment is to staff, where workers feel safe to reflect on and challenge the activities of the team.

Activity 2.5

What do you think makes a good working environment? Can you think of a time when you experienced such an environment and how this made you feel? Relate this to the women being cared for and how the environment can impact on them.

There are currently concerns around bullying cultures in the workplace (Barber 2012) and the impact that this can have on team working. This is not a phenomenon exclusive to the NHS and is often of multifactorial origin. Bullying has been defined as:

> …*repeated offensive behaviour through vindictive, cruel, malicious or humiliating attempts to undermine an individual or group of employees*…
>
> (Yildirim 2009, pp. 504–505)

This practice is illegal and all employers should have anti-bullying policies (Advisory, Conciliation and Arbitration Service (ACAS) 2013; DH 2013a) set up to protect practitioners and other workers. However, it can be difficult for people to speak up about such issues, particularly if the person is in a position of power. All practitioners need to examine their own behaviour and ensure that they are not using any 'bullying' tactics (Curtis et al. 2006; Keeling et al. 2006). They also need to articulate to others that this type of behaviour is unacceptable. Lewis (2006) describes how passive acceptance of verbal abuse by seniors to more junior members of staff, who tolerate this because they view it as 'just part of the job', normalises such behaviour, thus making it appear acceptable. The NHS Constitution (DH 2013a) is clear that bullying must not be tolerated.

There are strategies around conflict resolution, which can be used to mediate and address conflicts within teams (Lee et al. 2008; Trivedi et al. 2008). Brown et al. (2011) identified in their study the issue of conflict within teams. They looked at how conflict may have arisen and the factors involved in its resolution. They identified 'humility' as a key characteristic, which assists in preventing and resolving conflicts.

Activity 2.6

Read: Brown, J. Lewis, L. Ellis, K. Stewart, M. Freeman, T. Kasperski, M. (2011) Conflict on interprofessional primary healthcare teams – can it be resolved? *Journal of Interprofessional Care* 25, pp. 4–10.

Think about what this says about how conflict occurs, prevention and resolution of conflict.

Manley and McCormack (2008) highlighted the importance of culture in ensuring care is compassionate and women-centred. This is also a key component of the education of healthcare workers, which calls for the learning environment to emphasise the need for care and compassion in both practical and theoretical terms. This is identified by Perkins et al. (2012) as 'human flourishing'. Everyone needs to take responsibility for the environment in which they work, whether this is in the clinical environment or in university. It is important to ensure that everyone within a team reflects on how their behaviour affects other team members, both in a positive or negative way, to identify areas for development.

Communication

Effective communication is an essential component of high quality care and good team working. This is particularly important when the team includes multiprofessional disciplines and changing shift patterns. Two key points where communication is paramount are at handover and when there is a request for review of the patient's care.

There are tools and frameworks which can be used to assist in the process of effective handover and review, although the robustness of some of these has not been tested (Mayor et al. 2011; Staggers and Blaz 2012). Examples of communication tools used in midwifery practice are Situation, Background, Assessment and Recommendation (SBAR) (Raynor et al. 2012; NHS Institute for Innovation and Improvement 2008) and Reason, Story, Vital Signs and Plan (RSVP) (Featherstone et al. 2008). These have been designed in response to poor communication, affecting patient care and team working, with the intention of standardising elements of the handover to improve consistency in the approach and therefore less likelihood of missing important information. Johnson et al. (2012) also suggest the use of ICCCO for handovers, which relates to Identification of patient, Clinical risks, Clinical history/presentation, Clinical status, Care plan and Outcomes/goals of care. This was developed from their analysis of 126 handovers. This could also be a useful tool for teaching students and new staff the key issues required at handover.

Handover or transfer of care should be an opportunity to enhance consistent and effective care, but if not handled well can in fact compromise safety (Thomas et al. 2013). Staggers and Blaz (2012) identify the different types and context for handovers and how these differences are important. They identify that focusing on any one type of handover ignores the specific needs of different units and patients. Conversely, they recommend having some structure in the process, acknowledging that this can be a time when mistakes are made, leading to significant harm or near misses. The Australian Medical Association (2006) and British Medical Association (2004) give specific guidance on effective handovers and how these can protect the patient and staff. Structured handovers can also save time as information does not have to be repeated and assists in interprofessional or multidisciplinary working. There is also the opportunity to include the patient in the handover, giving attention to the place handover is carried out, to ensure confidentiality and privacy is respected.

A crucial element for success is identifying which tool works best for a particular team, taking into consideration the view and opinions of the members of the team as Johnson and Cowin (2013) found. Their research identified elements that can hamper effective handovers, including: a lack of focus; too many people involved; environment being too noisy and distracting; differences between handover information and records; and a lack of understanding of others roles. It also identified positive features around effective handovers of care in the information sharing between the team and patient, as well as a clear point at which the care moves from one team to another. Johnson et al. (2012) suggest that written handovers, eboards and other computer models may also help with this process.

Activity 2.7

Reflect on an effective and ineffective handover you have experienced and identify what the differences were between the two, in relation to both the handover and ongoing care.

Communication tools can also be used when reviewing patient's ongoing care. It is good practice to ensure that over a period of care, there is regular review of the situation to ensure that any developing risk factors or problems are identified in a timely manner. One review of care communication tool 'RSVP' already mentioned, relates to Reason, Story, Vital Signs and Plan when requesting action and advice related to a client; particularly useful when there has been deterioration in the patient's condition (Featherstone et al. 2008). Another tool widely used in maternity settings is 'SBAR' which stands for Situation, Background, Assessment and Recommendation; this has been developed to work with different disciplines and in other environments such as the military and aviation (Johnson, Jefferies and Nicholls 2012; Street et al. 2011).

Whichever framework is being used, it must be remembered that whilst it is there to provide structure, it should not constrain communication by missing out important questions and extra information which is specific to that particular patient or situation (Mayor et al. 2011).

The key elements around successful handovers and transfer of care are that they should:

- focus on the purpose of handovers
- focus on key elements
- not be overly long
- be objective
- be in an environment which facilitates listening
- involve the patient wherever possible
- not include jargon and abbreviations
- pay particular attention to structure and organisation
- be confidential.

Activity 2.8

Next time you attend a handover or transfer of care think about using a tool, or if one is used think about its effectiveness.

Whilst there are many different methods of communicating today, such as telephone; text; written records; verbal handovers and email, the key principles of the information that needs to be handed over is generally the same. Practitioners must however be mindful of information governance to ensure that if information is being passed electronically or in a form that could be accessed by someone other than the intended recipient; it is protected to ensure confidentiality (NMC 2008; NHS England 2013).The NMC has clear standards relating to record keeping within the Code (NMC 2008). All midwives and student midwives must be aware of what the Code says and adhere to these standards.

Clinical consideration

Remember that listening is an important skill in communication. Never forget that the woman is more in tune with herself than anyone else is, and her voice must be heard, her views respected and her contribution acknowledged and valued. This can be particularly challenging where women are hesitant or reluctant to participate in decision-making.

Collaboration

Downe and Finlayson (2011) argue that in order to facilitate effective interprofessional work, the focus should be on collaboration, rather than team working. Their view is that the act of trying to mould different groups into a team can be counterproductive and lead to the development of factions and hierarchies. These they argue hinder rather than foster team working. Downe and Finlayson (2011) discuss how this can happen in maternity services with doctors and midwives working in opposition to each other, rather than together. This conflict can occur due to misunderstandings around the aims of each discipline and justification for the plan of care. This distrust is well documented with maternity services worldwide (Gould 2008; McIntyre et al. 2012). By shifting the focus to collaborative working, for those involved in the care of a woman and her family, conflict and ineffective care can be reduced and women-centred, quality care facilitated. Through collaboration, practitioners put aside their differences and possible power struggles, with a direct correlation between high levels of collaboration and improved standards of care (Goodman and Clemow 2010). Collaborative working has been identified as being 'characterised by a shared vision, collective goal setting and a mutual understanding of roles' with an 'ethos of power-sharing' (Hutchings et al. 2003, p 35).

From clinical practice experience, it is crucial that this collaboration includes the woman and her family. The woman is a key team member and communication with her is vital. Relating to the rights of the woman, there should be a signing up to 'no decision about me, without me' (DH 2012a). Power struggles between professionals have been discussed, but there may also be a power struggle between the professionals and the woman. Many women have confidence in their ability to give birth and have strong views on how they will achieve this. The woman's view of how she will achieve her goal can be in conflict with that of the professionals involved in her care and can conflict within teams where there exists a lack of consensus. It is important to recognise that in some instances the woman may actually be the team leader. Hall (2013) puts forward the case for identifying an extra 'C' in compassionate care, which stands for 'centrality of the service user' and for the other C's to work around the user.

During emergency situations the dynamics and collaboration within teams is crucial, with each member of the team knowing their role during the event and working together seamlessly. There is a limited amount of time in which to make decisions and consult the woman and her partner about the necessary actions. Regular interprofessional training for all the members of the team can facilitate this. Gaining consent from a woman in such situations is a challenge, but with experience staff can develop methods of giving key information quickly and effectively. Any decisions made in such situations must take into account what is the best course of action and this will need to be justifiable and based on current evidence. It is essential that the woman and her partner are given the opportunity to debrief after the event, so that they can develop an understanding of the events and the thinking behind the decisions made. Depending on the nature of the event, other members of the team may also need some form of debriefing. It can be difficult for students to know what is happening and what their role is during these events. Therefore students should seek help from their mentor, Supervisor of Midwives or a midwifery lecturer to discuss situations they have been involved in.

Activity 2.9

Think about a woman and her family where you have participated in their care; identify how many people have been involved in this care. It may be useful to compare patients who are labelled as low and high risk.

What challenges does the number of people involved bring for collaborative working?

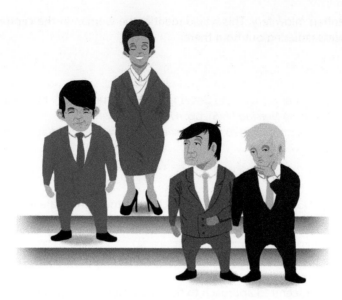

Figure 2.2   Unequal power and hierarchy. Source: Reproduced with permission from J. Green.

Power dynamics

As previously mentioned, one of the difficulties identified in team and collaborative working is unequal power within teams and hierarchies (Caldwell and Atwal 2003; see Figure 2.2). In order to fully collaborate, all members of the team must be treated as equal, particularly during decision-making processes. Hierarchies and lack of understanding of the roles of different team members can lead to misunderstanding around accountability. All professionals must remember that they are accountable for all their own acts and omissions. For all midwives it is essential to have a good working knowledge of the NMC Rules and Standards (NMC 2012) and the Code (NMC 2008) (see Chapter 1: 'To be a midwife', where this is discussed in more detail). Brown et al. (2011) recommend that leadership and good use of conflict resolution techniques can assist in effective team working and development of partnerships and collaboration within a team, so preventing the negative impact disempowerment can have on team working.

Team dynamics are related to power: who has the power and how is it used. The organisation of the NHS and other large institutions tends to involve hierarchy and an individual's position within this hierarchy tends to influence how much power a person will have. Power can be related to profession, experience and amount of time within the team.

There is a view that in the maternity setting doctors tend to see themselves as at the top of any hierarchy, with midwives below them and then the women (Downe and Finlayson 2011). Some midwives may also see themselves as lower down in a hierarchy, but others feel they are at the same level as the doctors. Downe and Finlayson (2011, p. 165) call this the *polarised culture of maternity care*' and Gould (2008) identifies 'professional dominance' as a threat to safe care and good team working. Since the woman knows herself better than anyone else does, it could be argued that she is in fact at the top of the hierarchy. Nothing can be done for her or to her without her consent. The power the professionals then wield is the manner in which they communicate with the woman to influence her decisions. This can be illustrated in the work of McCormack and McCance (2006) on person-centred nursing, which could just as easily be seen as person-centred midwifery. This would identify the woman in the centre of the framework, with the process radiating out from there.

Activity 2.10

Read: McCormack, B., McCance, T. (2006) Development of a framework for person centred nursing *Journal of Advanced Nursing* 56(5), pp. 472–479.

Look at the framework on page 476 and think about how you could apply this to your practice.

McCormack (2003) lists 29 'principles for action' of these there are four which are key:

1. Listen to women and allow them to tell their story as a legitimate part of assessment processes.
2. Suspend the use of prior knowledge about a woman and their social context until they have been enabled to tell their story.
3. Adopt a woman-centred approach to risk assessment and risk taking.
4. Help women to see beyond their own limited expectations of their involvement in care and their deference to others.

It is important to share power and knowledge appropriately. The issue is not whether there exists a hierarchy and power dynamic, but how this is managed and reflected in the care. Molyneux (2001) describes how a new team can be developed where team members work in a collaborative manner, with the importance of commitment, communication and development of a team working culture at the heart.

Activity 2.11

Think about where as a student midwife you fit within the midwifery team? What impact does this have on you day-to-day?

Regulation

Accountability

Key areas around effective team working include the culture within the team and leadership. The recent Francis Report (2013) talked about how the failure of the leadership of a Trust led to an environment where poor care became acceptable. Accountability is a key issue within all teams, but particularly within healthcare teams. Whilst leadership is important and can have a significant influence on how a team works, the people within the teams must be accountable for their own actions, and cannot pass this accountability on to others (NMC 2008; Griffith 2011). This is a fundamental principle of the role and responsibilities of the midwife. Richard Griffith has written several articles around accountability in midwifery, which discuss the key principles of who is answerable to whom (Griffith 2011; 2012a; 2012b; 2012c). He identifies the 'Pillars of Accountability', as society, the woman and baby, employer and profession (Griffith 2012a). The current focus on poor care in the press is related to an individual's accountability to society and the profession.

There has been justifiable outrage about the findings of the Francis Report (2013), and demand for professionals to go before their regulatory bodies, to be called to account and be prevented from practising.

A fundamental responsibility for the midwife is to ensure the mother, her baby and her partner remain the focus of all care and that any care given is always safe (NMC 2009). In order to provide women-centred care within a family environment, the needs of the mother, baby and her partner and family must be the midwives' first concern. Indeed the Department of Health indicates that the views of the patient must be paramount in any decisions made about their care (DH 2012a; 2012b). There should be a focus on seeking the views of patients, giving information and being honest and truthful. Such a philosophy can be challenging and difficult as Brass (2012) identifies occasions when women make choices against professional advice. This re-emphasises the role of the woman as the lead for effective team working and the importance of good communication for sound decision-making.

The NHS Constitution (DH 2013a, p. 128) makes clear its expectations of staff, stating that [you must] *'take responsibility not only for the care you personally provide, but also for your wider contribution to the aims of your team and the NHS as a whole'.* The NMC (2008) sets out standards for team working and patient inclusion: 'make the care of people your first concern'. This includes working effectively as part of a team and sharing information appropriately.

Escalating concerns

It is clear that anyone who works in the NHS must take action if they see inappropriate or poor care. The process for how midwives should do this is within the document raising concerns (NMC 2013), with which all midwives and student midwives should be familiar. It is not just about the care that a midwife herself gives, but also the care that she sees given by others. In order to protect and safeguard women and babies, it is essential that if there are concerns about the practice of others then we must act. Healthcare practitioners and students cannot sit back and think, 'My care is good; I am not responsible for anyone else's care.' Midwives are responsible for the environment in which they work, including the teams they are members of. This is where the importance of leadership and management of the team is crucial, since its leader and manager set the tone of the quality of the care offered by the team. Student midwives and midwives also have an extra support in the Supervisor of Midwives framework, which can assist in raising and dealing with concerns (NMC 2012). Students should find out who their named Supervisor of Midwives is in their area of practice. The NMC (2011a; 2013) also provide specific guidance to healthcare practitioners and students about how to deal with concerns about practice with which all practitioners and students should become familiar.

Further reading activity

Read: The NMC document Raising Concerns and think about how you would feel if you had to follow this process and where you could get support.

[Available online] http://www.nmc-uk.org/Nurses-and-midwives/Raising-and-escalating-concerns/

It is well documented what can happen if concerns are not expressed or are not managed appropriately (Francis 2013, DH 2013b). Therefore, it is essential that all healthcare workers and students take responsibility for expressing their concerns and taking appropriate action, as the

NMC states *'if you don't do something who will?'* (NMC 2011b). Courage is one of the 6 C's which is now part of the vision for the NHS; this is required when taking action about concerns that a healthcare worker or student might have about care (Cummings and Bennett 2012; DH 2012c).

Team player

A team of people working together in harmony towards a shared goal (see Figure 2.3), where the individual characteristics each team member brings complements those of others, is a powerful and effective entity. There can be much gained from team working, as members enjoy the support and comradeship of each other. The more positive staff feel about their team and their work the better their work is and this can have a positive effect on others around them. Bargagliotti (2011) terms this as *'work engagement'* and sees this as a state of mind that workers can have about their team and what they do (see Figure 2.4). The ability and opportunity to work with staff from other disciplines and backgrounds adds a richness to team working in the NHS which is interesting and exciting.

Activity 2.12

What characteristics can you bring to a team which will facilitate good team working? What can you do to develop these skills?

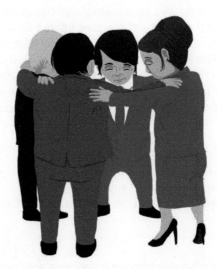

Figure 2.3   Team of people committed to a common goal. Source: Reproduced with permission from J. Green.

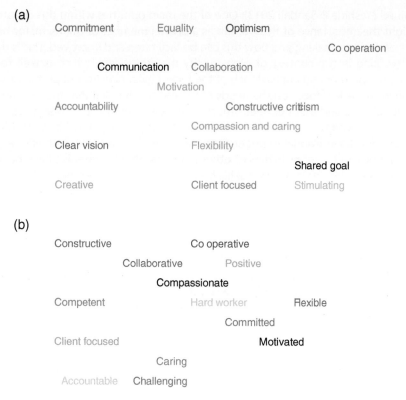

Figure 2.4   (a) Key principles of good team working and (b) key characteristics of a good team player.

Key points

- Women must be at the heart of everything that the NHS does in midwifery.
- Midwives must work in partnership with women and their families.
- The woman is key to all care decisions.
- Effective team working is crucial for good quality and safe care.
- Bullying must not be tolerated.
- It is everyone's responsibility to build an effective team and working environment.
- Communication is the foundation on which all care is built.
- Anyone who works in the NHS must raise any concerns they may have about inappropriate or poor care.

Conclusion

This chapter has examined the terms: team, manager and leader in the context of the NHS and particularly the maternity services. The importance of effective team working has been emphasised and how everyone has a responsibility to be a team player and facilitate collaborative working. Specific crucial points where team working is particularly important have been identified, for example around handovers, review of care and emergency situations. Tools which may assist in this process, have been examined. The benefits that students, midwives and other health professionals feel when enjoying working within a team and feeling valued, have been examined (Yoshida & Sandall 2013). One of the main priorities within this chapter has been to highlight the importance of the woman as a pivotal member of the team; for her to be at the centre of decision-making and how this can be facilitated and improved. This is the key to good team working in the context of high quality maternity care, which is well received by the woman, her partner and family. Much of the recent evidence around problems with care, have identified the lack of focus on the needs of the patient. A belief that the woman is the starting point for all care and that her needs must always be uppermost in everyone's minds is funda-mental to this chapter. In order to be a good team player, it has been established that it is important for the individual to understand their own role and responsibilities and how this fits with the roles and responsibilities of other team members. Strategies have been identified to assist in developing team working skills both for the student and the qualified midwife.

End of chapter activities
Crossword

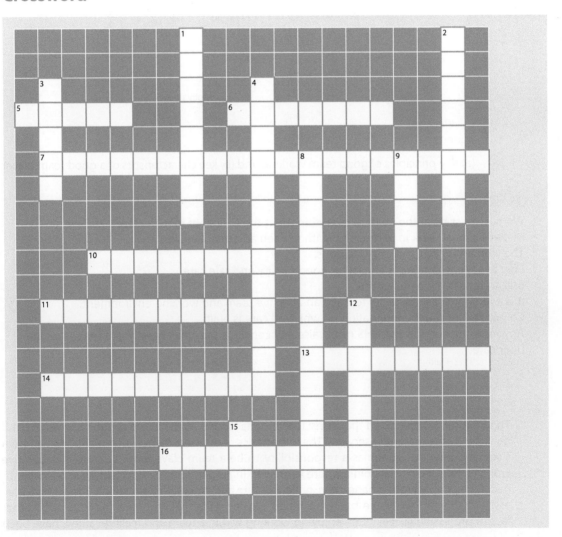

Across

5. The person who should be at the centre of all care
6. One of the C's
7. This is a crucial element of safe care
10. Communication event when information is passed from one care giver to another

11. A process to make things happen
13. Repeated offensive behaviour which attempts to undermine an individual
14. What you must do if you witness poor care
16. One of the key characteristics of a team player

Down

1. Modest estimate of own importance
2. One of the key principles of good team working
3. Something which should be shared
4. Working together

8. Taking responsibility for one's own actions and omissions
9. Communication tool
12. A person who sets a good example
15. The number of C's

Find out more

Below is a list of things you can find out about to enhance your knowledge of the issues and topics covered in this chapter. Make notes using the chapter content, the references and further reading identified, local policies and guidelines and discussions with colleagues.

1. Read section III of the NHS Constitution to find out more about complaints and the redress that is available to patients and their relatives if they are not happy with their care.

2. Read section IV of the NHS Constitution so that you can be aware of the expectations that the NHS has of staff.

3. It is important that you are aware of the structure of any organisation within which you work. A significant reorganisation of health and social care is currently underway. Use the references below to make sure you are up to date on how health and social care is structured. Also if you go to the Department of Health website there is an explanation of the structure of the NHS.

   Gardner, S. (2012) Centralising midwifery care *British Journal of Midwifery* 20(8), p. 536.

   Glasper, A. (2012) Caring for our healthcare future: The government White Paper. *British Journal of Nursing* 21(16), pp. 992–993.

   Sillett, J. (2012) Health and Social Care Bill: Health and Wellbeing boards. *British Journal of Nursing* 21(12), p. 710.

4. Read Yalden, B., McCormack, B. (2010) Constructions of dignity: a pre requisite for flourishing in the workplace? *International Journal of Older People Nursing* 5, pp. 137–147 and think about what implications this has for your practice and working within the maternity services.

5. Reflect on the care that you gave a particular woman; discuss this reflection with your mentor and a Supervisor of Midwives. Find out what other people think about your ability to work as part of a team. Ask the woman for feedback on your care; it might be useful to ask one of the women who are part of your caseloading to help you if this is not already part of your programme.

6. Use the 15 steps challenge to review your next placement area. Callard, L., Williams, A. (2012) The 15 Steps Challenge: A toolkit for Good Care. *Nursing Management* 19(8), pp. 14–18.

Glossary of terms

Accountability   Taking responsibility for one's own actions and omissions.

Bullying   Repeated offensive behaviour through vindictive, cruel, malicious or humiliating attempts to undermine an individual or group of employees.

Collaboration   To work together.

Compassion   Feeling for others, with a need to alleviate suffering.

Conflict resolution   Strategies which are used to try to overcome difficulties and challenges.

Consent   A client agrees to undergo a procedure after being giving the relevant information in which to make a decision.

Handover   Communication event, when information is passed from one care giver to another.

Hierarchy   System in which some people are seen as having more power or influence other others.

Humility   Modest estimate of own importance.

Integrity   To act with honesty.

Leadership   A process of social influence, concerned with the traits and styles and behaviours of individuals that causes others to follow them.

Management   The process of making things happens.

Resilience   Ability to cope with challenging situations.

Role model   A person who sets a good example.

Respect   To give value to something.

Team   A small number of people with complementary knowledge and skills who are committed to a common purpose.

References

Advisory, Conciliation and Arbitration Service (ACAS) (2013) *Bullying and Harassment at Work: A Guide for Employees*. London: ACAS.

Armstrong, M. (2012) *Armstrong's Handbook of Management and Leadership*. London: Kogan Page.

Australian Medical Association (2006) *Safe handover: Safe patients*. Australia: AMA.

Bargagliotti, L. (2011) Work engagement in nursing: a concept analysis. *Journal of Advanced Nursing* 68 (6), pp. 1414–1428.

Barber, C. (2012) Use of bullying as a management tool in healthcare environments. *British Journal of Midwifery* 21 (5), pp. 299–302.

Bayliss, J. (2009) *Working in a Team: A Workbook for Successful Dynamics*. London: Quay Books.

Belbin, R. (2010) *Management of Teams Why They Succeed or Fail*. Oxford: Butterworth-Heinemann.

Belbin, R. (2000) *Beyond the Team*. Oxford: Butterworth-Heinemann.

Bleakley, A. (2013) Working in 'teams' in an era of 'liquid' healthcare: What is the use of theory? *Journal of Interprofessional Care* 27, pp. 18–26.

Brass, R. (2012) Caring for women who go against conventional medical advice. *British Journal of Midwifery* 20 (12), pp. 898–901.

British Medical Association (2004) *Safe handover: safe patients*. London: BMA.

Brown, J., Lewis, L., Ellis, K., Stewart, M., Freeman, T., Kasperski, M. (2011) Conflict on interprofessional primary healthcare teams – can it be resolved? *Journal of Interprofessional Care* 25, pp. 4–10.

Bucknall, J., Forbes, H. (2009) There Is NO 'I' in TEAM: Working cooperatively to implement evidence into practice. *Worldviews on Evidence Based Nursing Fourth Quarter* pp. 187–189.

Caldwell, K., Atwal, A. (2003) The problems of interprofessional healthcare practice in hospitals. *British Journal of Nursing* 12 (20), pp. 1212–1218.

Carnell, R. (2013) The 10 essential qualities for leadership in the NHS http://www.theguardian.com/society/2013/feb/12/leadership-qualities-essential-in-nhs

Cummings, J., Bennett, V. (2012) *Compassion in Practice*. London: NHS England.

Curtis, P., Ball, L., Kirkham, M. (2006) Bullying and horizontal violence: Cultural or individual phenomena? *British Journal of Midwifery* 14 (4), pp. 218–221.

Day, J. (2013) *Interprofessional Working An Essential Guide for Health and Social Care Professionals*. Andover: Cengage Learning.

Department of Health (DH) (2007) *Maternity Matters: Choice, Access and Continuity of Care in a Safe Service*. London: DH.

DH (2013a) The Handbook to the NHS Constitution https://www.gov.uk/government/uploads/system/uploads/attachment_data/file/170649/Handbook_to_the_NHS_Constitution.pdf

DH (2013b) *Oral Statement on Morecombe Bay*. Gov.uk

DH (2012a) *Liberating the NHS: No Decision about Me without Me*. London: DH.

DH (2012b) *Respect and compassion at centre of new standards for NHS leaders*. https://www.gov.uk/government/news/respect-and-compassion-at-centre-of-new-standards-for-nhs-leaders

DH (2012c) *Compassion in Practice: Nursing, Midwifery and Care Staff Our Vision and Strategy*. London: DH.

Doody, O., Doody, C. (2012) Tranformational leadership in nursing practice. *British Journal of Nursing* 21 (20), pp. 1212–1218.

Downe, S., Finlayson, K. (2011) Collaboration: Theories, Models and Maternity Care. In: Downe, S., Bryom, S., Simpson, L. (eds) (2011) *Essential Midwifery Practice: Leadership, Expertise and Collaborative Working*. Chichester: Wiley Blackwell, pp. 155–179.

Featherstone, P., Chalmers, T., Smith, G. (2008) RSVP: a system for communication of deterioration in hospital patients. *British Journal of Nursing* 17 (13), pp. 860–864.

Francis, R. (2013) *Report of the Mid Staffordshire NHS Foundation Trust Public Inquiry Executive Summary*. London: The Stationary Office.

Fujita, N., Perrin, X., Vodounon, J., Gozo, M., Matsumtoto, Y., Uchida, S., Sugiura, Y. (2012) Humanised care and a change in practice in a hospital in Benin. *Midwifery* 28, pp. 481–488.

Glasper, A. (2010) Promoting wellbeing: Productive and healthy working conditions. *British Journal of Nursing* 19 (1), pp. 8–9.

Goodman, B., Clemow, R. (2010) *Nursing and Collaborative Practice*. Exeter: Learning Matters.

Gould, D. (2008) Professional dominance and subversion in maternity services. *British Journal of Midwifery* 16 (4), p. 210.

Griffith, R. (2011) Understanding accountability in midwifery practice: Key concepts. *British Journal of Midwifery* 19 (5), pp. 327–328.

Griffith, R. (2012a) Accountability in midwifery practice: answerable to society. *British Journal of Midwifery* 20 (7), pp. 525–526.

Griffith, R. (2012b) Accountability in midwifery practice: Answerable to the employer. *British Journal of Midwifery* 20 (10), pp. 753–754.

Griffith, R. (2012c) Accountability in midwifery practice: answerable to mother and baby. *British Journal of Midwifery* 20 (8), pp. 601–602.

Hall, J. (2013) Developing a culture of compassionate care – The Midwife's voice? *Midwifery* 29, pp. 269–271.

Healthcare Commission (2006) *Investigation into 10 Maternal Deaths at, or following delivery at, Northwick Park Hospital, North West London Hospital NHS Trust, between April 2002 and April 2005*. http://webarchive.nationalarchives.gov.uk/20060502043818/http://healthcarecommission.org.uk/_db/_documents/Northwick_tagged.pdf

Hutchings, S., Hall, J., Lovelady, B. (2003)*Teamwork A Guide to Successful Collaboration in Health and Social Care*. Bicester: Speechmark Publishing.

Hutchinson, M., Wilkes, L., Jackson, D., Vickers, M. (2010) Integrating individual, work group and organizational factors: testing a multidimensional model of bullying in the nursing workplace. *Journal of Nursing Management* 18, pp. 173–181.

Johnson, M., Cowin, L. (2013) Nurses discuss bedside handover and using written handover sheets. *Journal of Nursing Management* 21 pp. 121–129.

Johnson, M., Jefferies, D., Nicholls, N. (2012) Exploring the structure and organization of information within nursing clinical handovers. *International Journal of Nursing Practice* 18, pp. 462–470.

Keeling, J., Quigley, J., Roberts, T. (2006) Bullying in the workplace: What it is and how to deal with it. *British Journal of Midwifery* 14 (10), pp. 616–621.

Lewis, M. (2006) Nurse bullying: organizational considerations in the maintenance and perpetration of healthcare bullying cultures. *Journal of Nursing Management* 14, pp. 52–58.

Lee, L., Berger, D., Awad, S., Brandt, M., Martinez, G., Brunicardi, F. (2008) Conflict resolution: Practical principles for surgeons. *World Journal of Surgery* 32, pp. 2331–2335.

Mayor, E., Bangerter, A., Aribot, M. (2011) Task uncertainty and communication during nursing shift handovers. *Journal of Advanced Nursing* 68 (9), pp. 1956–1966.

Manley, K., McCormack, B. (2008) Person centred care. *Nursing Management* 15 (8), pp. 12–13.

McCormack, B. (2003) A conceptual framework for person-centred practice with older people. *International Journal of Nursing Practice* 9, pp. 202–209.

McCormack, B., McCance, T. (2006) Development of a framework for person centred nursing. *Journal of Advanced Nursing* 56 (5), pp. 472–479.

McIntyre, M., Francis, K., Chapman, Y. (2012) The struggle for contested boundaries in the move to collaborative care teams in Australian maternity care. *Midwifery* 28, pp. 298–305.

MENCAP (2009) *Death by Indifference: 74 deaths and counting. A progress report 5 years on.* London: MENCAP.

Molyneux, J. (2001) Interprofessional team working: what makes teams work well? *Journal of Interprofessional Care* 15 (1), pp. 29–35.

National Advisory Group on the Safety of Patients in England (2013) *A promise to learn – a commitment to act* https://www.gov.uk/government/uploads/system/uploads/attachment_data/file/226703/Berwick_Report.pdf

National Health Service (NHS) Institute for Innovation and Improvement (2008) *SBAR.* London: NHS Institute for Innovation and Improvement.

NICE (2009) *Promoting Mental Wellbeing Through Productive and Healthy Working Conditions: Guidance for Employers.* London: NICE.

Newson, P. (2006) Participate effectively as a team member. *Nursing & Residential Care* 8 (12), pp. 541–544.

NHS England (2013) Confidentiality Policy http://www.england.nhs.uk/wp-content/uploads/2013/06/conf-policy-1.pdf

Nursing and Midwifery Council (NMC) (2008) *The Code Standards of Conduct Performance and Ethics for Nurses and Midwives.* London: NMC.

Nursing and Midwifery Council (2009) *Standards for Pre Registration Midwifery Education.* London: NMC.

Nursing and Midwifery Council (NMC) (2011a) *Guidance for students of nursing and midwifery.* London: NMC.

Nursing and Midwifery Council (NMC) (2011b) *Update July 2011.* London: NMC.

Nursing and Midwifery Council (NMC) (2013) *Raising Concerns Guidance for Nurses and Midwives.* London: NMC.

Nursing and Midwifery Council (2012) *Midwives rules and Standards.* London: NMC.

Ortega, A., Sanchez-Manzanares, M., Gil, F., Rico, R. (2012) Enhancing team learning in nursing teams through beliefs about interpersonal context. *Journal of Advanced Nursing* 69 (1), pp. 102–111.

Perkins, B., Brady, M., Engelmann, L., Larson, J., Shultz, C. (2012) Human flourishing in Nursing Education. *Nursing Education Perspectives* 33 (5), p. 353.

Pinnock, D. (2012) The role of the ward manager in promoting patient safety. *British Journal of Nursing* 21 (19), pp. 1144–1149.

Professional Standards Authority (2012) *Press Release Compassion and respect at heart of new NHS Leaders standards* Professional Standards Authority http://www.professionalstandards.org.uk/docs/scrutiny-quality/121107-standards-for-nhs-leaders.pdf?sfvrsn=0

Raynor, M., Marshall, J., Jackson, K. (eds) (2012) *Midwifery Practice: Critical Illness, Complications and Emergencies Case Book.* Maidenhead: Open University Press.

Staggers, N., Blaz, J. (2012) Research on nursing handoffs for medical and surgical settings: an integrative review. *Journal of Advanced Nursing* 69 (2), pp. 247–262.

Street, M., Eustace, P., Livingston, P., Craike, M., Kent, B., Patterson, D. (2011) Communication at the bedside to enhance patient care: A survey of nurses' experience and perspective of handover. *International Journal of Nursing Practice* 17, pp. 133–140.

Thomas, M., Schultz, T., Hannaford, N., Runciman, W. (2013) Failures in transition: learning from incidents relating to clinical handover in acute care. *Journal for Healthcare Quality* 35 (3), pp. 49–55.

Tingle, J. (2012) Health Foundation report calls for better model of patient interaction. *British Journal of Nursing* 21 (15), pp. 936–937.

Trivedi, D., Singh, S., Hooke, R. (2008) Conflict resolution: a guide for the foundation year doctor. *British Journal of Hospital Medicine* 69 (8), p. M114.

Wright, A., Hawkes, G., Baker, B., Lindqvist, S. (2012) Reflections and unprompted observations by health-care students of an interprofessional shadowing visit. *Journal of Interprofessional Care* 26, pp. 305–311.

Wong, C., Laschinger, H. (2012) Authentic leadership, performance, and job satisfaction: the mediating role of the empowerment. *Journal of Advanced Nursing* 69 (4), pp. 947–959.

Yildirim, D. (2009) Bullying among nurses and its effects. *International Nursing Review* 56, pp. 504–511.

Yoshida, Y., Sandall, J. (2013) Occupational burnout and work factors in community and hospital midwives: A survey analysis. *Midwifery* 29, pp. 921–926.

Chapter 3

Sociology applied to maternity care

Mary Beadle

University of Hull, Hull, UK

Sarah Wise

Diana Princess of Wales Hospital, Grimsby, UK

Learning outcomes

By the end of this chapter the reader will be able to:

- identify relevant sociological perspectives
- define the terms gender and sexuality
- explore socially constructed concepts
- discuss the process of socialisation within families and society
- examine health, illness and wellbeing as concepts.

Introduction

The NMC (2009, p. 26) state that midwives must be able to:

> …*contribute to enhancing the health and social wellbeing of individuals and their communities' and 'practice in a way which respects, promotes and supports individuals' rights, interests, preferences, beliefs and cultures*…

This chapter identifies the knowledge necessary to undertake this role. It explains some of the key sociological theories and how these could relate to maternity care. This will assist in developing a sociological perspective and applying this to childbearing women and their families.

Overview of sociological perspectives

When studying sociology it is important to have a basic understanding of the theories behind this area of study. However, this is not a chapter on the theories of sociology and therefore it is

Fundamentals of Midwifery: A Textbook for Students, First Edition. Edited by Louise Lewis.
© 2015 John Wiley & Sons, Ltd. Published 2015 by John Wiley & Sons, Ltd.
Companion website: www.wileyfundamentalseries.com/midwifery

recommended that further reading is undertaken; this chapter aims only to apply some of the key sociological concepts to maternity care. As a way to start this process you should focus on a few of the key sociologists and their main ideas. These should include:

- Karl Marx – *class*
- Emile Durkheim – *division of labour, religion*
- Erving Goffman – *self in everyday life*
- Harriet Martineau – *study of institutions*
- Talcott Parsons – *sick role*
- Ivan Illich – *medical power*
- Max Weber – *social change – capitalism and religion*
- Anthony Giddens – *formation of social structures and identity*
- Simone De Beavoir – *feminism*
- Judith Butler – *doing gender*
- Sylvia Walby – *patriarchy*
- Peter Townend – *poverty.*

Further reading activity

Read about the main ideas from these sociologists in:

Giddens, A. (2009) *Sociology*, 6th edn. Chapter 3, Theories and perspectives in sociology, pp. 68–105. Cambridge: Polity.

Bradby, H. (2012) *Medicine, Health and Society*. Chapter 2, Social theory and the sociology of health and illness, pp. 2–40.

Hutchison, J. Parker, M. (eds) (2012) *Key Themes and Concepts in Applied Sociology*. London: Pearson.

Mik-Meyer, N. Obling, A. (2012) The negotiation of the sick role: General Practitioners classification of patients with medically unexplained symptoms. *Sociology of Health and Illness* 34 (7), pp. 1025–1038.

Giddens, A. Sutton, P. (eds) (2010) *Sociology: Introductory Readings*. Cambridge: Polity Press.

The following websites will also be useful:

http://www.newworldencyclopedia.org/entry/Sociology
http://www.sociosite.net/topics/sociologists.php
http://www.biography.com/people/groups/academics/sociologists

When looking at these sociologists views think about how these are relevant to healthcare.

Definition of society

Sociology has been defined as *'the scientific study of human life, social groups, whole societies and the human world'* (Giddens 2009, p. 6). The theory of social construction is also an important factor to discuss, as this has applications to healthcare and understanding childbearing within communities and cultures. Social construction is the idea that *'social reality is the product of interactions between individuals and groups'* (Giddens 2009, p. 38), rather than something that is just natural. In this way gender is something that tends to be viewed as natural, as it is to do with our physical appearance, but how we behave and how society relates to us depending on whether we are men or women is something constructed by our society. Each society has rules and beliefs which their members are expected to adhere to, with consequences for breaking these rules. These are often termed as 'social norms'; these change over time and may develop and adapt to different circumstances within society. An example of this would be what is classed as a normal family structure; this has changed significantly in some societies but not in others. These messages can be found in government policies and institutions; religious and cultural influences can also have significant influence. The reason why these issues are important to midwives is the impact that they can have on the lives of women and their families.

44

Activity 3.1

Think about what you would class as social norms.

The family

The family is a key institution within society and therefore has implications for the development of people's individual identities and beliefs. As McKie and Callan (2012, pp. 15,16) identify: *'families are the oldest and most enduring form of social grouping'*. They are *'formed, dissolved and reconfigured'*. There have been many changes over the last decades in family structures; these relate to the often termed 'ideal' family of a mother, father and two children. There are now many different types and make-up of families which are common and acceptable within society and the communities in which they live (see Figure 3.1). These include single-parent families, stepfamilies, children living in more than one family and couples living together but not married. Same-sex families are now more common but are not accepted by all sections of society.

The increase in divorce, separation and decline in marriage has also had an impact on the makeup of families. Different types of families have had an impact on the health and wellbeing of family members and the arrangements in which women give birth. Technological advances have also led to further complexities in relationships within families, for example; artificial insemination by donor, in vitro fertilisation, egg donation and surrogacy (see Chapter 5: 'Parent-hood', where variations of families are explored in more depth). This has changed the biological relationship to parents, in that there may be more than one family that a child belongs to, and there may be no biological, only a social connection to their family.

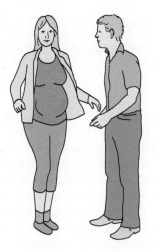
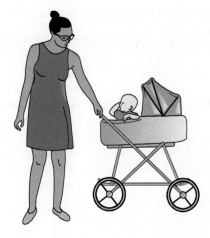

Figure 3.1   Variations in family structures.

There is a lack of clear definition for the different types of family which present within society; sometimes only terms such as traditional and non-traditional family structures are used (Farrell et al. 2012). These terms are not very helpful, as they can mean different things to different people. The key issue for midwives and other healthcare workers is to be aware of the diversity of family structures and the implications this can have, namely, the challenges and positive elements for the women and families they work with. It is essential not to make assumptions about relationships within families, as this can lead to inappropriate care and use of language, resulting in miscommunication and a loss of trust.

There are processes which happen within families which impact on the members' identities. James and Curtis (2010) explore the concept of 'family displays'; these are termed as 'everyday activities' in which family members communicate to each other and to those around them, that they are a family (James and Curtis 2010). This could be in the ways families communicate, where they live, their diet and habits. One of the key ways that this can occur is through the sharing of names; this is usually the last name or surname, which is passed down from generation to generation and is a way of signifying that this person belongs to this family. There can also be the use of specific names within families; this is particularly the case with boys, with many members of one family having the same first name. This tradition has been affected by the reduction of births within marriages, as the baby does not automatically take their father's surname unless they are named on their birth certificate. The non-traditional family can also lead to complexities in surnames, with children within the same family having different fathers and therefore surnames, as well as changing their surnames. This is effectively identified by Davies (2011) when one of the participants in the study had four surnames in the family, which was the norm for those children. This can have implications for midwives in that the baby's surname is not necessarily the one that is expected. People from outside the UK and other communities and cultures may have completely different naming systems which midwives need to be aware of, to be able to provide culturally sensitive care.

Activity 3.2

Can you think of a family display relevant to your family?

The characteristics of a 'family' relate to a formed identity, some form of economic contract, in which babies are born to form the next generation of that family, within which domestic and care work is undertaken (McKie and Callan 2012).

There are events within families which can have a negative impact on family members including children and women. These can include:

- poverty
- abuse
- substance misuse
- overcrowding
- mental illness
- physical illness.

There is current debate about the impact of certain types of families on society (Casey 2012). These have been labelled as 'troubled families' (Department of Communities and Local Government 2012; 2013). 'Troubled families' have been defined by recent government reports as households who:

- are involved in crime and anti-social behaviour
- have children not in school
- have an adult on out-of-work benefits
- cause high costs to the public purse.

(Department of Communities and Local Government 2012; 2013)

Further reading activity

Read: Donna and Jake's story on pages 17 & 18 of the *Listening to Troubled Families* report and think about how this family will be seen by the society in which they live. How could this label affect Donna, Jake and their children?

Casey, L. (2012) *Listening to Troubled Families*. London: Department for Communities and Local Government.

[Available online] https://www.gov.uk/government/uploads/system/uploads/attachment_data/file/6151/2183663.pdf

There has been criticism of the labelling of such families and the development of services based on the experiences of only a limited number of 'problem' families. Levitas (2012) is particularly critical of how the number of troubled families has been calculated and the impact of labelling them; how labels are then seized upon by the media to further stigmatise and vilify them.

Troubled families can be seen as being outside the cultural and societal norms or are seen as a drain on society. Some of the current changes to the welfare system could be seen to be aimed at these families, although other people within society may see the families and their members as vulnerable rather than troubled. Vulnerability is difficult to define and means different things to different people. Larkin (2009, p. 3) discusses how vulnerability can be assessed using criteria around how the person or group are '*marginalised, socially excluded, have limited opportunities and income and suffer abuse, hardship, prejudice and discrimination*'. Many elements of social exclusion can occur within the family and be a result of people being seen as outside of society's norms (Pierson 2010). These elements of exclusion can be found in the media and particularly the tabloids, stigmatising and sometimes demonising a certain type of person. Judgements can be made about people being good or bad parents, with a particular focus on mothers and pregnant women.

Activity 3.3

What do the stories below say about the media's view of a 'normal' family?

[Available online] http://www.thesun.co.uk/sol/homepage/features/4957397/Why-pick-on-Kate-when-Rod-had-eight-kids-by-five-women.html and http://www.telegraph.co.uk/news/celebritynews/10100935/Three-babies-by-three-fathers-will-it-be-third-time-lucky-for-Calamity-Kate-Winslet.html

Domestic abuse

There are messages within all societies around what is acceptable behaviour within families; these change over time and are linked to what is seen as the social norm. One particular message which affects the health and wellbeing of families is domestic abuse.

Domestic abuse is defined as:

...any incident or pattern of incidents of controlling, coercive, threatening behaviour, violence or abuse between those aged 16 or over who are, or have been, intimate partners or family members regardless of gender or sexuality...

The abuse can encompass, but is not limited to:

- psychological
- physical
- sexual
- financial
- emotional.

(Home Office 2013)

The definition of domestic abuse has changed over time, from relating solely to physical abuse to now incorporating all the above factors and specific campaigns around stalking and forced marriages. There is also a need to reflect the changes to family structures as previously discussed to include all the different variations. Historically in the UK it was seen as acceptable for a husband to physically punish his wife; this is now seen as unacceptable and a crime within the UK and many other countries, but not in all countries. However, this does not mean that domestic abuse does not happen; sadly the fact is that women are still living in fear and being murdered by their partners (Howard et al. 2013). Abuse is also experienced by men (ManKind Initiative 2013). This demonstrates that although something is seen as unacceptable by the majority of society and is deemed a crime, it will not necessarily stop the behaviour happening. It has been identified as the role of the midwife to identify and support women who are living with domestic abuse (see Chapter 11: 'Public health and health promotion', where domestic abuse is discussed in greater depth).

Safeguarding children and vulnerable adults

Domestic abuse is now also linked to safeguarding of vulnerable adults and children, as it is clear the emotional harm that can be caused to children who witness and live with domestic abuse. All societies cherish their children as the next generation; those who will care for their families as they grow older. However, there are still cases of those who step outside of the key social norms and abuse children. Powell and Uppal (2012) identify many different names of children whose treatment and deaths have led to changes in the law and practices in order to try to safeguard future children. The midwife is part of the safeguarding team for both vulnerable adults and children; it is also important to identify that it is possible to help families in order for them to care for their children in a more appropriate and safe way (see Chapter 8: 'Postnatal midwifery care', where safeguarding is discussed in greater depth).

Poverty

One of the issues within the family which has a profound impact on the health and wellbeing of the members is poverty. It has been well-recognised for decades that people with more income have better health and those with less have poorer health. This is classed as health inequalities, and these inequalities have been growing consistently over the years (Joseph Rowntree Foundation 2011; 2013). At this time of austerity, this divide is increasing: the rich are getting richer and the poor getting poorer. There is some debate around the definition of poverty and which one is used when developing policies and publishing statistics.

Activity 3.4

Think about what you would need to go without in order to make you feel that you were living in poverty. How would this be different if you lived in a least developed country?

There is a debate around how to define poverty and how to measure it in different contexts and communities.

Go to the website below and think about the different understandings of the term poverty.
[Available online] http://www.poverty.ac.uk/definitions-poverty

There are different definitions used such as absolute poverty which relates to the ability to survive. This tends to be linked to pictures on television of children from developing countries; however, it is stated that there are families in the UK today that are living in absolute poverty. There have been reports of increasing numbers of families relying on food banks in order to feed themselves, with some parents having to make difficult choices regarding what to go without. There is also relative or overall poverty, which relate to the ability to be able to participate in normal activities of the community in which a person lives (Poverty and Social Exclusion UK 2013). It has always been recognised that some families within the UK live in relative poverty. Reading Townend (1979) which is a seminal text around poverty, demonstrates how measurement of relative poverty has changed over the years, although some key elements have not. In his work, relative poverty is related to the ability to buy presents and have birthday parties, as well as eating a cooked breakfast.

There are other words used to describe poverty such as severe poverty which relates to the inability to afford to fund school trips, not having house insurance, being unable to repair any broken items in the house such as washing machines, and getting into significant debt to buy birthday and Christmas gifts (Witham 2012). However, this could also be termed relative poverty as these would probably be classed as normal day-to-day activities. There has been increasing concern about the rise in debt within families, and how this is being worsened by the use of loan companies, who charge exorbitant interest rates. These families become vulnerable to exploitation and therefore experience further difficulties with their budget. It could be that using the term deprivation is more relevant and is a more useful term to use. However, any label given to a person or family can lead to stigmatisation and discrimination.

It is well-documented that families living in poverty have poorer health and wellbeing; this is linked to the ability to afford good quality and fresh food, cost of exercise, poorer housing and living in unsafe neighbourhoods. The lack of opportunities and loss of hope, linked to the loss of the ability to meet their full potential and the mental health impact this has are recognised challenges for families living in poverty (Pierson 2010). The current focus on reductions in the welfare budget, and what some would say is a stigmatising of people living on benefits, will only lead to further difficulties and problems for this group.

Figures 3.2 and 3.3 illustrate the impact of poverty on the family and how these issues interlink with social exclusion.

The family is the structure in which we develop our identity, with specific elements outside the family influencing this development. There are key elements within our identity which impact on how we are viewed by society and what society expects of us. This chapter will now examine some of these key elements.

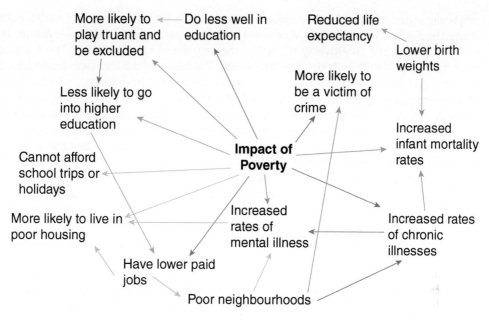

Figure 3.2　The impact of poverty on health.

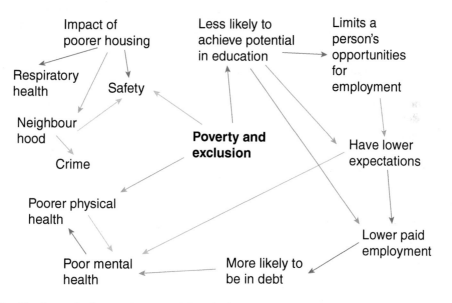

Figure 3.3　The impact of poverty on social exclusion.

Gender and sexuality

Gender and sexuality are terms which are sometimes used interchangeable or incorrectly, and are a key component of everyone's identity. The definitions which we will use in this chapter are that gender is a socially constructed identity (Marchbank and Letherby 2007) which is based around our biological sex. Sexuality is based around desire and is related to the people we are physically attracted to and have sexual intercourse with. Both these parts of our identities are related to displays within society. When and how these parts of our identity are formed is open to much debate and controversy, related to the nature and nurture debate. These discussions have developed significantly over the last decade. Previously all the focus was around the binary nature of gender and sexuality, with female and male and heterosexuality and 'other'; now this includes transgender, transsexual, bisexual, lesbian and gay (LGBT) communities (Equality Challenge Unit 2010). This is important in relation to power relations within society and what is termed as a social norm, and the consequences of stepping outside this norm. This has an impact on how certain groups within society can be excluded and discriminated against and therefore may not be happy to share information with healthcare workers. There is a particular impact on lesbian mothers, who have often not had the care they wanted or needed (Jackson 2003; Lee 2004; Dahl et al. 2013). Many lesbian couples do not tell their midwives about their sexuality, and this is their right; however, it can lead to inappropriate care being given and can affect the way that the woman's partner is treated. This is not surprising, though, in the face of prejudice or lack of under-standing displayed by society and NHS staff. The Department of Health (2009) has outlined how members of the LGBT community can be more effectively and fairly cared for. However, it is essential that there is not a heterosexual assumption within the maternity services, and that women are able to speak freely about their sexuality without fear of prejudice or discrimination; otherwise this group of women and their families will remain largely invisible.

Activity 3.5

Think about how you portray gender in your everyday life. What actions do you take which displays your gender to others. For example, deciding to use the male or female toilets.

Every society has roles, identities, expectations and characteristics which are assigned to people on the basis of their gender (Kane 2012). These tend to focus on two binary opposites of women and men and femininity and masculinity (Marchbank and Letherby 2007). However, there is some room for adaptation and development over time; for example, what are seen as feminine and masculine characteristics. The gender roles that people are socialised into have an impact on how the family works and what are seen as men and women's roles. These have changed over time as societies' and communities' views have changed and developed. This can lead to clashes between the generations as what was once seen as outside the social norm can now be identified as normal. An example of this would be the change in attitudes in the UK to pregnancy outside marriage; at one time an unmarried woman who had a baby was seen as a scandal and something to be frowned upon. This had a negative impact on her family. In the 21st century, for most families within the UK this is not now the case, and in fact in many communities this is the norm. In the past, women out of wedlock were hidden away in mental health institutions for stepping outside the norm; the mother and the baby may have lived there for the rest of their lives. This shame and guilt is still present in some cultures and communities and can lead to the woman's life being in danger, linked to so-called 'honour killings', although as one of the interesting gender differences, historically the man who was the father of the baby would mostly escape any punishment. This is evidence of the inequality between genders and how their behaviour is sanctioned and labelled as acceptable or unacceptable dependent on their gender. Kane (2012, p. 13) describes gender as a 'strict binary of two highly distinct categories, guiding people sometimes gently and sometimes coercively into one or the other'. This can be related to what are perceived as specific characteristics of femininity and masculinity, which are often seen as opposites, but in practice, can overlap.

Activity 3.6

Sit in a coffee shop or bar and watch the people; think about how you know whether the people are men or women.

How do you think you would feel if you could not identify their gender?

There is also a debate around the role of fathers and how this can often be marginalised and not fully explored, with the emphasis being on the role of the mother (Bainbridge 2008; Price 2012; Daniel 2005). This is often in terms of inequalities between the focus of care being on the woman rather than the father. The role of fathers has changed over time and is different depending on the family's culture and community. The changing attitude to fathers being present at the birth of their baby is evidence of how society's views can change and shape the families' experiences. It is made clear by the Nursing and Midwifery Council (NMC) (2009) and Department of Health (2007) that the focus of midwives' care should be on the whole family, not just the woman and the baby. Hansom et al. (2010) examined how services specifically aimed at young fathers can improve the health and wellbeing of all the family. The Royal College of Midwives (RCM) (2011) sets out guidance on how to help to involve fathers in maternity services and identifies the evidence which states that this will improve the health and wellbeing outcomes of all the family.

Ethnicity and race

There are other factors which can affect a person's health and wellbeing; these include race and ethnicity. It is well-documented that people from certain ethnic backgrounds have poorer health and wellbeing than the general population. This can be related to discrimination and racism which can have an impact on the person's mental and physical health. Although this does not explain all the differences, there are also genetic influences, with some groups having greater incidences of certain diseases. Practices within different communities can also influence the group's health in a positive and negative way: for example, having faith can improve a person's psychological wellbeing; female genital mutilation has a detrimental impact on girls and women (WHO 2013); the practice of marrying within a community can have genetic consequences with increased rates of infant mortality and congenital abnormalities. There are also health implications related to the age when people marry and start having children. This can vary significantly between cultures, communities and countries (Hepburn and Simon 2006).

It is important to be clear about what is meant by terms which are used to define people and groups of people. Bhopal (2004) discusses the difficulties in defining terms such as race and ethnicity and the fact that these terms are not necessarily 'fixed' or 'easily measured'. Bhopal (2004 p. 441) defines ethnicity as:

> ...a multifaceted quality that refers to the group to which people belong, and/or are perceived to belong, as a result of certain shared characteristics, including geographical and ancestral origins, but particularly cultural traditions and languages...

Bhopal (2004) also discusses the definition of race and its biological and social determinants, and identifies the difficulties of defining this term, although the study of discrimination of people due to their race is highlighted as being of key importance.

Activity 3.7

What race and what ethnicity would you identify yourself as and why?

Race and ethnicity are often seen as in terms of 'the other', the dominant race being 'white' within the UK. As can be seen with other types of discrimination this is related to difference from the majority and therefore the norm. Racism can be defined as:

> ...*a belief that some races are superior to others, used to devise and justify individual and collective actions that create and sustain inequality among racial and ethnic groups...*
>
> (Bhopal 2004, p. 444)

Aspinall (2010) discusses how trying to categories people into specific groups can be difficult, with the introduction of the 'mixed' ethnic or racial groups increasing this complexity. As Giddens (2009, p. 671) describes '*there are no clear cut characteristics by means of which human beings can be allocated to different races*'. Giddens (2009, p. 633) goes on to define ethnicity as '*cultural practices and outlooks of a given community of people which sets them apart from others*'. Burnett (2013) explores the sources of racial hatred and how this is shaped over time. He discusses how this hatred can be seen as normal by society, and can be reinforced by the media, giving the examples of asylum seekers and migrants, who are often seen as taking jobs and housing from the rest of the population and living on social benefits. This can tap into the fears of society, which can be around difference and are magnified during times of financial adversity.

Disability

A person has a disability if: '*they have a physical or mental impairment, the impairment has a substantial and long-term adverse effect on their ability to perform normal day-to-day activities*' (Equality Act 2010).

The key aspect of this definition is around the ability to carry out what are seen as normal day to day activities, this is a theme within the literature. Oliver (1996) identifies 'three core elements linked to the definition of disability: (a) the presence of impairment; (b) the experience of externally imposed restrictions; and (c) self-identification as a disabled person. This is well-applied to the concept of society affecting the opportunities of the disabled person as seen in the 'social model of disability', the presence of an 'impairment' linked to the medical model and the importance of how the person feels about being labelled as being disabled. As the term disability tends to be a negative one, people may want to reject this label and want to be viewed as an individual rather than a disability. There is also an 'affirmation model' (Swain and French 2000) which challenges society to see disability from a positive perspective; this can be seen in subcultures within disability, for example, the deaf culture (Sparrow 2010). This is interesting as there is controversy within this culture in how treatment for the disability is viewed, in that cochlear implants are seen as a way to wipe out the deaf culture (Sparrow 2010), to meet the medical model of disability within society. The assumption is that deaf people would want to become hearing. Walsh-Gallagher et al. (2012) have identified an affirmation model for pregnant women and mothers who have a disability, the key elements of 'celebration, achievement, bonding and confidence' identified from their interviews with women.

There is a debate around how society views disability and whether it is the parents' responsibility to ensure they do not have a disabled child requiring additional care and services from society which will be painful for them, the child and their family. As previously identified there are different models of disability (Brandon and Pritchard 2011; Larkin 2009). One of these is the 'social model of disability' (McDaniel 2013; Larkin 2009) which links disability to how society treats and views people with a disability, rather than focusing on the disability itself. This theory was developed in contrast and to challenge the medical view of disability, which focused on what was wrong and what could be done to make the person less disabled. The person is characterised by their disability, lives this experience, and is often not seen as anything else. This is followed by stigma and limitations and expectations of society, about what the disabled person can or cannot do (Barnes and Mercer 2010; Barnes et al. 2010; Burchardt 2010). This view has been challenged by activists from the disabled community, who challenge society to remove barriers which make the person disabled and for their members to have the same opportunities as others within society.

There has been some discussion around what the impact of the London Paralympics has been in relation to how society views those who are disabled, and how to change negative attitudes, some of which are based around prejudice and ignorance. It is unclear how much impact this will have in the future. Braye et al. (2012, p. 5) highlighted in their study the negative views of some disabled people to the Paralympic Games, with one of the participants stating that:

> ...the focus on elite Paralympians promotes an image of disabled people which is so far removed from the typical experiences of a disabled person that it is damaging to the public understanding of disability...

This has an impact on midwives as they are involved in caring for women who have disabilities, women who are having or have had a baby with a disability and their own emotions in relating to these families. This can also be viewed against the idea that the disabled body is one that is failing and has to be measured against the normal functioning body (Hughes 2009). From a childbearing viewpoint women and men who are infertile or have difficulty in conceiving could be viewed as failures; women who are unable to give birth naturally may view themselves as being less of a woman. This has obvious implications for a woman's self esteem and psychological wellbeing. The language that doctors and midwives use can also facilitate this feeling of failure. Harpur (2012) also discusses how behaviour outside of society's norms defines the person as disabled.

With advances in antenatal screening and diagnostic testing, women and their families are faced with making difficult and challenging decisions about what screening to have and what to do if there is likelihood of abnormality. Some of this is maybe linked to society's views of disability and the particular condition involved. Williams et al. (2002) discuss how screening for Down syndrome is sometimes explained by midwives, the implication being, that people with this condition have little to contribute to society and their family's lives.

Activity 3.8

Read Tom Bickerby's articles:

Bickerby, T. (2012) About a boy. *The Times* 18 June 2012, p. 7.
Bickerby, T. (2012) The letter I wish I'd read. *The Times* 16 July 2012, pp. 7–9.

Reflect on how you feel about the information in the articles.

Health and wellbeing

There are many different definitions of health, which vary from the lack of disease, to the ability to participate in the normal activities of life; there is currently more of a focus on wellbeing rather than just using the term health (Schickler 2005; Tomlinson and Kelly 2013). Health is one part of wellbeing and just because a person has a disease does not mean that they will auto-matically feel that their wellbeing has been negatively affected. This is important because if a person is 'labelled' as being ill this could have a negative affect on the person and also make them feel that their own experience and views have been disregarded. It is also important to recognise that this will vary between individuals, communities and cultures.

Activity 3.9

Read the article Schickler, P. (2005) Achieving health or achieving wellbeing? *Learning in Health and Social Care* 4(4), pp. 217–227.

Ask yourself the questions that the participants were asked about health and wellbeing; what does this tell you about how you view your own health and wellbeing?

This is relevant in relation to maternity care; midwives need to emphasise to women that pregnancy is not an illness and that the whole process of childbirth is one of normality. There has been an ongoing debate for many years about the medicalisation of childbirth and its impact on women and their babies. The view is that by putting women in hospitals to give birth and focusing on risk rather than normality, as well as the involvement of doctors, has meant that rather than see childbirth as a normal health event, Western society has seen it as one of risk and ill health (Scamell 2011; Barry and Yuill 2012). This has led to a loss of confidence in a woman's ability to give birth naturally, and to an increase in unnecessary intervention. The language that doctors and midwives use to describe pregnancy and childbirth events also has a psychological impact on the woman and her family; terms such as *'failure to progress'*, *'failed induction'*, *'lack of progress'*, all give an impression of the body as a machine which is malfunctioning (Walker 2012). Women may feel that this is their fault and that they somehow have control over this process. This can be related to the work of Illich (2012) who saw medicine as a *'threat to health'*; he describes how professionals *'assert secret knowledge about human nature, knowledge which only they have the right to dispense'* (Illich 1977, p. 19). Irving Zola (1977, p. 41) also describes how *'medicine is becoming a major institution of social control'*. He argued that the label of health and illness *'medicalises living'*.

With reference to childbearing, it is possible to see how the impact of reproductive technologies has led to the view that everyone has the right to have a child, and that there is the technology available to achieve this. Prior to this development women and men were accepting of the fact that difficulties with their fertility meant they would not be able to have a biological child, even though this would be met with sadness and psychological distress. Unfortunately in reality these advances will not lead to all couples having a baby, whether it is biologically related or not. There are also the financial implications of these technologies at a time of austerity, leading to inequalities of access to treatment dependent on post codes and wealth.

During the process of undertaking these technologies such as in vitro fertilisation (IVF) there can be a loss of health and wellbeing due to the physical and psychological impact of these treatments. This can be similar to how pregnant women feel about the process of childbirth and the many recorded physical and psychological side effects. For example; some disorders of pregnancy are labelled 'minor'. However, if a person who was not pregnant woke up every morning feeling nauseous and vomiting, and it continued throughout the day, one can be sure that they would not feel that this was a 'minor' illness. This identifies how all health and wellbeing needs to be viewed in context; for example, a person with multiple sclerosis may feel that they have a good level of wellbeing, but anyone else with the same symptoms would feel that they were unwell.

The implications and response to the pain of labour is an interesting factor in relation to health, illness and wellbeing. Pain is normally a physiological response of the body to a pathological process. The purpose of pain is normally to identify some problem with the functioning of the body. A normal social response to pain is to view it in a negative way, to see it as a warning that something is wrong and to want to find out what it is and to find ways to manage and cope with the pain.

There has been a great deal written about the 'sick role' (Giddens 2009; Mik-Meyer and Obling 2012) and how this impacts on a person's experience of illness and what society would see as their obligation to take action to get well. The link to pregnancy can be problematic as this is not seen as an illness, rather an identification of health, although it can be seen that some women do take on the sick role in order to manage their symptoms and in response to the views of their family and community. Midwives can encourage women to eat healthily and exercise normally, promoting good health for woman and baby, but some women feel that they need to 'eat for two' and that exercising is somehow dangerous for them and the pregnancy. This would appear to be further emphasised by the media with stories around what pregnant women should and should not do. It can be seen that pregnant women and mothers have responsibilities shaped by their community, which they are obliged to engage with in order to be seen as 'good mothers', with negative consequences if they falter outside of the expected cultural norms (Armstrong and Eborall 2012).

Activity 3.10

What does this story say about acceptable behaviour of women; what about their partners? Have a look at the NICE guidelines and see how accurate this story is.

[Available online] http://www.telegraph.co.uk/health/healthnews/10052282/Smoking-test-for -mothers.html

One of the messages that Western society gives is that members have a responsibility to their community to keep well and their activities should reflect this. This can be linked to what are seen as inappropriate behaviours; for example, messages around obesity, smoking and drug misuse (McDaniel 2013). Antenatal screening could also be seen as part of this message; there are increasing numbers of conditions that can be screened for and it can be viewed negatively if women and their partners do not want to have this screening, or once identified as at risk do not want to have diagnostic tests or treatment (Armstrong and Eborall 2012). The message around breastfeeding can be seen as confusing, the information from healthcare professionals is clear that breastfeeding is good, with clear health benefits for the mother and baby. However, the message from society is often around the need to breastfeed away from the public eye.

Activity 3.11

Go to the link below and think what message that this story gives to pregnant women about acceptable behaviour.

http://www.thesun.co.uk/sol/homepage/woman/4846871/I-ate-for-two-and-put-on-8-stone .html

Key points

- The society in which we live has a significant impact on our lives.
- Society's views and social norms can label people as being deviant.
- Midwives have a role to play in protecting vulnerable people within society.
- It is essential that midwives put aside their own views and beliefs in order to be caring and compassionate.

Conclusion

Some key sociological theories and how they can be applied to childbearing and maternity services have been explored and linked to appropriate issues. Sociology has been identified as a key area of knowledge which is required by student midwives and healthcare practitioners (NMC 2009). The circumstances in which people live and into which they are born have a significant impact on their lives, hopes and aspirations. There has been a discussion on how society views specific groups and behaviours and how this can lead to stigma and discrimination which in turn links to ill health and reduced life chances. There are many elements within a society which can impact on a person's health; this chapter has identified and explored some of these issues and how they can affect the woman and her family. The family has been identified as a key structure within everyone's life which can have negative and positive implications. Historical changes in family structures have been examined and how these have impacted on reproduction and the lives of family members. The activities within the chapter should have helped you to examine your own views and experiences within society to help gain a better understanding of how these can impact on women and their families.

End of chapter activities
Crossword

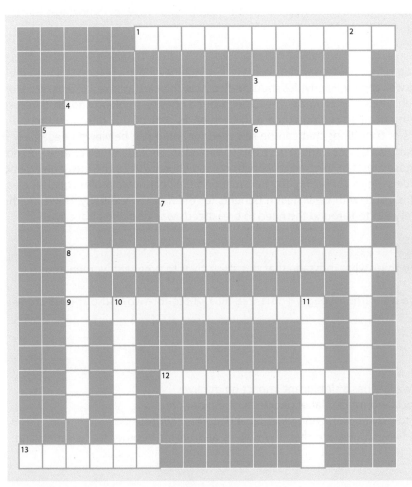

Across

1. A society in which men are the most powerful and influential
3. A social group which share certain financial, cultural or social characteristics
5. A group of people related by common descent or heredity
6. Key institution of society
7. The view that one person is inferior to another due to a particular characteristic

8. Treating a person less favourably than another due to a particular characteristic
9. Rules and beliefs which members of any society are expected to adhere to
12. Shared characteristics which can be geographical including cultural traditions and languages
13. A socially constructed identity

Down

2. Circumstances which mean that a person does not have the means for survival
4. Everyday activities in which family members communicate with each other and to those around them that they are a family

10. A lived experience
11. A group of people connected together by a shared culture

Find out more

Below is a list of things you can find out about to enhance your knowledge of the issues and topics covered in this chapter. Make notes using the chapter content, the references and further reading identified, local policies and guidelines and discussions with colleagues.

1. Find out how you would report any safeguarding concerns you had about a member of a family you were caring for. Who would you go to for support?

2. Look at the census information [available online] http://www.ons.gov.uk/ons/guidemethod/census/2011/index.html paying particular attention to health inequalities and lifestyle and behaviours. If you compare the life expectancy measures for Cornwall and Glasgow City you can see significant differences. Why do you think this is? Have a look at your area and compare that to an area with a lower or higher rate.

3. Think about the following questions:

    What is the role of a woman; does this change when she becomes pregnant and then a mother?
    What is the role of a man; does this change when he becomes a father?
    If pregnancy is not an illness, how can midwives explain all the treatments, appointments and screening which are expected?
    What events and experiences have formed your identity? What impact have these had on your life?
    Do you believe that infertility is an illness? Is it the right of all couples to have a baby regardless of cost?

4. Draw a family structure diagram and think about how this has changed over the generations.

5. Read the article: Oliver, M. (2013) The social model of disability: thirty years on. *Disability & Society* 28(7), pp. 1024–1026. Do you agree with his views regarding the welfare reforms?

6. In order for society to be protected against infectious diseases then a certain number of people need to be vaccinated or immunised against the disease. Read the article below and think about how parents who do not participate in these programmes are viewed by the rest of society.

    Griffith, H. (2013) Wales measles: 1200 MMR jabs given at drop in clinics. http://www.bbc.co.uk/news/uk-wales-22048635

Glossary of terms

Class　A social group which share certain financial, cultural or social characteristics.

Culture　A lived experience within a specific group.

Disability　A physical or mental impairment; the impairment has a substantial and long-term adverse effect on their ability to perform normal day-to-day activities.

Domestic abuse　Any incident or pattern of incidents of controlling, coercive, threatening behaviour, violence or abuse between those aged 16 or over who are, or have been, intimate partners or family members regardless of gender or sexuality.

Ethnicity　A multifaceted quality that refers to the group to which people belong, and/or are perceived to belong, as a result of certain shared characteristics, including geographical and ancestral origins, but particularly cultural traditions and languages.

Family　Form of social grouping.

Family displays　Everyday activities in which family members communicate to each other and to those around them that they are family.

Feminism　View that women should have equal rights to men and that everyone is equal.

Gender　A socially constructed identity which is based around a person's biological sex.

Patriarchy　Society in which men are the most powerful and influential.

Race　A group of people related by common descent or heredity.

Sexual orientation　General attraction a person feels towards one sex or the other (or both).

Sexuality　Sexual characteristics, meanings and social practices.

Social construction　Social reality is the product of interactions between individuals and groups.

Social norms　Rules and beliefs which members of any society are expected to adhere to.

Society　A group of people connected together by a shared culture.

Sociology　Scientific study of human life, social groups, whole societies and the human world.

Transgender　People who live part or all of their lives in their preferred gender role.

References

Armstrong, N., Eborall, H. (2012) The sociology of medical screening: past present and future. *Sociology of Health and Illness* 34 (2), pp. 161–176.

Aspinall, P. (2010) Concepts, terminology and classifications for the 'mixed' ethnic or racial group in the United Kingdom. *Journal of Epidemiology and Community Health* 64, pp. 557–560.

Bainbridge, J. (2008) Modern man battles to be included. *British Journal of Midwifery* 16 (5), p. 319.

Barry, A., Yuill, C. (2012) *Understanding the Sociology of Health*. London: Sage Publications.

Barnes, C., Mercer, G. (2010) *Exploring Disability: A Sociological Introduction*. Cambridge: Polity.

Barnes, C., Mercer, G., Shakespeare, T. (2010) The Social Model of Disability. In: Giddens, A. Sutton, P. (eds) (2010) *Sociology: Introductory Readings*, 3rd edn. Cambridge: Polity, pp. 161–167.

Bickerby, T. (2012) About a boy. *The Times* 18 June 2012, p. 7.

Bickerby, T. (2012) The letter I wish I'd read. *The Times* 16 July 2012, pp. 7–9.

Bhopal, R. (2004) Glossary of terms relating to ethnicity and race: for reflection and debate. *Journal of Epidemiology and Community Health* 58, pp. 441–445.

Brandon, T., Pritchard, G. (2011) Being fat: a conceptual analysis using three models of disability. *Disability & Society* 26 (1), pp. 79–92.

Braye, S., Dixon, K., Gibbons, T. (2012) A mockery of equality: an exploratory investigation into disabled activists views of the Paralympic Games. *Disability & Society* Published online 21 December 2012, http://dx.doi.org/10.1080/09687599.2012.748648

Burnett, J. (2013) Britain: racial violence and the politics of hate. *Race & Class* 54 (5), pp. 5–21.

Burchardt, T. (2010) Capabilities and disability: the capabilities framework and the social model of disability. *Disability & Society* 19 (7), pp. 735–751.

Casey, L. (2012) *Listening to Troubled Families*. London: Department for Communities and Local Government.

Daniel, L. (2005) Children need fathers too: Helping fathers to get involved. *British Journal of Midwifery* 13 (12), p. 759.

Davies, H. (2011) Sharing surnames: children, family and kinship. *Sociology* 45 (4), pp. 554–569.

Dahl, B., Fylkesnes, A., Sorlie, V., Malterud, K. (2013) Lesbian women's experiences with healthcare providers in the birthing context: A meta-ethnography. *Midwifery* 29, pp. 674–681.

Department of Communities and Local Government (2012) *The Troubled Families Programme* DCLG. https://www.gov.uk/government/uploads/system/uploads/attachment_data/file/11469/2117840.pdf

Department of Communities and Local Government (2013) *The Fiscal Case for Working with Troubled Families* DCLG https://www.gov.uk/government/uploads/system/uploads/attachment_data/file/79377/20130208_The_Fiscal_Case_for_Working_with_Troubled_Families.pdf

Department of Health (2007) *Maternity Matters*. London: DH.

Department of Health (2009) *Sexual Orientation a practical guide for the NHS*. London: DH.

Equality Challenge Unit (2010) *Trans Staff and Students in Higher Education*. London: ECU.

Equality Act (2010) access online http://www.legislation.gov.uk/ukpga/2010/15/section/6

Farrell, B., VandeVusse, A., Ocobock, A. (2012) Family change and the state of family sociology. *Current Sociology* 60 (3), pp. 283–301.

Giddens, A. (2009) *Sociology*. Cambridge: Polity.

Hansom, J., Nur Young, N. (2010) Who cares about teenage dads? Role of a young fathers' worker. *British Journal of Midwifery* 18 (2), pp. 106–109.

Harpur, P. (2012) From disability to ability: changing the phrasing of the debate. *Disability & Society* 27 (3), pp. 325–337.

Hepburn, S., Simon, R. (2006) Women's roles and statuses the World over. *Gender Studies* Spring 2006, pp. 62–68.

Home Office (2013) *Domestic Violence and Abuse*. https://www.gov.uk/domestic-violence-and-abuse

Howard, M., Laxton, C., Musoke, P. (2013) *Women's Aid Annual Survey 2013*. Bristol: Women's Aid Federation of England.

Hughes, B. (2009) Wounded/monstrous/abject: a critique of the disabled body in the sociological imaginary. *Disability & Society* 24 (4), pp. 399–410.

Illich, I. (2012) Ivan Illich on medical nemesis. *Nurse Education Today* 32, pp. 5–6.

Illich, I. (1977) Disabling professions. In: Illich, I., Zola, I., McKnight, J., Caplan, J., Shaiken, H. (eds) *Disabling Professions*. London: Marion Boyars, pp. 11–39.

Jackson, K. (2003) Midwifery care and the lesbian client. *British Journal of Midwifery* 11 (7), pp. 434–437.

James, A., Curtis, P. (2010) Family displays and personal lives. *Sociology* 44 (6), pp. 1163–1180.

Joseph Rowntree Foundation (2013) *Poverty, Participation and choice* http://www.jrf.org.uk/publications/poverty-participation-and-choice

Joseph Rowntree Foundation (2011) *Monitoring poverty and social exclusion 2011*. York: JRF.

Kane, E. (2012) *Rethinking Gender and Sexuality in Childhood*. London: Bloomsbury.

Larkin, M. (2009) *Vulnerable Groups in Health and Social Care*. London: Sage Publications.

Lee, E. (2004) Lesbian users of maternity services: appropriate care. *British Journal of Midwifery* 12 (6), pp. 353–358.

Levitas, R. (2012) *There may be trouble ahead: What we know about those 120,000 'troubled' families Poverty and Social Exclusion in the UK* http://www.poverty.ac.uk/system/files/attachments/WP%20Policy%20Response%20No.3-%20%20%27Trouble%27%20ahead%20%28Levitas%20Final%2021April2012%29.pdf

ManKind Initiative (2013) Types of domestic abuse [online] Available: http://www.mankind.org.uk/typesdomesticabuse.html

Marchbank, J., Letherby, G. (2007) *Introduction to Gender: Social Science Perspectives*. London: Pearson Education.

McDaniel, S. (2013) Understanding health sociologically. *Current Sociology* 61 (5–6), pp. 826–841.

McKie, L., Callan, S. (2012) *Understanding Families A Global Introduction*. London: Sage.

Mik-Meyer, N., Obling, A. (2012) The negotiation of the sick role: General Practitioners' classification of patients with medically unexplained symptoms. *Sociology of Health and Illness* 347, pp. 1025–1038.

Nursing and Midwifery Council (2009) *Standards for pre-registration midwifery education*. London: NMC.

Oliver, M. (1996) *Understanding Disability: From Theory to Practice*. Basingstoke: MacMillan.

Pierson, J. (2010) *Tackling Social Exclusion*. London: Routledge.

Price, C. (2012) Fatherhood and maternity care. *British Journal of Midwifery* 20 (12), p. 910.

Poverty and Social Exclusion (PSE) (2013) Absolute and overall poverty http://www.poverty.ac.uk/definitions-poverty/absolute-and-overall-poverty Accessed 10th July 2013.

Powell, J., Uppal, E. (2012) *Safeguarding Babies and Young Children*. Maidenhead: Open University Press.

Royal College of Midwives (2011) Reaching out: Involving fathers in maternity care http://www.rcm.org.uk/college/policy-practice/government-policy/fathers-guide/

Schickler, P. (2005) Achieving health or achieving wellbeing? *Learning in Health and Social Care* 4 (4), pp. 217–227.

Sparrow, R. (2010) Implants and ethnocide: learning from the cochlear implant controversy. *Disability & Society* 25 (4), pp. 455–466.

Swain, J., French, S. (2000) Towards an affirmation model of disability. *Disability & Society* 15 (4), pp. 569–582.

Tomlinson, M., Kelly, G. (2013) Is everybody happy? The politics and measurement of national wellbeing. *Policy & Politics* 41 (2), pp. 139–157.

Townend, P. (1979) *Poverty in the United Kingdom*. http://www.poverty.ac.uk/definitions-poverty/absolute-and-overall-poverty

Walker, S. (2012) Mechanistic and Natural body metaphors and their effects on attitudes to hormonal contraception. *Women & Health* 52 (8), pp. 788–803.

Walsh-Gallagher, D., Sinclaire, M., McConkey, R. (2012) The ambiguity of disabled women's experiences of pregnancy, childbirth and motherhood: A phenomenological understanding. *Midwifery* 28, pp. 156–162.

Williams, C., Alderson, P., Farsides, B. (2002) What constitutes 'balanced information in the practitioners' portrayals of Down's Syndrome? *Midwifery* 18, pp. 230–237.

Witham, G. (2012) *Child Poverty in 2012 It Shouldn't Happen Here*. Manchester: Save The Children.

World Health Organization (2013) *Female Genital Mutilation* http://www.who.int/mediacentre/factsheets/fs241/en/

Zola, I. (1977) Healthism and disabling medicalization. In Illich, I., Zola, I., McKnight, J., Caplan, J. (eds), *Disabling Professions*. London: Marion Boyars.

Chapter 4

Psychology applied to maternity care

Julie Jomeen

University of Hull, Hull, UK

Lynda Bateman

University of Hull, Hull, UK

Learning outcomes

By the end of this chapter the reader will be able to:

- identify the main theoretical models of psychology
- discuss why the study of psychology helps to understand behaviour or individual responses to a given situation
- recognise how psychology can help midwives relate to the women in their care and their families
- recognise that midwifery practice can be enhanced by understanding psychology.

Introduction

Psychological health is important with respect to how we function and adapt. Its relevance to childbearing women is clear when we acknowledge the significant transition and adaptation that women go through in their journey from conception through to motherhood. Understanding psychology in relation to pregnancy, birth and the postnatal period will afford midwives insight into the complexity of a woman's experience and enable a more perceptive consideration of her emotional needs. Midwives are key to assuring the quality of women's experiences across the perinatal period and hence can be central to women's emotional health and wellbeing. How they communicate and interact with women can have both momentous and enduring consequence. This chapter will explore the study of how psychology can help midwives relate to the women in their care and their families.

Fundamentals of Midwifery: A Textbook for Students, First Edition. Edited by Louise Lewis.
© 2015 John Wiley & Sons, Ltd. Published 2015 by John Wiley & Sons, Ltd.
Companion website: www.wileyfundamentalseries.com/midwifery

Defining psychology

Psychology is concerned with the thoughts, feelings and motivations underlying behaviour. Psychology is the scientific study of behaviour and mental processes which emerged as a distinct discipline around 150 years ago (Hewstone et al. 2005). There are many diverse sub-fields within psychology and whilst it could be argued that all these sub-fields relate to childbearing women, midwifery and maternity care provision in some way, some have a more direct and lucid relevance. These include:

Developmental psychology: Change in behavioural and mental processes over the lifespan.
Social psychology: The reciprocal influence of the individual and their social context.
Family psychology: The family as a system and the relationships within that system.
Abnormal psychology: The nature and development of abnormal behaviours, thoughts and feelings associated with distress or impaired functioning that is not a culturally expected response to an event.
Health psychology: The identification and psychological causes and correlates of health and illness, psychological aspects of health promotion and prevention and treatment of disease.

Psychology is a combination of specialities which place differing degrees of emphasis on understanding varying elements of the person and potentially make *psychology a wide-reaching subject with rather fuzzy boundaries*' (Hewstone et al. 2005, p. 5). The five major historical approaches to psychology will be described, which have led to the evolution of many of the different sub-fields of psychology, including those described above. More contemporary approaches, including social constructionism and feminist psychology have also been highlighted as valuable within a maternity care context (Raynor and England 2010). Feminist approaches emphasise how most of the influential theories within psychology are based on the study of men and then applied to women. Men's behaviour becomes the standard against which women's behaviour is judged, ignoring the role of socially constructed ideas of women and their place within society and as mothers. The social constructionist paradigm takes into account the effects on a person of society, culture, politics, environment and economics. Ways of talking about the world vary, but so do subjective experiences of living, which are constituted in and from those ways of speaking. Psychological knowledge is socially, culturally and hence historically specific.

An understanding of different approaches within psychology can meaningfully contribute to our understanding of women's psychological responses to pregnancy, birth and early motherhood.

Theories of psychology

To acknowledge the importance of psychology to midwifery it is important to look at psychological theories and how they can be applied to clinical practice. While midwives are not expected to replace the work of psychologists, psychiatrists, therapists and counsellors, they need to have grounding in psychological theories to enable them to engage with women and their families to support them and enhance their effectiveness when confronted with challenging situations. Five major approaches to psychology are discussed below together with their impact on psychological understanding.

Social constructionist approach

This is not further explored in this chapter; for further reading see Crombie and Nightingale (1999) *Social Constructionist Psychology*.

Behaviourist approach

The Behaviourists theorised that behaviour could be changed by conditioning and reinforcement of behaviour. The famous 'Pavlov's dog' is an example of conditioning changing behaviour. When an individual is rewarded for a behaviour, it will impact positively on the individual and will strengthen the behaviour (positive reinforcement: Skinner 1976). A conditioned change of behaviour requires a process of association. For example a baby learns that smiling at the mother is rewarded with attention, therefore will continue smiling to gain more attention – the behaviour has been *positively reinforced* by the attention; the baby is *conditioned* to smile and associates smiling with reward. Moreover, there is benefit for the mother as when she gives attention to her baby she too is rewarded by smiles.

Freudian approach

Freud was the founder of psychoanalytic psychology which has impacted on all psychological theory. Freud defined three basic structures of personality – the id, the ego and the superego (Stevens 2008). He proposed that unconscious, destructive behaviour, when analysed and brought into consciousness could be resolved. For example, a woman continually fails to attend the antenatal clinic at the General Practitioners (GP). When questioned by the midwife, the woman discloses that the 'smell' of the GP surgery reminds her of an uncomfortable experience as a child: being chastised by her mother for incontinence (due to a recurrent kidney infection) in front of the GP. The smell of the surgery brings back uncomfortable memories and thus the woman does not attend her midwife's appointment.

Cognitive approach

Cognitive psychologists by contrast are interested in the scientific study of the mind, in particular, the elements of thinking and reasoning, language, learning and memory, perception, attention and consciousness. For example, a midwife may observe that a woman's pulse is elevated following birth and a trickle of blood exits from the genital tract. The midwife calls for help and will 'automatically' commence uterine palpation and administer an oxytocic preparation, as she is cognisant with the predisposing factors of a post-partum haemorrhage (see Chapter 16: 'Emergencies in midwifery', where postpartum haemorrhage is discussed in more depth). Her behaviour is not based on positive reinforcement or unconscious memory; it is a function of acting from memory and reasoning whereby she has the 'data' on how to manage a post-partum haemorrhage and acts accordingly.

Humanistic approach

Humanistic Psychology developed by Carl Rogers and Abraham Maslow is a 'softer', less analytical and rationalist approach and heralded a move from analytical psychology to therapeutic person-centred psychology. The emphasis in person-centred psychology is that the individual is valued for who they are, without judgement and are accepted unreservedly (Rogers 1961). Thus three key conditions emerge: empathy, congruence and unconditional positive regard, which are an essential aspect of midwifery practice.

Bio-psychological approach

The final psychological approach is bio-psychological, which incorporates neuroscience and psychology, noting the impact of neurobiology on psychology (Pinel 2011). This approach marries the biological response with the psychological response and examines the biological reasons for behaviour. Thus a woman's behaviour can be impacted by neurological phenomena which may not have a rational basis. An example is the function of the endocrine system whereby a lactating woman can experience an oxytocin-mediated milk-ejection reflex merely by thinking of her baby. The biophysical response is triggered by thought alone and not by the baby sucking at the breast, which is the normal activator of the endocrine response during lactation.

A bio-psychosocial model recognises that psychological health is best understood through the combination of physical, psychological and social factors, rather than working to a medical model aimed at identifying and categorising disease. This model acknowledges the importance of an interdisciplinary approach, the complexity of the constructs being defined and the uniqueness of the childbearing experience, thus aiding the conceptualisation of psychological health in the perinatal period.

Summary

Notwithstanding the psychological theories above, it is also important to note that the woman is situated within a social and cultural context. The woman's perception of herself within her socio-cultural context will inform and impact on her decision-making during her childbearing experience. Midwives' practice within a cultural context determined by local and national guidelines and their individual experiences are also societally mediated, sometimes in conflict with personal beliefs which potentially can create tensions in practice.

Midwives will bring their own psychology and socio-cultural influences to the maternity setting and the challenge to midwives is to develop self-awareness and sensitivity to those influences and the concomitant influence on women.

Psychology and public health in maternity care

Public health is concerned with helping people to stay healthy and protecting them from threats to their health. Government policy seeks to support people to be able to make healthier choices, regardless of their circumstances, and to minimise the risk and impact of illness and adverse health outcomes. Health psychology considers the relationship between health and illness and between the mind and the body. Its approach reflects the bio-psychosocial model that health and illness are the product of a combination of factors including the biological (genetics), behavioural (lifestyle, stress, health beliefs) and social (family/social support and cultural influence). The individual is not merely the passive victim of some external factor but has individual responsibility for their own health behaviours.

Marks et al. (2005) suggest that this first requires a definition of health and have amended the World Health Organization's definition of health to account for what they see as missing elements. They define health as '… *a state of well-being with physical, cultural, psychosocial, economic and spiritual attributes*, not simply the absence of illness …' (p. 4). In a maternity care context, there is very clear evidence that health of the mother and the fetus is not only dependant on medical conditions, but on environmental conditions and lifestyle choices during pregnancy. Midwives are providers of care, but are also in a position to facilitate the empowerment of women to increase control over their health to make healthier decisions. There are some key public health issues within contemporary maternity care that are well evidenced to result in poorer health outcomes for mother and/or baby (see Chapter 11: 'Public health and health promotion', where these are discussed in further depth). However, despite the apparently clear evidence of harm, women continue to engage in behaviours that are detrimental to their health. It is therefore of value to understand the psychology that underpins healthy versus unhealthy behaviour.

Further reading activity

For further information access the GOV.UK website [Available online] https://www.gov.uk/government/topics/public-health

Health beliefs and behaviours

Strong evidence now underpins the belief that health behaviours are important in predicting morbidity and mortality (Stringhini et al. 2011). In psychology the role of health beliefs have been considered as predictors of behaviour.

Health locus of control

Health locus of control (HLoC) has been suggested as important as to whether or not we change our behaviour and/or adhere to recommendations by a health professional. HLoC proposes that individuals differ in whether they regard their health as controllable (internal HLoC) or uncontrollable (external HLoC) by them. Wallston and Wallston (1982) developed a measure to evaluate HLoC to determine whether an individual believes their health is:

- controllable by them (internal)
- not controllable by them and down to fate/luck (external chance)
- under the control of powerful others, such as healthcare professionals (external powerful others).

Clearly those with an internal HLoC are more likely to believe that their own behaviours can influence health outcomes. Studies in maternity care have shown links between HLoC and behaviour (for example see, Martin and Jomeen 2004; Jomeen and Martin 2008a).

Unrealistic optimism

Other authors have suggested that the reason people continue to practise unhealthy behaviours are inaccurate perceptions of risk (Weinstein 1983; 1984). Weinstein called this phenomenon unrealistic optimism, and proposed four cognitive factors that contribute:

- lack of personal experience with the problem
- the belief that the problem is preventable by individual action
- the belief that the problem has not yet appeared, so it will not appear in the future
- the belief that the problem is infrequent.

Weinstein suggested that individuals show selective focus, in that they ignore their risk increasing behaviours and focus on risk decreasing behaviour.

Clinical consideration

A pregnant woman who is overweight may think that it is important, but think 'At least I have given up alcohol.' Individuals, as a consequence of egocentricism, then focus on the risk increasing behaviour of others and ignore the risk decreasing behaviour.

Table 4.1   Summary of the stages of change model

Pre-contemplation	I am happy being overweight and don't intend to do anything about it
Contemplation	I am pregnant and being overweight can be harmful for my baby, perhaps I will consider losing weight
Preparation	I will stop eating fattening foods and start to exercise
Action	I have started eating more healthily and doing gentle exercise
Maintenance	I have kept my weight gain during pregnancy within recommended levels and intend to maintain my behaviour post birth

The stages of change model

The stages of change model is a synthesis of 18 therapies, describing processes involved in behavioural change, developed in 1982 by Prochaska and DiClemente (cited in Hewstone et al. 2005). This model of change has been applied to several health related behaviours including smoking, alcohol use and screening. The model suggests the stages shown in Table 4.1.

This model suggests behaviour change as dynamic, and highlights that individuals can move backward and forward before reaching the maintenance stage, and may still slip back over time. It examines how individuals weigh up costs and benefits of particular behaviours. The motivation of pregnancy may be an additional factor in weighing up costs and benefits of altering behaviours.

Social cognition models

These different perspectives have been integrated into Social Cognition Models (SCM) which aims to develop theories to explain the relationship between knowledge, attitudes and behaviour. It is believed that there is a close relationship between these elements and a person's intentions to act in a particular way. Two well utilised SCM theories include the Health Belief Model (HBM: Rosenstock 1966; Becker et al. 1977) and the Theory of Planned Behaviour (TPB: Ajzen 1985; 2002a; 2002b).

Health Belief Model

In the Health Belief Model (HBM) a pregnant woman who smoked would be asked to consider:

- her own susceptibility to lung cancer and the implications for the baby such as stillbirth, miscarriage and low birth weight
- the seriousness of these conditions and consequences
- the positive effects and value of giving up smoking
- the potential negative consequences of giving up smoking.

The HBM also acknowledges the role of cues, which might be internal, such as a smoker's cough, or external such as meeting someone with lung disease, as well as their own motivation. In pregnancy, it might be evidence that their baby is growth retarded or the placental flow is inadequate, hence, how important to them is their health and the health of their baby. The HBM suggest these core beliefs can successfully predict health behaviours. Following criticism, the

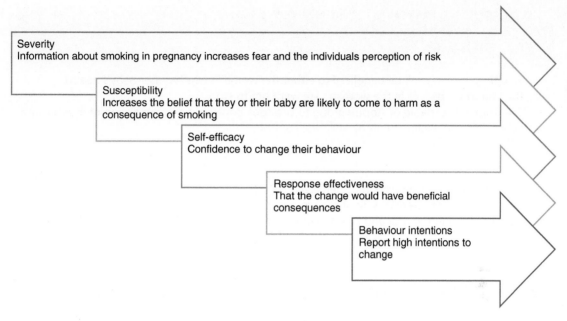

Figure 4.1 An adaptive coping response.

model was revised to include health motivation – readiness to be concerned about health matters – and perceived control – belief in personal ability to enact the behaviour (Becker and Rosenstock 1987).

The protection motivation theory developed by Rogers (1975; 1983; 1985) extended the HBM to include additional aspects. This theory describes five components: severity, susceptibility and fear as relating to 'threat appraisal'; response effectiveness and self-efficacy as relating to 'coping appraisal'. There are two types of information source:

1. Environmental: such as verbal persuasion, observational learning.
2. Intrapersonal: such as prior learning.

This information influences the five components outlined in Figure 4.1 which then elicit an adaptive (behavioural intention) or a maladaptive (avoidance/denial) coping response.

Theory of Planned Behaviour

The Theory of Planned Behaviour (TPB) proposes that behaviour is informed by attitudes and behavioural intentions. Three factors predict behavioural intentions, which then link to behaviour itself:

- Attitude towards a behaviour – positive or negative evaluation and beliefs about the outcome.
- Subjective norms – the beliefs of important others and the individuals motivation to comply.
- Perceived behavioural control – can the individual carry out the behaviour in light of internal and external control factors.

Using the same example as above, a woman would have high intentions to stop smoking if she believes the following factors (Box 4.1).

Box 4.1   Theory of planned behaviour applied to practice

- Stopping smoking will be beneficial to either the woman's heath or her baby's health.
- The important people in the woman's life want her to stop.
- The woman is capable of stopping due to previous behaviour and evaluation of internal and external control factors (high behavioural control).

The model also predicts that perceived behavioural control can predict behaviour without the influence of intentions. So if the woman does not believe she can stop smoking because she has tried in the past and failed then intention becomes less relevant.

Activity 4.1

Many pregnant women continue to smoke even though they know smoking is bad for them – using the above models of behaviour think about the potential reasons why this might be?

Summary

Psychology clearly has a role to play in helping to understand how childbearing women engage with the public health agenda in a maternity care context. This agenda tends to assume several things, first that achieving good health is a shared objective; second there is agreement on what being healthy means; third there is scientific consensus on the behaviours necessary to facilitate good health.

Understanding why people engage in unhealthy behaviours and the psychological aspects relating to cessation or behaviour change is significant for practitioners who are applying health promotion and support interventions. The theories presented above help to explain why sometimes women might not change unhealthy behaviours, despite the evidence presented to them that certain health behaviours are harmful.

Emotions across the childbearing experience

The onset of pregnancy heralds a period of physiological and psychological transition (Darvill et al. 2010). While the physiological transitions can be obvious for example, changing body shape, nausea, fatigue, the psychological changes may not be as transparent or expected by women. It is important therefore that midwives are aware of the emotional challenges in pregnancy to differentiate between normal anxieties and abnormal pathological psychiatric conditions, for example, tocophobia – a morbid fear of pregnancy and childbirth – which can impact on the woman's daily functioning (Hofberg and Ward 2003).

Antenatal considerations

Primiparous women are faced with the transition from 'maid to mother' and the complexities involved with physiological adaptations and changes in identity and social status. Equally, multiparous women will have their own transitions and may have negative echoes from their previous experiences, which they carry into their present pregnancy. While many women report great joy at the onset of pregnancy, for some, it results in tensions, which have their basis in fear and anxiety. These can include:

- fear of pregnancy
- tocophobia (fear of childbirth)
- fear of pain and access to analgesia
- fear of enforced analgesia
- fear of clinical intervention
- fear of their own death
- fear of fetal damage or demise
- fear of the ability to cope postnatally. (Maier 2010)

Anxieties may arise for many reasons and psychological, social and emotive issues can impact on maternal wellbeing. These may include: weight gain, altered body image (Nicholson et al. 2010), mood swings, the impact of physiological changes (such as hyperemesis and fatigue), financial worries, and identity renegotiation. Whilst many women will adapt to these changes normally, for others they create a state of psychological vulnerability (Raynor and England 2010).

Psychological factors in the antenatal period

Beck (2001) identifies that the strongest predictors of postnatal depression (PND) are depression in the antenatal period, particularly if the woman has low self-esteem or stress related to child-care or antenatal anxiety. Furthermore Misri et al. (2010) noted a correlation between antenatal depression (AND) and postpartum parenting stress. This highlights how the emotional journey for women begins early in the perinatal period and forms part of a continuum across the spectrum of childbirth (Alderdice et al. 2013).

In the context of relationships, couples may have concerns about the financial impact of having a baby, lack of a support network and their own ability to parent, which can result in stress within the relationship and impact on the pregnancy (Raynor 2006; Salonen et al. 2009; Zachariah 2009).

Psychosocial factors in the antenatal period

Marital conflicts may surface in the antenatal period and it is well documented that domestic violence increases in pregnancy, with negative impact on the woman and fetal wellbeing, with an increased risk of preterm delivery and antepartum haemorrhage. This can, in some incidences, lead to miscarriage or maternal death (Field et al. 2010; Shah and Shah 2010).

Clinical consideration

In the general population, one in three women will have been abused by an intimate partner; the onset of pregnancy increases the risk of domestic violence with one in four pregnant women reporting abuse (Keeling and Mason 2011).

This could in part be related to the raised anxiety and depression levels that have been noted for both partners in the first and third trimester (Teixeira et al. 2009). Noteworthy, was that greater anxiety in the third trimester was identified in multiparous women and their partners; the authors suggest that this could be related to previous birth experience. These authors highlight the need for interventions by health professionals to reduce antenatal anxiety, to promote maternal, paternal and fetal wellbeing.

The UK National Institute for Health and Care Excellence (NICE) guidelines on Antenatal and Postnatal Mental Health (2007), which will be discussed in more detail in Chapter 13, give midwives a clear remit with regard to the prediction and detection of mental health illness at the booking appointment.

The Nursing and Midwifery Council (NMC) 2012 states that the midwife should provide safe, responsive, compassionate care in an appropriate environment to facilitate her physical and emotional care through the childbearing period. This aims to facilitate the identification of women with both a pre-existing severe psychological condition, for example, schizophrenia or bipolar disorder, and those who develop psychological distress during pregnancy. Identification then enables referral to appropriate services.

The impact of antenatal stressors on postnatal outcomes has been reported but women still report on their voices not being heard, with midwives being 'too busy to care' (Green 2012). The significance of psychological status has been well-documented, with implications for clinical obstetric outcomes, long-term mental health of the mother and the quality of the mother–infant relationship all well-acknowledged (Jomeen and Martin 2008b). Fransson et al. (2011) identify that women experiencing antenatal depression are at greater risk of preterm birth. Furthermore, antenatal depression and anxiety can result in low birth weight, complications in childbirth and poor fetal outcomes compared to women with positive mental states who experience better fetal and maternal outcomes (Hernandez-Martinez et al. 2011). Jomeen (2004) noted increased epidural analgesia, assisted deliveries and neonatal admissions, together with the risk of spontaneous abortion, fetal malformations and pre-eclampsia in women with antenatal depression.

Antenatal depression can impact postnatally with women experiencing difficulty interacting with their infant (Alhusen 2008; Hayes et al. 2013). However it has been noted that when a women has a positive pregnancy experience it can be empowering and can positively impact on the woman's self-esteem and bonding with her baby (Clement 1998).

Birth

The birth of a baby is a life-changing experience for a woman and it can impact positively or negatively on her psychological wellbeing. Some of the negative factors include: loss of control, fear and pain. The sense of being in control is woven through childbirth literature. Bandura (1997) describes being in control as 'self-efficacy', which increases when women believe and know, at a fundamental psychological and physiological level, that they have the ability to cope with labour.

Bandura notes that 'self-efficacy predicts the use of behavioural and cognitive strategies to relieve pain' and can 'lessen the extent to which painful stimulation is experienced as conscious' (Bandura 1997, p. 268).

O'Hare and Fallon (2011) noted that women reported a high degree of self-efficacy when taking control and mastering their breathing through labour. By contrast, women reporting negative birth experiences describe feeling violated, vulnerable, excluded, cheated, frightened, undignified and depersonalised (Mercer et al. 2012).

Fear of childbirth is well-documented and can be attributed to physiological (pain) and psychological (stress, anxiety) functions. The number of Caesarean sections (CS) on maternal request has risen and this is partly due to psychosocial factors, such as convenience and body image. It can also be associated with previous birth trauma, sexual abuse or lack of self-efficacy (D'Souza 2012). However some women request CS due to a pathological fear of childbirth, known as tocophobia, and incidence has been reported as high as 1:5 pregnant woman. Television programmes like 'One Born Every Minute' in the UK, have focused, in the main, on painful medicated controlled childbirth and Talbot (2012) suggests that 'catastrophising' labour pain increases the woman's sense of helplessness and fear of labour. Salomonsson et al. (2013) state the midwife could identify and promote strategies and behaviours to support women to consider vaginal birth and enhance self-efficacy. Goodin and Griffiths (2012) suggest that women requesting CS should be referred to psychological services with the caveat that where the woman has severe tocophobia, denial of a CS could lead to post-traumatic stress disorder (PTSD).

Postnatal considerations

The transition to parenthood heralds a major change in a woman's life and most women will experience the birth of a baby as a joyous experience; however some women experience conflicting emotions ranging from despair to euphoria. In the postnatal period, women need to adapt to the challenging physical, emotional and psychological demands of motherhood, the immediate postnatal period, especially notable in first-time mothers, creates new situations for women to navigate and are reflected in Box 4.2.

Box 4.2   Physical, emotional and social changes in the immediate postnatal period

- Change of role and responsibilities
- Change in employment status
- Loss of income
- Isolation
- Physical and mental exhaustion
- Emotional lability
- Feeling overwhelmed caring for a new baby
- Loss of control
- Abandonment
- Changes in self/body image
- Physical impact on body
- Loss of identity
- Vulnerability
- Feeling unprepared
- Sleep disturbances/deprivation
- Loss of independence

Table 4.2   Differences between baby blues and postnatal depression

Baby blues	Postnatal depression
Transient low mood – peaks 4–5 days postnatally, usually disappears by 4 weeks	Can occur at any time in the early or late postnatal period
Women may experience: • fatigue • feeling overemotional, tearfulness • mood swings • low spirits, • anxiety, • forgetfulness and muddled thinking • depression • confusion • headache • insomnia irritability • emotional lability Does not usually require intervention	Women may experience: • an inability to experience pleasure • depressed mood • loss of interest or pleasure • significant increases or decreases in appetite • insomnia or hypersomnia • psychomotor agitation or retardation • fatigue or loss of energy • feelings of worthlessness or guilt • diminished concentration • recurrent thoughts of suicide Requires healthcare interventions (see Chapter 13: 'Perinatal mental health' for further detail) (NICE 2006)

Baby blues and postnatal depression

It is common for women to experience the 'baby blues', a fluctuation of emotions and low mood (Table 4.2). This emotional phenomenon is transitory, commencing between 4–5 days postnatally and lasting for less than a month. Postnatal depression (PND) in contrast, differs from the baby blues in that it can occur at any time during the postnatal period including up to one year postnatally and has a significant impact on the women's physical and psychological recovery following birth (NICE 2006); with an incidence of 10–15% (Royal College of Psychiatrists 2014).

A smaller percentage of women will report symptoms commensurate with PTSD, which are often mistaken for PND and thus the treatment process may not fit the disease (Peeler et al. 2013) (see Chapter 13: 'Perinatal mental health', where both PND and PTSD will be discussed in more detail).

Other factors influence women's psychological status and may contribute to psychological distress such as difficulty breastfeeding, coping with crying, unsettled babies and fatigue (Taylor and Johnson 2010). However, this is not inevitable and midwives can contribute to maternal psychological wellbeing by giving practical support relating to infant feeding and building women's confidence in their mothering skills (Marshall et al. 2007).

Some women will attempt to mask depression (see Figure 4.2); the 'rigging' of responses to the Edinburgh Postnatal Depression Scale due to difficulty expressing 'maternal ambivalence' and desires to conceal their actual reality of motherhood has been demonstrated (Miller 2011). One explanation may be the concept of 'blissful parenthood', still embedded in society's expectations of motherhood, which can relegate women with PND to the status of 'bad mother' (Buultjens and Liamputtong 2007). Women have reported feeling that they should be able to cope with motherhood; the inability to cope conflicting with their pre-birth perception of 'self' as a competent woman (Buultjens and Liamputtong 2007).

Relationships can be critical in terms of psychological wellbeing, yet Bateman and Bharj (2009) highlight the impact of the birth of a baby on marital satisfaction and authors have found a correlation between maternal and paternal PND (Goodman 2004; Ramchandani et al. 2005).

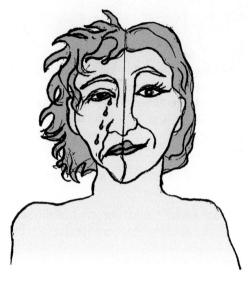

Figure 4.2   Some women may mask their true feelings in motherhood. Source: Reproduced with permission from P. Alexander.

This has implications on the quality of the family relationship if both parents are depressed. Women suffering psychological distress describe support from other mothers as invaluable because it normalises the emotional lability of the postnatal experience and affords permission to express negative emotions (Darvill et al. 2010). The role of the midwife can also play a critical role in supporting women through periods of emotional turmoil of psychological distress, as discussed later in this chapter.

The postnatal period is an emotional journey, where women adapt to the role and demands of motherhood and renegotiate their identity. A labile, emotional journey is both inevitable and normal and evidence illustrates that improved postnatal physical recovery is paralleled with an improved psychological profile (Jomeen and Martin 2008a); indeed a study by McKenzie and Carter (2013) found that the transition to parenthood can result in improvements in psychological distress and mental health once the immediate postnatal period is traversed. Some women, however, will enter the postnatal period in a vulnerable psychological state which began antenatally or during birth. Kitzinger (2012) notes that women who felt powerless in labour report a sense of loss, of having missed out on the experience of birthing their babies and will report feelings of 'failure' which can impact self-esteem and mental wellbeing.

Summary

The midwife will be involved in caring for women within normal physiological parameters of childbearing who can bring their psychological pathology to pregnancy. Most women will go through a range of differing and undulating emotions in pregnancy, birth and the postnatal period and that is normal and expected. Midwives have a key role to play in supporting women through their emotional journey being mindful of the myriad of challenges they may experience. While the midwife is not expected to be a psychologist/psychiatrist or counsellor, awareness and recognition of normal emotional reactions versus abnormal are critical.

Women and midwives: relationships and communication

One of the most characterising aspects of being human is that they are social, affected by the presence of other people, have strong needs to affiliate and form relationships with others and behave in certain ways towards members of their own and other groups. Amongst others, one of a person's motives for affiliation is anxiety reduction and information seeking (Hewstone et al. 2005). Therefore, a positive relationship with the midwife can be critical to women.

Mavis Kirkham writes

> …The midwife relationship of maternity services: for many women that relationship is the service … (Kirkham 2010, p. xiii)

When a relationship is 'done well' it undoubtedly benefits all parties and enhances feelings of self-worth, wellbeing and satisfaction. Poor relationships on the other hand can be damaging to women in terms of self-esteem, feelings of control and quality of experience and for midwives in terms of job satisfaction and emotional labour.

The psychological importance of the woman–midwife relationship

For women

Childbearing is a complex experience. Midwives need to both understand this complexity, but also be able to build effective relationships with women while they are in pain, distracted, anxious and fearful or disadvantaged in some way (Raynor and England 2010) and offer the support women need.

The stimuli experienced by a woman through pregnancy, labour, birth and in making the transition to motherhood, are exceptional. Women are required to appraise emotion producing events within a constantly changing environment, which is largely driven by psychological and biological components. It is also strongly influenced, however, by social conditions, which are created through the presence of those who surround the woman at that time and the relationships that are formed within that context.

This highlights the significant role that the midwife has in creating women's childbearing context and experience. While most women appraise the events around childbirth satisfactorily and make the transition to motherhood smoothly, the successful dealing with and processing of maternal emotions is critical. White (2005) suggests that failure to process emotions successfully could explain the emergence of conditions such as PND depression or post-birth traumatic stress. Little direct information exists about how interaction with care givers might support emotional processing *per se*, but evidence does suggest that how the midwife deals with emotion can have a significant impact on women. This can be in terms of women's decision-making (Edwards 2009) and level of anxiety at the time (Byrt et al. 2008; Hunter et al. 2008), but it is also suggested that the midwife–woman relationship is an important aspect of satisfaction. This is linked to the level at which women feel involved in and have some control over, the process of their care (Slade et al. 1993; Tinkler and Quinney 2001). Evidence suggests that a woman's feelings of being 'in control' are impacted on by the positive attitudes of the midwives caring for them, information giving during pregnancy and labour and being able to make and be included in decision-making during labour (Gibbins and Thomson 2001; see Chapter 3: 'Antenatal midwifery care', where decision-making is examined in greater depth). This could be defined as supportive care, which has been identified both qualitatively and quantitatively as an important variable with regard to more positive experiences for women (Waldenström et al. 2004; Kitzinger 2006; Kirkham 2010). Conversely, reduced levels of control and satisfaction have been linked to more enduring negative psychological consequences for women, such as PTSD and depression (Czarnocka and Slade 2000; Nilsson and Lundgren 2009) and poorer adjustment to motherhood (Dimatteo and Khan 1997).

The psychological impact on women of the way that midwives interact with them seems clear, but equally important is how midwives manage their own emotions.

For midwives

Emotional work is a feature of all human relationships and is about dealing with our own and other people's emotions. Interactions between midwives and women as already suggested are social encounters, but ones that often happen in non-ordinary circumstances and involve intimate procedures and personal information. Midwives need to manage their feelings so that they are appropriate to the situation they are in (Deery and Hunter 2010); however this can be at cost to the worker who must maintain a professional demeanour (Edwards 2009). The requirement for midwives to give the right emotional response to the clinical situations that emerge has been reported in several studies as challenging and stressful (Deery and Kirkham 2006; 2007; Earle et al. 2007). Billie Hunter (2006) writes about four key situations which midwives encounter; these include balanced exchanges, rejected exchanges, reversed exchanges and unsustainable exchanges. The latter three exchanges require high levels of 'emotion work' by the midwife, whilst balanced exchanges, where there is 'give and take' on both sides, are more emotionally rewarding for the midwife. This highlights the clear significance of positive relationships for midwives as well as women, which can happen even in the face of adverse outcomes where a supportive relationship has enabled the situation to be as good as possible in the circumstances (Deery and Hunter 2010).

> … When a meaningful relationship is created, emotion work is not experienced as hard work
> but is something akin to a gift…
>
> (Bolton in Deery and Hunter 2010)

Often, however, midwives employ strategies to remain detached. Ruth Deery (Deery and Hunter 2010) describes:

Technical detachment: The fragmentation of a woman's care into manageable tasks in order to maximise the midwife's control of clinical decision-making.
Emotional detachment: Aimed to protect against over-involvement with women, often engaged in times of high anxiety, which might have short-term benefits for the midwife.

Whilst these types of strategies are most often engaged to enable midwives to cope, they inevitably create boundaries and distance from women. Strategies also include stereotyping women as a way of discounting needs that cannot be met (Deery and Kirkham 2007). The problem with such approaches is that they lead to a task-oriented, de-personalised approach, low morale, stress and burn-out (Hunter 2004; Deery and Kirkham 2007). Those relationships that are emotionally positive, underpinned by mutuality, trust and genuineness contribute not only to job satisfaction, but also the midwives sense of self, as a person not a role (McCourt and Stevens 2009). Where midwives keep their *'emotional lids'* on (Deery and Kirkham 2007, p81), women tend to take their cues from that and do the same (Edwards 2009) and the opportunity to achieve a balanced exchange (Hunter 2006) is inevitably lost.

It is valuable to consider how and why meaningful relationships develop in some circumstances and situations but not in others. A number of things come into play, such as individual personalities. We cannot all instantaneously build rapport with everyone; some relationships may take a little more emotion work and create the need to draw on communication skills.

Individuals are not all the same in their ability to communicate, and capacities for empathy and trust also vary (Deery and Hunter 2010). The model within which care is delivered may also facilitate or restrict the development of relationships (for examples see McCourt and Stevens 2009; Dykes 2009; Kirkham 2010). Unfortunately, research evidence continually suggests that communication within maternity care is an area of dissatisfaction for women (Edwards 2004; Jomeen 2010; Jomeen and Redshaw 2012) and something we could 'do' better.

Activity 4.2

Can you think of situations in clinical practice where you have engaged in emotional labour?

- How did your behaviour affect the women you were caring for?
- How did your behaviour affect you?
- What might you have done differently?

Initiating, building and maintaining relationships

So if the key is the potential to create a meaningful relationship, we might ask: How this can be achieved?

Central to any relationship is effective communication. Communication is complex and about more than just the imparting of information. Essentially communication falls into two groups; verbal and non-verbal, but we communicate in three ways, through the content of our speech, our body language and the tone of our voice.

Verbal communication: Refers to using speech and writing to share thoughts, feelings and ideas with other people.

Non-verbal communication: Includes all other ways that people share their thoughts, feelings and ideas:
- facial expressions
- touch
- gestures such as nods of the head
- silence
- the way people sit or stand
- the space they maintain between them. (Arnold and Boggs 2007; Sully and Dallas 2010)

First impressions

The context within which midwives and women meet for the first time will inevitably have an impact on the initiation of the relationship. Early impressions, especially those gleaned from non-verbal communication are often the most influential and enduring and can be negative or positive. Initial inferences (non-verbal or verbal) can be corrected, but require greater emotional work on behalf of both parties and sometimes may not be remedied (Raynor and England 2010).

Building and/or maintaining a woman–midwife relationship

Once an impression has been formed people look for evidence that reinforces their initial conclusions. Women have highlighted the characteristics of midwives that shape either close or distant relationships. Nicholls and Webb (2006) state the attributes of a 'good' midwife that are important to women. These are midwives who are: friendly, kind, smiling, caring, approachable, non-judgmental, have time, are respectful, provide support and companionship and are good communicators. 'Good' midwives establish rapport and create a relationship of a social nature (Bharj and Chesney 2010). 'Bad' midwives are unhelpful, insensitive, abrupt, officious, fail to listen and lack concern (Nicholls and Webb 2006), fail to respond to women's support needs and are perceived as disrespectful and insensitive, leaving women feeling disempowered (Jomeen and Redshaw 2012).

Midwives themselves recognise that they are not always able to form an emotional relationship with a woman; in these cases they form a professional relationship through which they attend to the physical aspects of care (McCrea and Crute 1991). Whilst women have profiled 'bad' midwives this is most often based on the midwife's attitude, attributes and the lack of a relationship, rather than a failure to provide physical care (Bharj and Chesney 2010). What this demonstrates is how valuable the midwife–woman relationship is in women's experiences of care. A combination of verbal and non-verbal communication behaviours underpin women's assessments of a midwife's attributes. Poor communication when described by women is consistently linked to the behaviours and characteristics that midwives display (Jomeen and Redshaw 2012).

There will be levels of communication which range from superficial to deep which are perfectly normal and a functional part of human relating (Raynor and England 2010). Even if there is no strong sense of connection, midwives can still draw on communication skills to create rapport (Deery and Hunter 2010). Sometimes, for example, women adopt aggressive or passive communication styles, which can result in a strong temptation for the midwife to pull away. Raynor and England (2010) argue that this is a mistake because *it nurtures a psychological void* (p. 91) and believe such behaviour actually requires sustained contact, continuity and assertive communication, which facilitates the midwife to express appropriate thoughts in a transparent and authentic way, that does not result in psychological expense to the woman.

Concepts that underpin effective communication and the woman–midwife relationship

Listening

It is fundamental in any relationship to be heard (Kirkham 2010), yet listening is a difficult skill to develop because it takes time (Raynor and England 2010). This is affected by several elements:

- Women do not like to ask because midwives are busy.
- Midwives working in fragmented, busy environments may see little point in listening to women who they are never going to meet again.
- Midwives focus on tasks not women, which prevents them from hearing women.
- Midwives are more concerned with giving information and advice, because they know better.

Being heard is important to a woman, it means she is being taken seriously and her thoughts and feelings matter. Care can be 'smiley' but if it is still formulaic (Kirkham 2010), it prevents midwives listening, inhibits the woman who might wish to express her wishes and promote her decisions and hence prevents the development of an effective relationship (Kirkham 2010; Raynor and England 2010).

Listening is more than just letting someone talk; it is an active activity. The listener must pay attention, concentrate on what the woman has to say and be present. Empathy, for example, requires listening skills to understand others' feelings of anxiety and self-doubt. This in turn then requires *an emotional shift* (Raynor and England, p. 94) from thinking to feeling, where the midwife then is able to communicate a sincere non-judgmental understanding of the woman's experience.

Presence

The offering of presence and time is a powerful form of psychosocial support. Presence is 'being with' rather than 'doing to' and can be particularly valuable when words become redundant (Raynor and England 2010).

Trust

Trust rests on common value, not necessarily on common viewpoints, but the midwife must have respect for the woman's values and priorities (Kirkham 2010). When a mother feels safe in her relationship with her midwife, a positive relationship is much more likely to develop because the mother feels acknowledged and valued. This is in direct opposition to a midwife who exerts authority, offers choice but then proffers personal opinions, either through her verbal or non-verbal communication, or gate-keeping through the withholding of information. The notion of choice and the woman as an active decision-maker then becomes largely illusory, which can have implications for women's psychological health (Jomeen 2010).

Summary

Women clearly believe that good relationships with their midwives are central to their experiences of childbirth; many midwives hold similar beliefs. Verbal and non-verbal cues are critical in first impressions and establishing and maintaining relationships. Good relationships are built on trust, mutuality and empathy. All of these aspects require an active not passive approach and can be emotionally demanding, but when achieved are also immensely rewarding for both parties. Awareness that the development and establishment of relationships can be both challenging and emotionally demanding, and attentiveness to barriers, both real and perceived, are critical to ensure that both women and midwives do not suffer negative emotional consequences.

Bonding and attachment

Bonding and attachment are vital for the maternal–child relationship and the wellbeing of the infant. It is important to differentiate between 'bonding' and 'attachment' as the terms are often used interchangeably (Redshaw and Martin 2013). The origins of attachment are predominantly based on Bowlby's development of Attachment Theory (Bowlby 1969).

Defining bonding and attachment

Bonding describes the *maternal–infant relationship*, that is, the *mother's* relationship with her infant.

Attachment describes the *infant–maternal relationship* – the *infant's* connection with its mother/caregiver.

Attachment theory has informed our understanding of the importance of the infant–maternal bond, the 'secure base' (Bowlby 1988), for the psychological and physiological wellbeing of the neonate. Attachment, as stated above, is used to define the infant's connection with a caregiver. Bonding, as described by Altaweli & Roberts (2010) is a complex phenomenon which defines a deep, enduring emotional attachment between mother and fetus in utero, which progresses to bonding with the neonate post-birth. However, there is a lack of conceptual clarity regarding the maternal–fetal relationship during pregnancy, and whether bonding is an appropriate term in this context (Redshaw and Martin 2013).

Further reading activity

For further reading on the antenatal maternal–fetal relationship, see Walsh, J., Hepper, E.G., Bagge, S.R., Wadephul, F., Jomeen, J. (2013) Maternal–fetal relationships and psychological health: emerging research directions. *Journal of Reproductive and Infant Psychology* 31(5), pp. 490–499.

Laxton-Kane and Slade (2002) also note that attachment and bonding differ in that (postnatal) bonding is reciprocal – the infant will relate directly with the mother. However, it is important for neonatal/infant physical sensory and cognitive development that this reciprocal relationship is acknowledged by the mother to enable a secure attachment from the infant (Canadian Paediatric Society Position Statement 2004).

The importance of bonding

Bonding increases through the course of pregnancy (Della Vedova et al. 2008; Cannella 2005) and is positively related to early fetal movements (Hjelmstedt et al. 2006). Antenatal bonding has been linked to postnatal parent–infant relationships, infant development and maternal and child psychological health (Figueiredo and Costa 2009; Della Vedova et al., 2008), as well as improving health behaviours in pregnancy and formation of maternal identity (Della Vedova et al. 2008). However, it has also been proposed that reduced bonding during pregnancy can act as a protective mechanism against loss (Clement 1998).

Early research on bonding by Kennell et al. (1974) focused on the post-birth context and described mothers who were given immediate contact post-birth, and extended contact thereafter and found these women displayed significant differences in 'attentiveness and responsiveness' towards their infants from birth to one year.

Critiques have been made about the concept of bonding both postnatal (Eyer 1994) and antenatal (Mitchell 2001). Eyer (1994) suggested that bonding was misappropriated and turned into a 'rigid doctrine' which necessitated bonding in the first hour at a woman's peril, with the onus placed on women to ensure that their infants emerged psychologically sound. Mitchell (2001) reinforces this argument suggesting that bonding with the fetus is a cultural construct related to the impact of a woman's behaviour on the baby's development.

Whilst this is an important consideration in terms of maternal consequences, evidence indicates a 'sensitive' period does indeed exist post-birth (Bystrova et al. 2009), which is enhanced by immediate skin to skin, breastfeeding and rooming in. But bonding is more than proximity; bonding utilises all the senses, including the smell, taste, touch and sound of the baby.

The importance of attachment

Bowlby (1988) defined different forms of attachment, notably secure and insecure attachment and found that infants displaying secure attachments with their caretakers were more

Box 4.3   Secure attachment behaviour

- Self-reliant
- Self-confident
- High self-esteem
- Resilience
- Flexible
- Curious and exploring
- Able to regulate behaviour
- Able to form relationships
- Persistence
- Socially competent
- Empathic
- Socially assured

self-reliant. Secure attachments (see Box 4.3) require maternal psychological availability to relate to the infant. Sroufe (2005) noted that for infants with a secure maternal attachment, in later life they demonstrated more flexibility, resilience, curiosity and exploratory behaviours, could moderate their behaviour, were more self-assured, socially competent and could develop healthy adult romantic relationships. Conversely, the insecure (disorganised) attached individuals displayed dissociative behaviours and self-harm.

The US National Institute of Child Health and Human Development (NICHD) Study of Early Child Care and Youth behaviour (2006) noted the quality of the maternal–infant interactions were *'the most important and consistent predictors of child cognitive and social development'* and that better outcomes were noted when the mother was *'sensitive, responsive, attentive, and cognitively stimulating'.* A meta-analysis into disorganised attachment and later behaviour problems found that attachment insecurity was associated with behavioural problems which were more prevalent in boys (Fearon et al. 2010). While it is important to note the impact of secure and insecure attachment on the social, emotional and cognitive development of the infant, it is equally important to examine factors which can impact on attachment and how women who are not bonding with their infants can be recognised and supported.

Potential factors influencing attachment and bonding

Ultrasound scans and bonding

Early suggestions that ultrasound could enhance bonding have been embraced by many authors Campbell (2006). However, empirical evidence overall is scant, though many women and their partners report that the baby feels more real and like a member of the family after a scan (Molander et al. 2010). Roberts (2012) reports the duality of the scan experience: the sonographer's task to view and measure the fetus from a clinical perspective; and the parents, who perceive the scan as an opportunity to 'see the baby'. She reports that behavioural, personality and physical characteristics are projected onto the fetus with imaginative interpretations of the features of the scan to create a fetal identity. However, the quality of the scan's bonding experience is dependent on the sonographer's sensitivity and feedback (Roberts 2012). There is some evidence that having seen the fetus on a scan can make loss more difficult for some women (Black 1992). More recently the commercial introduction of non-diagnostic 3D and 4D scans to promote bonding has encouraged parents to 'meet' with and engage with the fetus pre-birth. Early speculation regarding the potential psychological effects of 3/4D scans was based on emotional reactions to these scans (Campbell 2002). Some studies have reported a positive bonding impact (Roberts 2012; de Jong-Pleij et al. 2013), whilst others have shown no effect (Lapaire et al. 2007). The evidence to support the psychological benefits of scanning and bonding remains tenuous; the scan is here to stay and it is important that sonographers approach their description of the fetus thoughtfully and that the midwife appreciates the importance of the scan in terms of its impact on the mother, whether negative, positive or ambivalent.

Maternal psychosocial status

Factors within the family, for example, maternal depression, low income, domestic violence or lack of social support can impact on the bonding process. When the mother feels insecure in her social setting this insecurity may result in an insecure attachment for the infant. Furthermore where a disjunct exists between the antenatal representation of the infant by the mother, which may emerge in part from the scan and the 'real' infant, there is potential for discordant bonding (Huth-Bocks et al. 2011). Whilst the promotion and support of bonding is important, bonding is not always instantaneous and practitioners should be mindful not to create standards for women which are both unrealistic and unattainable, within the context of their lives and the continuum of motherhood transition.

Neuroscience research has revealed interesting developments in the physiological impact on bonding and attachment. Studies have found that particular areas of the brain and discrete hormones are stimulated during the maternal–infant interaction. However, maternal depression and substance abuse can inhibit these activities and hence bonding (Swain et al. 2007; Strathearn 2011).

Summary

The relationship between the mother and the baby is the foundation for all future relationships. It is essential for survival of the infant who will instinctively attach to its caregiver and is a powerful, instinctive, emotional and biological activity in women which occurs in the antenatal and postnatal period. Donald Winnicott coined the term 'good enough' mother whom he defined as the ordinary devoted mother, arguably a mother who had bonded with her child (Winnicott 1953). Bonding and attachment theory are clearly defined and discussed in the literature and the midwife's role is to navigate through pregnancy and the postnatal period with the woman, promoting every opportunity for the mother to develop a deep, meaningful relationship with her infant. This may require an interprofessional approach and referral to additional services, to ensure mothers have the support they need to determine a secure base for themselves and their infant.

Key points

- The perinatal period is a period of physical and social change and is therefore inevitably characterised by emotional lability.
- Psychological health and wellbeing is not merely the absence of mental illness or psychological distress.
- Psychological understanding enables midwives to consider what is normative and how women cope with the challenges of pregnancy.
- Psychological theory can inform health professionals about factors that influence people's lifestyles and what motivates certain health-related behaviours.
- An understanding of the psychology of communication enables ways of optimising the midwife–mother relationship.

Conclusion

Childbearing presents women with challenges and sometimes adversities. Women will experience fluctuating mood states, negative and positive emotions affected by a multitude of factors; women's responses will inevitably be as individual as women's experiences. Midwives are ideally placed to support women through the normative emotional adjustment that embodies this period in women's lives but are equally well placed to identify the triggers that may signal psychological distress.

End of chapter activities
Crossword

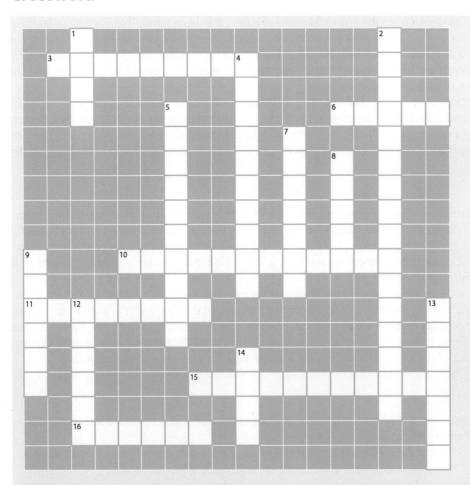

Across

3. Coined the term 'good enough mother'
6. Of control sounds like a flying insect?
10. A connection between the midwife and woman
11. One of the Freudian structures of personality
15. A woman who has had more than one child
16. Talkative Communication

Down

1. A UK organisation which sets guidelines for the childbearing continuum
2. The first stage of change
4. Fear of Childbirth
5. Scientific study of behaviour and mental processes
7. A cause of low birth weight

8. One of the senses. Non-verbal?
9. One of the humanistic psychologists
12. End of love without a vowel creates a salivating dog
13. Key public health issue in maternity
14. Colour relating to postnatal baby experience?

Find out more

Activity	Background reading
Look at NICE guidelines to develop your understanding of the midwife's role in caring for a woman's psychological needs. Consider how a woman's psychological needs may differ in pregnancy, labour and in the postnatal period.	National Institute for Health and Clinical Excellence (2007) *Antenatal and Postnatal Mental Health Guideline*. London: NICE.
Reflect on your experience of midwives in practice – what have you seen to underpin your understanding of the midwife-mother relationship?	Kirkham, M. (2010) *The Midwife–Mother Relationship*. Basingstoke: Palgrave Macmillan. McCrea, H., Crute, V. (1991) Midwife/client relationship: Midwives perspectives. *Midwifery* 7(4), pp. 183–192. Tinkler, A., Quinney, D. (2001) Team midwifery: the influence of the midwife-woman relationship on women's experiences and perceptions of maternity care. *Journal of Advanced Nursing* 28(1), pp. 30–35.
Winnicott coined the term 'good enough mother' What is your understanding of a 'good enough mother'?	Alhusen, J.L. (2008) A literature update on maternal–fetal attachment. *Journal of Obstetric, Gynecologic & Neonatal Nursing* 37(3), pp. 315–328. Bowlby, J. (1988) *A Secure Base. Clinical Applications of Attachment Theory*. London: Routledge. Winnicott, D. (1953) The theory of the parent–infant relationship. *International Journal of Psychoanalysis* 41, pp. 585–595.
How can you develop your understanding of healthy and unhealthy behaviours based on theoretical models discussed in the text?	Becker, M.H., Rosenstock, I.M. (1987) Comparing social learning and the health belief model. In: Ward, W.B. (ed.) *Advances in Health Education and Promotion*. Greenwich, CT: JAI Press. Hewstone, M., Fincham, F.D., Foster, J. (2005) *Psychology*. Oxford: BPS Blackwell. Rogers, R.W. (1985) Attitude change and information integration in fear appeals. *Psychological Reports* 56, pp. 179–182. Wallston, K.A., Wallston, B.S. (1982) Who is responsible for your health? The construct of health locus of control. In: Sanders G.S., Suls, J. (eds) *Social Psychology of Health and Illness*. Hillsdale, NJ: Lawrence Erlbaum and Associates. Weinstein, N.D. (1983) Reducing unrealistic optimism about illness susceptibility. *Health Psychology* 2, pp. 11–20.

Glossary of terms

Antepartum haemorrhage   A blood loss from the genital tract of 500 mL or more during pregnancy.

Attribution theory   A theory based on how individuals perceive and attach meaning to self or others behaviour.

Congruence   The ability to be authentic and genuine in relationships, acknowledging the other person.

Edinburgh Postnatal Depression Scale   A measure that can be used to determine risk of post-natal depression.

Egocentrism   Self-centred, focus on self

Empathy   The ability to recognise and understand another's emotions.

Hyperemesis   Nausea and vomiting, especially noted in early pregnancy.

Meta-analysis   An analysis of research from several studies on the same subject comparing and contrasting results.

Morbidity   The unhealthy or diseased state of the individual.

Mortality   The demise (death) of an individual or death rates within a population.

Multiparous   A woman who has given birth more than once.

Neurological   Relating to nerves or the nervous system.

Oxytocin   A hormone produced in the posterior pituitary gland which stimulates breast milk ejection and uterine contractions.

Parous   A woman who has given birth one or more times.

Perinatal   The period surrounding birth – from 24 weeks gestation and the first month post-birth.

Post partum haemorrhage   A significant blood loss from the genital tract of 500 mL or more post-birth.

Primiparous   A woman experiencing her first pregnancy.

Psychoanalytic psychology   A psychological theory based on Freudian psychology which focuses on analysing behaviour retrieved from the unconscious mind via dreams or association.

Qualitative   Research studying the 'lived experience' within its natural setting to make sense of and understand the lived phenomena and the meanings that people attribute to their experience.

Quantitive   Research based on statistical analysis of data.

References

Ajzen, I. (1985) From intentions to actions: A theory of planned behavior. In: J. Kuhl, J. Beckman (eds) *Action-Control: From Cognition to Behaviour*. Heidelberg: Springer.

Ajzen, I. (2002a) Perceived behavioural control, self-efficacy, locus of control, and the theory of planned behavior. *Journal of Applied Social Psychology* 32, pp. 665–683.

Ajzen, I. (2002b) Residual effects of past on later behaviour: Habituation and reasoned action perspectives. *Personality and Social Psychology Review* 6, pp. 107–122.

Alderdice, F., Ayers, S., Darwin, Z., Green, J., et al. (2013) Measuring psychological health in the perinatal period: workshop consensus statement. *Journal of Reproductive and Infant Psychology* 31 (5), pp. 431–438.

Alhusen, J.L. (2008) A literature update on maternal-fetal attachment. *Journal of Obstetric, Gynecologic & Neonatal Nursing* 37 (3), pp. 315–328.

Altaweli, R., Roberts, J. (2010) Maternal infant bonding: a concept analysis. *British Journal of Midwifery* 18 (9), pp. 552–559.

Bharj, K.K., Chesney, M. (2010) Pakistani Muslim women-midwives relationships: what are the essential attributes. In Kirkham, M. (ed.) *The Midwife-Mother Relationship*. Basingstoke: Palgrave Macmillan.

Bandura, A. (1997) *Self Efficacy: The Exercise of Control*. New York: W.H. Freeman.

Bateman, L., Bharj, K. (2009) The impact of the birth of the first child on a couple's relationship. *Evidence Based Midwifery* 7 (1), pp. 16–23.

Beck, C.T. (2001) Predictors of postpartum depression: an update. *Nursing Research* 50, pp. 275–285

Becker, M.H., Maiman, L.A., Kirscht, J.P., Haefner, D.P., Drachman, R.H. (1977) The health belief model and prediction of dietary compliance: a field experiment. *Journal of Health and Social Behavior* 18 (4), pp. 348–366.

Becker, M.H., Rosenstock, I.M. (1987) Comparing social learning and the health belief model. In Ward, W.B. (ed.) *Advances in Health Education and Promotion*. Greenwich, CT: JAI Press.

Black, R.B. (1992) Seeing the baby: the impact of ultrasound technology. *Journal of Genetic Counselling* 1 (1), pp. 45–54.

Bowlby, J. (1969) *Attachment, Separation and Loss*. New York: Basic Books.

Bowlby, J. (1988) *A secure Base. Clinical Applications of Attachment Theory*. London: Routledge.

Byrt, R., Hart, L., James-Sow, L. (2008) Patient Empowerment and Participation: Barriers and the Way Forward. In: Kettles, A.M., Woods, P., Byrt, R. (eds) *Forensic Mental Health Nursing: Competencies, Roles, Responsibilities*. London: Quay Books.

Buultjens, M. and Liamputtong, P. (2007) When giving life starts to take the life out of you: women's experiences of depression after childbirth. *Midwifery* 23, pp. 77–91.

Bystrova, K., Ivanova V., Edhborg, M., et al. (2009) Early contact versus separation: effects on mother–infant interaction one year later. *BIRTH* 36 (2), pp. 97–109.

Canadian Paediatric Society Position Statement (2004) Maternal depression and child development [available online] http://www.cps.ca/documents/position/maternal-depression-child-development.

Campbell, S. (2002) 4D, or not 4D: that is the question. *Ultrasound in Obstetrics & Gynecology* 19, pp. 1–4.

Campbell, S. (2006) 4D and prenatal bonding: still more questions than answers. *Ultrasound in Obstetrics & Gynecology* 27 (3), pp. 243–244.

Cannella, B.L. (2005) Maternal-fetal attachment: an integrative review. *Journal of Advanced Nursing* 50 (1), pp. 60–68.

Clement, S. (1998) *Psychological Perspectives on Pregnancy and Childbirth*. Edinburgh: Churchill Livingstone.

Crombie, J. and Nightingale, D.J. (1999) *Social Constructionist Psychology*. Buckingham: Open University Press.

Czarnocka, A.J. & Slade, P. (2000) Prevalence and predictors of posttraumatic stress symptoms following childbirth. *British Journal of Clinical Psychology* 39, pp. 35–51.

Darvill, T., Skirton, H., Farrand, P. (2010) Psychological factors that impact on women's experiences of first-time motherhood: a qualitative study of the transition. *Midwifery* 26, pp. 357–366.

Deery, R., Kirkham, M. (2006) Supporting midwives to support women. In: Page, L.A., McCandlish, R. (eds) *The New Midwifery: Science and Sensitivity in Practice*. London: Elsevier Health Sciences.

Deery, R., Kirkham, M. (2007) Drained and dumped on: the generation and accumulation of emotional toxic waste in community midwifery. In: Kirkham, M. (ed.) *Exploring the Dirty Side of Women's Health*. London: Routledge.

Deery, R., Hunter, B. (2010) Emotion work and relationships in midwifery. In: Kirkham, M. (ed.) *The Midwife–Mother Relationship*. Basingstoke: Palgrave Macmillan.

de Jong-Pleij, E.A.P., Ribbert, L.S.M., Pistorius, L.R., Tromp, E., Mulder, E.J.H., Bilardo, C.M. (2013) Three-dimensional ultrasound and maternal bonding, a third trimester study and a review. *Prenatal Diagnosis* 33 (1), pp. 81–88.

85

Della Vedova, A.M., Dabrassi, F., Imbasciati, A. (2008) Assessing prenatal attachment in a sample of Italian women. *Journal of Reproductive & Infant Psychology* 26 (2), pp. 86–98.

DiMatteo, M.R., Khan, K.L. (1997) In: S.J. Gallant, K.G. Puryear & R. Royal Schaler (eds) *Health Care for Women: Psychological, Social and Behavioural Influence.* Washington: American Psychological Association.

D'Souza, R. (2012) Caesarean section on maternal request for non-medical reasons: Putting the UK National Institute of Health and Clinical Excellence guidelines in perspective. *Obstetrics and Gynaecology* 27 (2), pp. 165–177.

Dykes, F. (2009) 'No time to care': Midwifery work on postnatal wards. In: Hunter, B., Deery, R. (eds) *Emotions in Midwifery and Reproduction.* Basingstoke: Palgrave Macmillan.

Earle, S., Komaromy, C., Foley, P., Lloyd, C. (2007) Understanding reproductive loss: Part 2: the moment of death. *The Practising Midwife* 10 (7), pp. 27–30.

Edwards, N.P. (2004) Why can't women just so say? And does it really matter? In: Kirkham, M. (ed.) *Informed Choice in Maternity Care.* Basingstoke: Palgrave Macmillan.

Edwards, N.P. (2009) Women's emotion work in the context of current maternity services. In: Hunter, B., Deery, R. (eds) *Emotions in Midwifery and Reproduction.* Basingstoke: Palgrave Macmillan.

Eyer, D.E. (1994) Mother–infant bonding: a scientific fiction. *Human Nature* 5 (1), pp. 69–94.

Fearon, R.P., Bakermans-Kranenburg, M.J., Van IJzendoorn, M.H., Lapsley, A., Roisman, G.I. (2010) The significance of insecure attachment and disorganization in the development of children's externalizing behavior: a meta-analytic study. *Child development.* 81 (2), pp. 435–456.

Field, T., Diego, M., Hernandez-Reif, M., et al. (2010) Comorbid depression and anxiety effects on pregnancy and neonatal outcome. *Infant Behaviour Development* 33 (1), pp. 23–29.

Figueiredo, B., Costa, R. (2009) Mother's stress, mood and emotional involvement with the infant: 3 months before and 3 months after childbirth. *Archives of Women's Mental Health* 12 (3), pp. 143–153.

Fransson, E., Ortenstrand, A., Hjelmstedt, A. (2011) Antenatal depressive symptoms and preterm birth: a prospective study of a Swedish national sample. *BIRTH* 38 (1), pp. 10–16.

Gibbins, J., Thomson, A.M. (2001) Women's expectations and experiences of childbirth. *Midwifery* 17 (4), pp. 302–313.

Goodin, M., Griffiths, M. (2012) Caesarean section on demand. *Obstetrics, Gynaecology & Reproductive Medicine* 22 (12) pp. 368–370.

Goodman, J.H. (2004) Paternal postpartum depression, its relationship to maternal postpartum depression, and implications for family health. *Journal of Advanced Nursing* 45 (1), pp. 26–35.

Green, J.M. (2012) Integrating women's views into maternity care research and practice. *BIRTH* 39 (4), pp. 291–295.

Hayes, L.J., Goodman, S.H., Carlson, E. (2013) Maternal antenatal depression and infant disorganized attachment at 12 months. *Attachment & Human Development* 15 (2), pp. 133–153.

Hjelmstedt, A., Widström, A.M., Collins, A. (2006) Psychological correlates of prenatal attachment in women who conceived after in vitro fertilization and women who conceived naturally. *Birth* 33 (4), pp. 303–310.

Hewstone, M., Fincham, F.D., Foster, J. (2005) *Psychology.* Oxford: BPS Blackwell.

Hernandez-Martinez, C., Val, V.A., Murphy, M., Busquets, P.C., Sans, J.C. (2011) relation between positive and negative maternal emotional states and obstetrical outcomes. *Women & Health* 51 (2), pp. 124–135.

Hofberg, K., Ward, M.R. (2003) Fear of pregnancy and childbirth. *Postgraduate Medical Journal.* 79, pp. 505–510.

Hunter, B. (2004) Conflicting ideologies as a source of emotion work in midwifery. *Midwifery* 22 (4), pp. 308–322.

Hunter, B. (2006) The importance of reciprocity in relationships between community based midwives and mothers. *Midwifery* 22 (4), pp. 308–322.

Hunter, B., Berg, M., Lundgren, I., Olafsdottir, O.A., Kirkham, M. (2008) Relationships: The hidden threads in the tapestry of maternity care. *Midwifery* 24 (2), pp. 132–137.

Huth-Bocks, A.C., Theran, S.A., Levendosky, A.A., Bogat, G.A. (2011) A social-contextual understanding of concordance and discordance between maternal prenatal representations of the infant and infant–mother attachment. *Infant Mental Health Journal.* 32 (4), pp. 405–426.

Jomeen, J. (2004) The importance of assessing psychological status during pregnancy, childbirth and the postnatal period as a multidimensional construct: A literature review. *Clinical Effectiveness in Nursing* 8 (3/4), pp. 143–155.

Jomeen, J. (2010) *Choice and Control in Contemporary Childbirth: Understanding through Women's Experiences*. London: Radcliffe.

Jomeen, J., Martin, C.R. (2008a) The impact of choice of maternity care on psychological health outcomes for women during pregnancy and the postnatal period. *Journal of Evaluation in Clinical Practice* 14 (3), pp. 391–398.

Jomeen, J., Martin, C.R. (2008b) Reflections on the notion of post-natal depression following examination of the scoring pattern of the women on the EPDS during pregnancy and in the post-natal period. *Journal of Psychiatric and Mental Health Nursing* 15, pp. 645–648.

Jomeen, J., Redshaw, M. (2012) Ethnic minority women's experience of maternity services in England. *Ethnicity and Health* [available online: http://dx.doi.org/10.1080/13557858.2012.730608]

Keeling, J., Mason, T. (2011) Postnatal disclosure of domestic violence: comparison with disclosure in the first trimester of pregnancy. *Journal of Clinical Nursing* 20 (1/2), pp. 103–110.

Kennell, J.H., Jerauld, R., Wolfe, H., Chester, D., Kreger, N.C., McAlpine, W., Steffa, M., Klaus, M.H. (1974) Maternal behavior one year after early and extended post-partum contact. *Developmental Medicine and Child Neurology* 16 (2), pp. 172–179.

Kirkham, M. (2010) *The Midwife–Mother Relationship*. Basingstoke: Palgrave Macmillan.

Kitzinger, S. (2006) *Birth Crisis*. Abingdon: Routledge.

Kitzinger, S. (2012) Rediscovering the social model of childbirth. *BIRTH*. 39 (4), pp. 301–304.

Lapaire, O., Alder, J., Peukert, R., Holzgreve, W. and Tercanli, S. (2007) Two- versus three-dimensional ultrasound in the second and third trimester of pregnancy: impact on recognition and maternal–fetal bonding. A prospective pilot study. *Archives of Gynecology and Obstetrics* 276 (5), pp. 475–479.

Laxton-Kane, M., Slade, P. (2002) The role of maternal prenatal attachment in a woman's experience of pregnancy and implications for the process of care. *Journal of Reproductive and Infant Psychology*. 20 (4), pp. 253–266.

Maier, B. (2010) Women's worries about childbirth: making safe choices. *British Journal of Midwifery* 18(5), pp. 293–299.

Marks, D.E., Murray, M., Evans, B., Willig, C., Woodall, C., Sykes, C.M. (2005) *Health Psychology: Theory, Research and Practice*. London: Sage.

Marshall, J.L., Godfrey M., Renfrew, M.J. (2007) Being a 'good mother': Managing breastfeeding and merging identities. *Social Science and Medicine* 65, pp. 2147–2159.

Martin, C.R., Jomeen, J. (2004) The impact of clinical management type on maternal locus of control in pregnant women with pre-labour rupture of membranes at term. *Health Psychology Update* 13, pp. 3–13.

McCourt, C., Stevens, T. (2009) Relationships and reciprocity in caseload midwifery. In: Hunter, B., Deery, R. (eds) *Emotions in Midwifery and Reproduction*. Basingstoke: Palgrave Macmillan.

McCrea, H., Crute, V. (1991) Midwife/client relationship: Midwives perspectives. *Midwifery* 7 (4), pp. 183–192.

McKenzie, S.K., Carter, K. (2013) Does transition into parenthood lead to changes in mental health? Findings from three waves of a population based panel study. *Journal of Epidemiology Community Health* 67, pp. 339–345.

Mercer, J., Green-Jervis, C., Brannigan, C. (2012) The legacy of a self-reported negative birth experience. *British Journal of Midwifery* 20 (10), pp. 717–723.

Miller, T. (2011) Transition to first-time motherhood. *The Practising Midwife* 14 (2), pp. 12–15.

Misri, S., Kendrick, K., Oberlander, T.F., Norris, S., Tomfohr, L., Zhang, H., Grunau, R.E. (2010) Antenatal depression and anxiety affect postpartum parenting stress: a longitudinal, prospective study. *Canadian Journal of Psychiatry* 55 (4), pp. 222–228.

Mitchell, L.M. (2001) *Baby's First Picture. Ultrasound and the Politics of Fetal Subjects*. Toronto: University of Toronto Press.

Molander, E., Alehagen, S., Berterö, C.M. (2010) Routine ultrasound during pregnancy: a world of possibilities. *Midwifery* 26 (1), 18–26.

National Institute for Health and Care Excellence (2006) *Postnatal care. Routine postnatal care of women and their babies*. [Available online] http://nice.org.uk.

National Institute for Health and Clinical Excellence (2007) *Antenatal and Postnatal Mental Health Guideline*. London: NICE.

National Institute of Child Health and Human Development (NICHD). (2006) *The NICHD Study of Early Child Care and Youth Development*. [Available online] https://www.nichd.nih.gov.

Nicholls, L., Webb, C. (2006) What makes a good midwife? An integrative review of methodologically diverse research. *Journal of Advanced Nursing* 56 (4), pp. 414–429.

Nicholson, P., Fox, R., Heffernan, K. (2010) Constructions of pregnant and postnatal embodiment across three generations: mothers', daughters' and others' experiences of the transition to motherhood. *Journal of Health Psychology* 15, pp. 575–585.

Nilsson, C., Lundgren, I. (2009) Women's lived experience of fear of childbirth. *Midwifery*, 25 (2), pp. e1–e9. [Available online] http://www.scopus.com/record/display.url?eid=2-s2.0-61749088458&origin=inwar d&txGid=54DFCDB0CF81AA536BA232DA8FD1DD9B.zQKnzAySRvJOZYcdflziQ%3a2

Nursing and Midwifery Council (NMC). (2012) *Midwives Rules and Standards*. London: NMC.

O'Hare, J., Fallon, A. (2011) Women's experience of control in labour and childbirth. *British Journal of Midwifery* 19 (3), pp. 164–169.

Peeler, S., Chung, M.C., Stedmon, J., Skirton, H. (2013) A review assessing the current treatment strategies for postnatal psychological morbidity with a focus on post-traumatic stress disorder. *Midwifery* 29 (4), pp. 377–188.

Pinel, J.P.J. (2011) *Biopsychology* (8th edn). Boston: Pearson.

Ramchandani, P., Stein, A., Evans, J., O'Connor, T.G. (2005) Paternal depression in the postnatal period and child development: a prospective population study. *Lancet* 365 (9478), pp. 2201–2205.

Raynor, M. (2006) Social and psychological context of childbearing. *Women's Health Medicine* 3 (2), pp. 64–67.

Raynor, M., England, C. (2010) *Psychology for Midwives: Pregnancy, Childbirth and Puerperium*. Maidenhead: Open University Press.

Redshaw, M., Martin, C.R. (2013) Babies, 'bonding' and ideas about parental 'attachment'. *Journal of Reproductive and Infant Psychology* 31 (3), pp. 219–221.

Roberts, J. (2012) 'Wakey wakey baby': narrating four-dimensional (4D) bonding scans. *Sociology of Health & Illness* 34 (2), pp. 299–314.

Rogers, C. (1961) *On Becoming a Person: A Therapist View of Psychotherapy*. New York: Mariner Books.

Rogers, R.W. (1975) A protection motivation theory of fear appeals and attitude change. *Journal of Psychology* 91, pp. 93–114.

Rogers, R.W. (1983). Cognitive and physiological processes in fear appeals and attitude change: A revised theory of protection motivation. In: Cacioppo, J., Petty R. (eds) *Social Psychophysiology*. New York: Guilford Press.

Rogers, R.W. (1985) Attitude change and information integration in fear appeals. *Psychological Reports* 56, pp. 179–182.

Rosenstock, I.M. (1966) Why people use health services. *The Milbank Memorial Fund Quarterly* 44 (3), pp. 94–127.

Royal College of Psychiatrists (2014) *Postnatal Depression* [Available online] http://www.rcpsych.ac.uk/healthadvice/problemsdisorders/pnd-keyfacts.aspx

Salomonsson, B., Berterö, C., Alehagen, S. (2013) Self-efficacy in pregnant women with severe fear of childbirth. *Journal of Obstetric, Gynecologic & Neonatal Nursing* 42 (2), pp. 191–202.

Salonen, A.H., Kaunonen, M., Astedt-Kurki, P., Järvenpää, A., Isoaho, H., Tarkka, M. (2009) Parenting self-efficacy after childbirth. *Journal of Advanced Nursing* 65 (11) pp. 2324–2336.

Shah, P.S., Shah, J. (2010) Maternal exposure to domestic violence and pregnancy and birth outcomes: a systematic review and meta-analyses. *Journal of Women's Health* 19 (11), pp. 2017–2031.

Skinner, B.F. (1976) *About Behaviourism*. New York: Vintage Books.

Slade, P., MacPherson, S., Hume, A., Maresh, M. (1993) Expectations, experiences and satisfaction with labour. *British Journal of Clinical Psychology* 32, pp. 469–483.

Sroufe, L.A. (2005) Attachment and development: A prospective, longitudinal study from birth to adulthood. *Attachment & Human Development* 7 (4), pp. 349–367.

Stevens, R. (2008) *Sigmund Freud: Examining the Essence of his Contribution*. Basingstoke: Palgrave Macmillan.

Strathearn, L. (2011) Maternal neglect: oxytocin, dopamine and the neurobiology of attachment. *Journal of Neuroendocrinology* 23, pp. 1054–1065.

Stringhini, S, Dugravot, A., Shipley, M., Goldberg, M., Zins, M., Kivimäki,M., Marmot, M., Sabia, S., Singh-Manoux, A. (2011). Health Behaviours, Socioeconomic Status, and Mortality: Further Analyses of the British Whitehall II and the French GAZEL Prospective Cohorts. *Plos Medicine* [Available online] http://www.plosmedicine.org/article/info%3Adoi%2F10.1371%2Fjournal.pmed.1000419. DOI: 10 .1371/journal.pmed.1000419

Swain, J.E., Lorberbaum, J.P., Kose, S., Strathearn, L. (2007) Brain basis of early parent–infant interactions: psychology, physiology, and *in vivo* functional neuroimaging studies. *Journal of Child Psychology and Psychiatry* 48 (3–4), pp. 262–287.

Talbot, R. (2012) Self-efficacy: women's experiences of pain in labour. *British Journal of Midwifery* 20 (5), pp. 317–321.

Taylor, J. and Johnson, M. (2010) How women manage fatigue after childbirth. *Midwifery* 26, pp. 367–375.

Teixeira, C., Figueiredo, B., Conde, A., Pacheco, A., Costa, R. (2009) Anxiety and depression during pregnancy in women and men. *Journal of Affective Disorders* 119 (3), pp. 142–148.

Tinkler, A., Quinney, D. (2001) Team midwifery: the influence of the midwife-woman relationship on women's experiences and perceptions of maternity care. *Journal of Advanced Nursing* 28 (1), pp. 30–35.

Waldenström, U., Hildingsson, I., Rubertsson, C., Rådestad, I. (2004) A negative birth experience: prevalence and risk factors in a national sample. *Birth*, 31 (1), pp. 17–27.

Wallston, K.A., Wallston, B.S. (1982) Who is responsible for your health? The construct of health locus of control. In: Sanders G.S., Suls, J. (eds) *Social Psychology of Health and Illness*. Hillsdale, NJ: Lawrence Erlbaum and Associates.

Weinstein, N.D. (1983) Reducing unrealistic optimism about illness susceptibility. *Health Psychology* 2, pp. 11–20.

Weinstein, N.D. (1984) Why it won't happen to me: perceptions of risk factors and susceptibility. *Health Psychology* 3, pp. 431–457.

White, G. (2005) *Postnatal Moods: Emotional Changes Following Childbirth*. Auckland: Random House.

Winnicott, D. (1953) The theory of the parent–infant relationship. *International Journal of Psychoanalysis* 41, pp. 585–595. [Available online] http://nonoedipal.files.wordpress.com/2009/09/transitional-objects-and-transitional-phenomenae28094a-study-of-the-first-not-me-possession.pdf

Zachariah, R. (2009) Social support, life stress, and anxiety as predictors of pregnancy complications in low-income women. *Research in Nursing & Health* 32 (4) pp. 391–404.

Chapter 5

Parenthood

Olanma Ogbuehi

University of Hull, Hull, UK

Jacqui Powell

Women and Children's Hospital, Hull, UK

Learning outcomes

By the end of this chapter the reader will be able to:

* explain different definitions of mother and father and describe different family structures
* define the role of the midwife in support of mothers and fathers
* explain key health and social considerations in childbearing across the lifespan of women
* describe major contributing factors to the health of the population of childbearing women and their babies
* recognise and respond to different parenting styles using sound evidence.

Introduction

This chapter offers a brief overview of parenthood and its centrality to midwifery practice. The scope of midwifery practice as it relates to motherhood and parenthood in general is explained. The focus is on motherhood, with some consideration of fatherhood. Definitions of parenthood and the boundaries of parenthood are discussed, in terms of biology capability and assisted reproduction. Different family structures are described, into which babies are born, in the United Kingdom. Challenges faced by younger mothers, older mothers and disabled parents are considered. Different parenting styles are also described. The role of the midwife in supporting parents through the childbearing period is discussed throughout, in relation to the main areas of content.

Midwifery, by definition, focuses on the role of women at that stage in life when they embark on motherhood. A midwife is:

> ...*a responsible and accountable professional who works in partnership with women to give the necessary support, care and advice during pregnancy, labour and the postpartum period,*

Fundamentals of Midwifery: A Textbook for Students, First Edition. Edited by Louise Lewis.
© 2015 John Wiley & Sons, Ltd. Published 2015 by John Wiley & Sons, Ltd.
Companion website: www.wileyfundamentalseries.com/midwifery

*to conduct births on the midwife's own responsibility and to provide care for the newborn
and the infant…*

(International Confederation of Midwives (ICM) 2011)

The United Kingdom's (UK) Nursing and Midwifery Council (NMC) (2012, p. 15) determines
that midwives should ensure the primacy of the *'needs of the woman and her baby'*, and work in:

*…partnership with the woman and her family providing safe, responsive, compassionate
care in an appropriate environment to facilitate her physical and emotional care throughout
childbirth…*

'Childbirth' covers the antenatal, intrapartum and postnatal periods (NMC 2012) encompassing the care of the baby. Midwives use their '… skills to refer to and coordinate between any
specialist services that may be required …' (Department of Health/Partnerships for Children,
Families and Maternity 2007, p. 15). Furthermore, the midwife's scope of practice incorporates
'preparation for parenthood' (ICM 2011). Therefore, parenthood and more specifically, motherhood is the core focus of midwifery and fundamental to midwifery practice.

Parenthood

A parent is either a person who biologically brings forth offspring and has a relationship of
nurturance towards them during their development to maturity and social independence, or a
parent is someone who takes on the role of nurturance of a child through maturation to social
independence, at some point following their birth. Parenthood has biological, social, ethical and
legal dimensions and is a subset of a larger whole – the family – itself a subset of society. Smith
(2010) considers that parenting constitutes a significant life transition in the majority of people
which begins either prior to, or during pregnancy and continues throughout life. It is acknowledged that the word *'family'* may have a number of definitions (see Chapter 3: 'Sociology applied
to maternity care', where family and society are discussed in greater depth). Giddens' (2009)
definition of a family as a group of people bonded by ties of kinship, in which adults care for
children, is helpful. Kinship between individuals may be established through genetic descent:
that is blood relations – fathers, mothers, siblings and offspring (consanguines), or through
marriage (affines) (Giddens 2009; Chambers 2012).

A traditionalist model of the family is centred on marriage between a man and a woman
(Fulcher and Scott 2007; see Figure 5.1). Historically, sociological ideas about the family and
kinship in the mid 1800s were drawn from anthropology, which was predominantly concerned
with ideas of biological relatedness (Chambers 2012). In Western Europe and America these
views of marriage and family life were heavily influenced by the Judeo-Christian worldview: the
1662 Anglican Book of Common Prayer explains marriage as a creation ordinance given by God,
for purposes including the procreation and nurture of children, closeness, companionship and
exclusive sexual intimacy between a man and a woman (Christian Institute nd; Church of
England, 2014).

Sociologically, by the 1850s, marriage was conceived as an institution biologically determined
to meet the needs of procreation and childrearing; this involved a protracted period of depend-
ence on parents by their offspring, within marriage, where the nurturance and training of these
children would occur (Chambers 2012). In the mid 20th century, sociologists favoured the
concept of the 'nuclear family' (see Figure 5.2) comprising of a married couple – mother, father
and their children – for the period of time in which the offspring lived at home (Cheal 2002).
The boundaries of this family were formed by the walls of their accommodation and societal

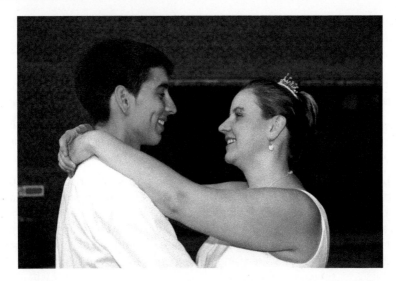

Figure 5.1   Marriage was the foundation of the 'traditional' nuclear family in the Western world.

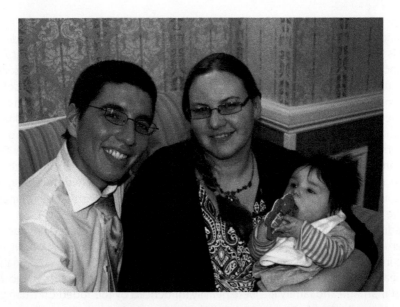

Figure 5.2   A traditional, nuclear family unit, consisting of father, mother and child.

consensus agreements not to interfere with these private arrangements. Such households were considered to be the basic units of production, including food preparation (Cheal 2002). Bottero (2011) argues that the North West European pattern of marriage (excepting Ireland), between the 14th and mid-18th centuries was characterised by:

- A commonly held belief within the culture that couples would only marry when they achieved the ability to set up, financially viable households, independently of their parents.
- A comparatively late age of marriage; 25–26 for women and 27–28 for men (in early 1700s England).

- Strong societal censure of extramarital sexual intercourse, with resultant stigma and penalties which reduced fertility outside marriage.

The industrial revolution led to a relaxation of certain social restrictions on sexual relationships, due to the changing pattern of work and residency of adults (fewer household servants or tied workers): this was accompanied by a population explosion, and high levels of illegitimacy (Bottero 2011). However, arguably, the nuclear family was already an established 'norm' in North West Europe.

This portrayal of the traditional nuclear family is tempered with a broader vision of family life that represents the diversity of social arrangements in 21st century Britain. Longstanding variations exist from the notion of nuclear family, for example, the *extended family* defined by Bradley and Mendels (1978, p. 381) is '... *when a household is composed of one person and some other kin in addition to spouse or child.*' Although the extended family model may be assumed to be more prevalent among certain ethnic groups, in the UK, they exist throughout society. Socioeconomic factors, such as national recession may create more extended family households and somewhat heighten their importance (Byrne et al. 2011). Extended family members, such as the baby's grandparents, aunts and uncles may prove supportive and influential to parents. Family structures are also shaped by the marital status of the parents. The Office for National Statistics (ONS 2013a) report from the General Lifestyle Survey (GLS) for Great Britain (GB) showed that 49% of women aged over 16 were married; 21% of these women were single, 11% were cohabiting, and 10% were divorced or separated (Table 5.1). ONS (2013b) reported a declining trend in the proportion of first marriages for both partners between 1966 and 2011. A total of 82% of religious marriages were between partners who had never married before in 2011 compared with 60% of civil marriages. However, 88% of couples who married in civil ceremonies and 78% of those who had religious ceremonies had cohabited prior to marriage (ONS 2013b). When parents remarry, it is considered that '... *stepchildren and joint biological children who live together ... belong to a "blended" family*' (Ginther and Pollak 2004, p. 4). In 2012, about 48% of live births were registered to parents who were either cohabiting, living separately, or who were single parents (ONS 2013c). Therefore midwives can expect to care for married, cohabiting and single mothers, within the varying family contexts. Occasionally, the baby may also be cared for by a single father.

Table 5.1   Marital status of women aged 16 or over in England and Wales 2011 (ONS 2013a)

	Percentage of the population of women aged 16 or over
Married	49
Civil partnership	0
Cohabiting	11
Single	21
Widowed	9
Divorced	7
Separated	2

A more focused discussion of how the meaning of parenthood has evolved through the use of reproductive technologies and legislation on surrogacy arrangements, civil partnerships and same-sex marriage in the UK, now follows. Different definitions of parenthood and the relational bonds between mothers, fathers and babies are discussed below.

Motherhood and fatherhood

Gutteridge (2010, p. 73) has eloquently expressed that:

> …Motherhood brings with it expectations and dreams; it is a social proclamation of female maturity and an opportunity to pass on our knowledge, skills and stories of womanly experiences…

A deep-rooted belief persists in contemporary societies that motherhood reflects *'feminine gender identity'* (Gillespie 2003, p. 122); it delineates women's social roles and is both sought-after and gratifying for women. By contrast Gutteridge (2010, p. 73) describes fatherhood as merely *'a social construct,'* setting motherhood apart as something physically embodied in women. Whilst women do possess unique biological capacity to house and nurture their developing offspring, during pregnancy and then postnatally through lactation (Murray and Hassall 2009; Coates 2010; Lawrence and Lawrence 2011), reducing fatherhood to a social construct is to deny the significance of the biological and relational investment of men in their children.

Draper (2002a,b) found fathers physically involved in pregnancy, through 'body mediated movements' (e.g. pregnancy test confirmation and physically feeling the babies' movements within their mother's wombs) and medical imaging. A child could be seen as the embodiment of a prior intimate union between a man and a woman – without whom there would be no child. The Fatherhood Institute (2008) note that a father's initial level of involvement in his baby's life before, during and after the birth predicts the level and likelihood of his continued involvement in the child's later life. Supportive fathers also foster improved experiences of mothers and babies during birth and in the early postnatal weeks and months. Therefore, midwives should respectfully support both mothers and fathers and provide compassionate care towards them (see Chapter 8: 'Postnatal midwifery care', where fatherhood is discussed in greater depth). Parental status can be seen as a powerful motivation for people to nurture, protect and provide for children.

Defining parents

Christian ethicist, Professor Oliver O'Donavan (1984) asserts that the differentiation of the sexes in humankind enables them to engage in natural reproduction:

> …It is because we stand over against one another, as men and women, as equal but complementary members of one human race, that we can, as a race, be fruitful…
>
> (O'Donavan 1984, p. 15)

Men and women combine through their biological uniqueness and complementary function to produce offspring. Since the late 20th century there has been an increasing ability to separate reproduction from sexual intercourse between a man and a woman (Ber 2000). This contradicts what Wyatt (2009) describes as the 'original human design' (p. 100), in which 'making love and making babies' are inseparable, so that the genetic material deoxyribonucleic acid (DNA) is:

> …the means by which a unique love between a man and a woman can be converted physically into a baby…
>
> (Wyatt 2009, p. 100)

However, the development of extremely effective and well-tolerated contraceptive methods, from the mid-20th century, concurrent with increasing scientific understanding of reproduction and therapeutic techniques to modify it, have increasingly isolated sexual intercourse from reproduction (Ber 2000; Velde and Pearson 2002). Sexual intercourse can be mainly recreational, with conception being a planned outcome (Benagiano et al. 2010). Furthermore, conception, itself, may now arise devoid of any physical relationship or social connection between '*mothers*' and '*fathers*'. These developments necessitate a re-definition of parenthood (Ber 2000). Griffith (2010) therefore, rightly emphasises the importance of midwives being familiar with current legislation affecting parental status to ensure that they treat the appropriate persons as a child's parents. These changes have been enacted via the Surrogacy Act 1985, Human Fertilisation and Embryology Acts, 1990, 2008 and legal redefinitions of what constitutes legitimate spousal relationships (Marriage [Same Sex] Couple's Act 2013). In the following section, these definitions are discussed.

Genetic, biological and social parents

A genetic parent is one who has provided the gametes – the mature sex cells of males and females – which are the source of the fertilised ovum (the zygote) from which the baby develops: the spermatozoon comes from the man and the ovum from the woman (Tiran 2008; Martin 2010). At a minimum each child must have:

- a genetic mother
- a genetic father.

The exceptions to this rule would be reproductive cloning, currently illegal in most countries and use of mitochondrial replacement therapy (Human Reproductive Cloning Act, 2001; Wyatt, 2009; Human Fertilisation and Embryology Authority [HFEA], 2013). Traditionally, parents would have been in a social contract of marriage and the child would have been carried in the womb of his genetic mother, being the progeny of both his genetic mother and genetic father, who would also be responsible for his nurture (see Figure 5.3).

A *biological parent* is one with whom the child has a direct biological connection; either through their gametes, or through being carried in a woman's uterus during pregnancy (Ber

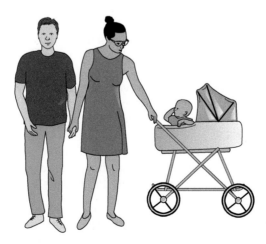

Figure 5.3   A traditional nuclear family: husband, wife and baby.

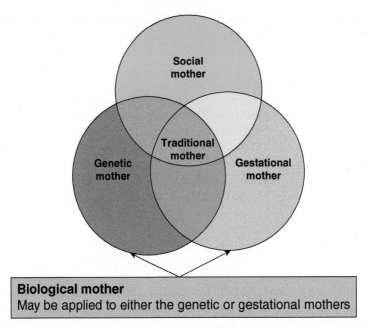

Figure 5.4   Venn diagram illustrating the division of social and biological mothering in gestational surrogacy (Ber 2000; Erin & Harris 1991; FIGO Committee for the Ethical Aspects of Human Reproduction and Women's Health 2008).

2000). Figures 5.4–5.9 are essentially the same Venn diagram used to illustrate different facets of the mothering role as it exists today. Each diagram emphasises a different aspect of mother-hood. A *biological mother* (see Figure 5.4) may, therefore, be considered to be:

* the woman who provides the ovum for conception (genetic mother), or
* the woman who carries the pregnancy to term (gestational mother).

Due to surrogacy arrangements and more traditionally, adoption and fostering arrangements *gestational mothers* may be subdivided into one of the following categories:

* A *genetic mother*, who has conceived a child through natural means of sexual intercourse with the genetic father, or through artificial insemination by husband, male partner, or by sperm donor. In partial surrogacy (see Figure 5.6) the genetic mother also acts as the gestational mother who will relinquish the child.
* A woman who has conceived through in-vitro fertilisation, using donor gametes (oocyte or sperm, or a donor embryo), who intends to be the social mother of this child. Her biological connection to the child is through containing, maintaining and sustaining him or her through pregnancy (see Figure 5.9).
* A woman who has conceived through in-vitro fertilisation, using donor gametes (or a donor embryo), who intends to relinquish the child after birth – a *gestational (full) surrogate mother* (see Figure 5.9); her biological connection to the child is also through pregnancy.

Those parents who fulfil the nurturing role for the child during pregnancy and beyond, or only after birth can be called the *social parents* (Ber 2000): social parents may have no genetic connection to the child. In a surrogacy arrangement they would be known as the commission-ing parents. A child may have at least one social parent, who may be:

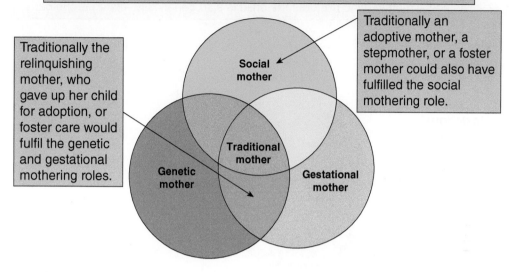

A traditional mother is the source of the egg, carries the pregnancy and nurtures the baby after birth, fulfilling genetic, gestational and social roles

Traditionally the relinquishing mother, who gave up her child for adoption, or foster care would fulfil the genetic and gestational mothering roles.

Traditionally an adoptive mother, a stepmother, or a foster mother could also have fulfilled the social mothering role.

Social mother

Traditional mother

Genetic mother

Gestational mother

Figure 5.5   Venn diagram illustrating the social and biological roles of traditional mothers (Ber 2000; Erin & Harris 1991; FIGO Committee for the Ethical Aspects of Human Reproduction and Women's Health 2008).

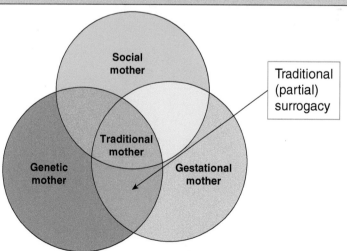

Partial or traditional surrogacy is where the gestational mother is the source of the egg and carries the pregnancy, but another social mother nurtures the baby after birth. The baby is genetically related to the surrogate.

Social mother

Traditional (partial) surrogacy

Traditional mother

Genetic mother

Gestational mother

Figure 5.6   Venn diagram illustrating the division of social and biological mothering in traditional surrogacy (Ber 2000; Erin & Harris 1991; FIGO Committee for the Ethical Aspects of Human Reproduction and Women's Health 2008).

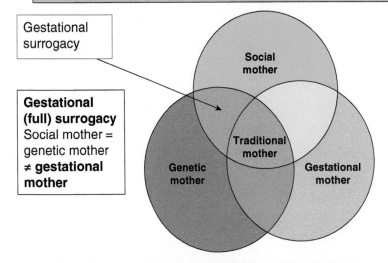

In gestational surrogacy the social mother may provide the egg, the gestational mother conceives through in vitro fertilization (IVF) and carries the baby to term. The social mother, who nurtures the child is also genetically related to the baby.

Gestational surrogacy

Gestational (full) surrogacy
Social mother = genetic mother ≠ **gestational mother**

Social mother

Traditional mother

Genetic mother

Gestational mother

Figure 5.7   Venn diagram illustrating the division of social and biological mothering in gestational surrogacy where the social mother is also the genetic mother (Ber 2000; Erin & Harris 1991; FIGO Committee for the Ethical Aspects of Human Reproduction and Women's Health 2008).

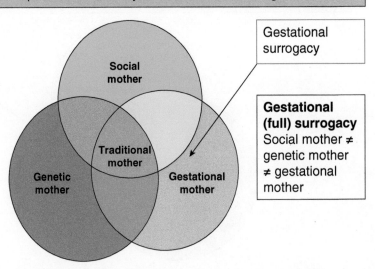

A further form of gestational surrogacy is where one woman is the genetic mother, or egg donor, the gestational mother carries the baby to term, and another woman, the commissioning mother, acts as the social mother. There is no genetic relationship between the baby and the social or surrogate mothers.

Gestational surrogacy

Social mother

Traditional mother

Genetic mother

Gestational mother

Gestational (full) surrogacy
Social mother ≠ genetic mother ≠ gestational mother

Figure 5.8   Venn diagram illustrating the division of social and biological mothering in gestational surrogacy where the social mother is not the genetic mother (Ber 2000; Erin & Harris 1991; FIGO Committee for the Ethical Aspects of Human Reproduction and Women's Health 2008).

A final category is women who conceive using a donor embryo, who are both the
gestational mother and the social mother. This is not a surrogacy arrangement.

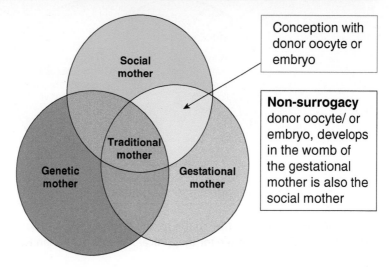

Figure 5.9   Venn diagram illustrating the social and gestational mother intersection, when a
woman conceives by ovum or embryo donation (Ber 2000; Erin & Harris 1991; FIGO Committee for
the Ethical Aspects of Human Reproduction and Women's Health 2008).

- a *social mother* (see Figure 5.5)
- a *social father* (see Figure 5.10).

A child may also legally have two social parents of the same gender (Griffith 2010).
A social mother may be:

- A *traditional mother* (see Figure. 5.5): a woman who fulfils all three roles the genetic mother,
gestational mother and the social mother.
- A woman (the *commissioning mother*) who intends to raise a child carried by a surrogate
mother (the gestational mother). She may also be the genetic mother, whose ovum was
fertilised to become the embryo implanted in the womb of the gestational (surrogate)
mother.
- A woman who legally takes on responsibility for the nurture of a child, through adoption,
foster care, or a parental order, or alternatively, through marriage as a stepmother.

The International Federation of Gynaecology and Obstetrics (FIGO) (2008) define surrogacy
as:

> …*where a woman carries a pregnancy and delivers a child on behalf of a couple where the
> woman is unable to do so, because of congenital or acquired uterine abnormality or serious
> medical contraindication to pregnancy…*

(FIGO 2008, p. 312)

Brazier et al. (1998) define surrogacy as:

> …*the practice whereby one woman (the surrogate mother) becomes pregnant, carries and
> gives birth to a child for another person(s) (the commissioning couple) as the result of an*

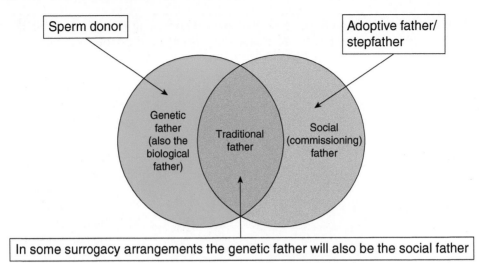

Sperm donor

Adoptive father/ stepfather

Genetic father (also the biological father)

Traditional father

Social (commissioning) father

In some surrogacy arrangements the genetic father will also be the social father

Figure 5.10 Venn diagram illustrating the nature of biological and social fatherhood (Ber 2000; Erin & Harris 1991; FIGO Committee for the Ethical Aspects of Human Reproduction and Women's Health 2008).

agreement prior to conception that the child should be handed over to that person after birth…

(Brazier et al. 1998, Annexe A)

The latter definition does not preclude commercial surrogacy arrangements for example. Brazier et al. (1998) further defined a surrogate mother as:

…The woman who carries and gives birth to the child … or 'surrogate'. She may be the genetic mother ('partial' surrogacy) – i.e. using her own egg – or she may have an embryo – which may be provided by the commissioning couple -implanted in her womb using in-vitro fertilisation (IVF) techniques…

('host' or 'full' surrogacy [see Figure. 5.7]; Brazier et al. 1998, Annexe A)

Adoptive mothers and foster mothers are more familiar variants of the social mothering role (see Figure 5.5) with whom midwives may also interact. The main difference is that a surrogacy arrangement is a contract, which is entered, prior to conception, for the benefit of the commissioning parents, whilst adoption and fostering are arrangements undertaken post-conception mainly for the benefit of the children (Wyatt 2009). Regardless of mode of conception, or identity of the genetic parents, it is important that midwives grasp that UK law and the midwife's sphere of practice recognises only the childbearing woman (gestational mother) as the mother during pregnancy and the postnatal period (ICM 2011 and NMC 2012. That is:

…the woman who is carrying or has carried a child as a result of the placing in her of an embryo or of sperm and eggs, and no other woman…

(Human Fertilisation and Embryology Act 2008)

This is only superseded by the completion of a parental order, or through legal adoption (Griffith 2010). Parental orders take effect after six weeks postpartum; prior to this a surrogate mother may decide not to relinquish her baby (Human Fertilisation and Embryology Act 2008; Griffith 2010).

Midwives normally rely on childbearing women to identify their babies' fathers. Sometimes, none is identified. In the traditional model of families, or the nuclear family, the husband is both the genetic father and the social father (see Figure 5.10), where a:

- *Genetic father* is the man who provides the spermatozoon for fertilisation of the ovum.
- *Social father* is the man who provides nurture and care for the child following birth.

The social father is a role shared by the traditional father, the commissioning father in a surrogacy arrangement, and also by stepfathers and adoptive fathers. The *traditional father* would have fulfilled both the social and biological roles.

Illustrated in Figures 5.11 and 5.12 are some potential combinations of non-traditional families in which a midwife could be involved, via surrogacy arrangements.

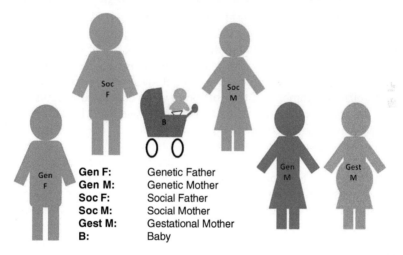

Gen F:	Genetic Father
Gen M:	Genetic Mother
Soc F:	Social Father
Soc M:	Social Mother
Gest M:	Gestational Mother
B:	Baby

Figure 5.11   A surrogacy arrangement with heterosexual commissioning parents who are not genetically related to the baby.

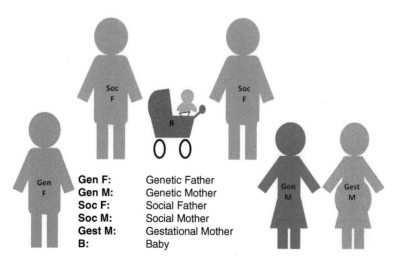

Gen F:	Genetic Father
Gen M:	Genetic Mother
Soc F:	Social Father
Soc M:	Social Mother
Gest M:	Gestational Mother
B:	Baby

Figure 5.12   A surrogacy arrangement with same-sex commissioning parents, neither of whom is genetically related to the baby.

Midwives must act as advocates for gestational mothers and their babies, remembering to '...*listen to the people in*...' their '...*care and respond to their concerns and preferences*' (NMC 2008, p. 3). However, they must negotiate and communicate sensitively with the family, as they choose to define themselves. Midwives are primarily concerned with supporting child-bearing women and babies whilst appreciating the diversity of parenting roles they may encounter.

Conception across the lifespan

Parenthood may occur at different stages in a person's lifespan. From a biological perspective, a woman may be no more than adolescent at first conception, or she may be on the cusp of menopause (Tiran 2008; Blackburn 2013). Men are also capable of fathering children from the time they reach sexual maturity; this effect is attenuated to a lesser extent with ageing in men, as many remain fertile well beyond the age of 40 (Ledger and Cheong 2011). The timing of conception may be controlled through the use of family planning and contraceptive strategies (see Chapter 12: 'Contraception', where family planning is discussed in greater depth), but also increasingly through assisted reproductive technology. Anxieties are often expressed about the health and welfare of women and their offspring when conception occurs in mothers at either extreme of the age spectrum for natural fertility. Midwives must be prepared to provide sensitive and supportive care for childbearing women across this age spectrum.

Trends for conceptions by maternal age are pictured in Figure 5.13. The majority of conceptions consistently occur in the 20–24 year age group, with the fewest being among women aged 40 years and over. For women, there are boundaries to their '*fertility*' or '*fecundity*'. Women's childbearing years begin, during puberty, with the development of secondary sexual characteristics, marked by the onset of hormonally regulated reproductive cycles, known as menarche.

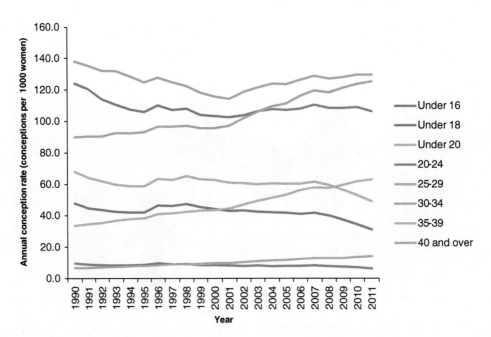

Figure 5.13   Annual conception rates (conceptions per 1000 women in age group (ONS 2013d).

Menarche usually occurs between 9 to 12 years of age (Tiran 2008; Thain 2009; Blackburn 2013) and is indicated by the onset of menstruation in the adolescent girl. The cessation of female fertility is marked by the menopause or the climacteric which is the gradual process by which a woman transitions from a reproductive to a non-fertile state. The climacteric describes the changes that occur from the perimenopausal, through the menopausal, to postmenopausal stages (Blackburn 2013). From around 37.5 years of age, women experience accelerated atresia (degeneration) of ovarian follicles; ovaries become less responsive. Menopause can occur anytime from the middle thirties to the mid-fifties (median age is 51). Natural menopause is diagnosed retrospectively, after 12 consecutive months of amenorrhea (Martin 2010). However, the upper age limits for pregnancy may be increased, by the use of assisted reproductive technologies and other health and lifestyle interventions.

Adolescent parents

Adolescent parenthood seems to concern health professionals and policy makers which can be deduced from policy drives such as the Teenage Pregnancy Strategy (Social Exclusion Unit 1999) which aimed to halve the rate of conception in under-18s and establish a clear downward trend in under-16 conceptions. The terms 'teenager' and 'adolescent' are often used synonymously, but need definition. Martin (2010) gives a clinical definition of adolescence as the developmental stage that occurs from the time of puberty to adulthood, between 12 to 19 years old in girls, and 14 to 19 years old in boys. The World Health Organization (WHO) (2004, p. 5) defines adolescent pregnancy as, 'pregnancy in a woman aged 10–19 years'. The Office for Nationals Statistics (ONS 2013a) discusses teenage conception in terms of, 'under-18 conceptions.' Figures are sometimes cited as pregnancies among 15–17 year olds. In 2011 the under-18 conception rate continued to decline; reaching its lowest level since 1969 at 30.9 conceptions per 1000 women aged 15–17. In 2010 the conception rates among the under 20s were the only ones which decreased as a whole compared to the remainder of age groups of childbearing women, and in 2011, conception rates declined in all women under 25 (ONS 2013b). The Abortion Statistics, England and Wales (DH/ONS, 2013) suggest that has been a decline in teenage abortion rates (under 16 and under 18), in recent years. The Teenage Pregnancy Independent Advisory Group (2010) reported that between 1998 and 2008, there was a decline of 13.3 % in teenage conceptions overall, although some areas that had been more consistent in applying the 'Teenage Pregnancy Strategy' had achieved declines of up to 45%.

Young parenthood raises the spectre of early sexual activity, linked with moral objections and sometimes concerns regarding safeguarding of children. Young adolescent girls may have been subject to non-consensual sexual intercourse (rape) or coercive sexual intercourse which resulted in pregnancy, via partners of similar ages or significantly older (Barter et al. 2009). Young fathers are also more likely than older fathers and other young men to have been subjected to violence or sexual abuse (Barter et al. 2009). Midwives and other health professionals must use their professional judgement to decide whether it is right to maintain confidentiality for adolescent girls who have conceived under the age of 16, or whether there is cause to intervene because abuse is suspected, where significant risks to the welfare of children outweigh their right to privacy (Department for Schools, Children and Families and DH 2009). In such instances locally agreed safeguarding protocols must be observed and implemented.

Teenage pregnancy indicates unprotected sexual intercourse, which is a risky behaviour, in the context of transient and/or multiple partnerships. Statistics for the occurrence of sexually transmitted infections (STIs) support this. The report 'HIV and Other Sexually Transmitted Infections in the United Kingdom' (The UK Collaborative Group for HIV and STI Surveillance 2006) found that young people were overrepresented in the statistics for the incidence of genital

Table 5.2 Teenage pregnancies: health outcomes for women and babies

Teenage/adolescent study group	Comparison group	Health concerns among the study group (teenage mothers)	Authors
Mothers aged 11–19	Mothers aged (20–29)	Greater neonatal and infant mortality	Gilbert et al. (2004)
		Increased risk of adverse obstetric outcomes among teenage pregnancies, despite a lower caesarean section rate	
Mothers aged 13–19 years	Mothers aged 20–34 years	Increased risk of congenital anomalies of central nervous system, gastrointestinal and muskoskeletal/integumentary systems in babies	Chen et al. (2007)
Teenage mothers who smoked	Adult mothers who smoked	Babies born to teenage mothers who smoked were significantly more likely to be born at a low birth weight	Dewan et al. (2003)

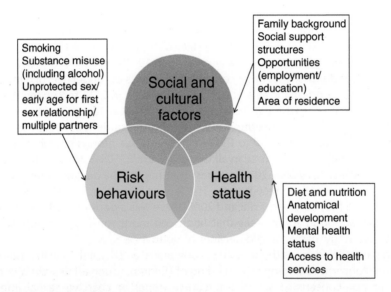

Figure 5.14 Context of teenage pregnancy.

Chlamydia infections, gonorrhoea and genital warts. The highest rates of genital warts appeared among the 16–19 years age-group in women and in the 20–24 years age group in men: diagnoses of these and other STIs (such as Herpes simplex) have risen in frequency in recent years (Public Health England 2013). These diseases are potentially deleterious to the short and long-term health of mothers, babies and their exposed sexual partners. Teenage pregnancy has been linked to a number of poor outcomes for the health of women and babies (see Table 5.2). However, growing evidence suggests that the problems are more attributable to complex social factors than merely young maternal age. The relationship between the context of teenage pregnancy (see Figure 5.14) and its outcomes needs to be considered by midwives and the interprofessional team. Risk factors significantly associated with conception by 16 years and for

Table 5.3 Risk for teenage pregnancy (Sloggett and Joshi 1998; McCulloch 2001; WHO 2004; Allen et al. 2007; Smith 2010)

Category of risk factor	Specific risks for teenage pregnancy
Social circumstances	• Living in non-privately owned housing • Living in an economically inactive household • Social deprivation
Aspirations	• No expectation of being in further/or higher education (by age 20 years)
Beliefs	• Belief that >50% of peers are sexually active
Behaviours	• Being drunk at least once a month at age 13 • Pregnant teenagers are also more likely to engage in other 'risk behaviours' such as substance misuse and smoking. Five out of nine drug dependant mothers who committed suicide in the latest Confidential Enquiry into Maternal and Child Health (2006–2008) were teenagers (CMACE 2011).
Experiences	• Prior experience of physical and sexual abuse

teenage pregnancy, generally, are listed in Table 5.3. This suggests socioeconomic and personal factors may be more significant than age alone in influencing the short and long-term outcomes for adolescent parents and their children. Macvarish (2010) argues that concerns about young pregnancy are possibly symptomatic of hypocritical moralising in a society which largely approves of and promotes premarital sex, but disapproves of its visible consequences. These concerns tend to negate the idea of young mothers being rational, moral agents who choose motherhood (Macvarish 2010).

Ethnic group may influence the prevalence and acceptability of teenage pregnancy. For example, in Europe there are significantly higher rates of teenage pregnancy in England than comparable European Union (EU) states (Aspinall and Hashem 2010). The Millennium Cohort Study showed wide variations of percentages of mothers from different ethnic groups in England who were teenagers at the birth of their first baby. The study showed that 34% of Bangladeshi mothers, 25% of Black Caribbean mothers, 18% of Pakistani mothers, 17% of white mothers, 13% of Black African mothers and 6.1% of Indian mothers gave birth for the first time as teenagers (Jayaweera et al. 2007). Multiple factors could influence these variations, including cultural approval or encouragement of early marriage and childbearing (Higginbottom et al. 2006) and the relative importance attached to further and higher education of young women. Adolescent pregnancy must be considered in its socioeconomic and cultural contexts to interpret its significance.

Midwives must consider that adolescent pregnancy may be planned and desirable for mothers and families; they must also seek to understand, explore and address potential challenges for young mothers and their babies. Family Nurse Partnerships (FNPs) exist to provide an intensive programme of nurse home-visiting services and support from early pregnancy through the first two years of the child's life, for young pregnant mothers and fathers (with consent from mothers) (Department for Education n.d.; Birkbeck University 2012).

Family nurses work alongside existing health and social services such as midwives and social workers, to support young parents. Further means of support include Doulas, such as the Goodwin Volunteer Doula Project in Hull, East Yorkshire which supports women with complex social factors throughout the childbearing period (Sandall et al. 2011). Positive collaboration between midwives, family nurses and Doulas can produce a supportive network and plan of care to meet the needs of teenage mothers. Teenage parenthood may present opportunities for positive life transformation and may therefore be seen as a positive life choice by the mother (Sawyer 2012). An example of good practice is a scheme called 'the Schoolgirl Mum's Unit' in Kingston-Upon-Hull, which aims to provide education, opportunity, and support for young mothers and their babies to gain independence and increase future options (The Boulevard Centre n.d.); this project received an outstanding commendation for:

> '…promoting the achievement of girls and young women and in developing their future economic well-being…'

> (Ofsted 2009)

Appropriate support, education and opportunities may reap rewards in helping young parents to be successful in parenting and making future, positive life choices and changes.

Further reading activity

Read the following items to learn more about the role and purpose of the Family Nurse Partnership:

- Family Nurse Partnership programme to be extended [Available online] https://www.gov.uk/government/news/family-nurse-partnership-programme-to-be-extended
- Family Nurse Partnership [Available online] http://education.gov.uk/commissioning-toolkit/Content/PDF/Family%20Nurse%20Partnership%20FNP.pdf
- Eligibility for the Family Nurse Partnership programme: Testing new criteria. [Available online] http://www.iscfsi.bbk.ac.uk/projects/files/Eligibility-for-the-Family-Nurse-Partnership-programme-Testing-new-criteria.pdf

Listen to the broadcast by Miranda Sawyer (2012) The Teenage Pregnancy Myth. Available: http://www.bbc.co.uk/programmes/b01dhhpq.

Older mothers

At the other end of the fertility spectrum are older mothers. Women's fertility probably ends around 10 years before the menopause, or sometime in their mid-forties (Velde and Pearson 2002; American Society of Reproductive Medicine 2012). The optimum age for women to bear children is between 20 and 35 years of age, according to the Royal College of Obstetricians and Gynaecologists (RCOG 2011); this partly reflects the steep decline in women's ability to produce offspring, observed after age 35 (Menken et al. 1986; see Figure 5.15). Whilst the use of assisted reproductive technologies has extended the age at which many women are able to conceive, there are still health concerns attendant with conception and pregnancy at advanced maternal age (see Table 5.4, for definitions). Some key concerns regarding health of women of advanced maternal age and their babies are shown in Figure 5.16. Historically, the phenomenon of older mothers was associated with women of lower socioeconomic status and higher parity, but more recently there has been a shift so that older mothers are more commonly women of higher socioeconomic status and lower parity (Velde and Pearson 2002; Chan and Lao 2008; Carolan et al. 2011).

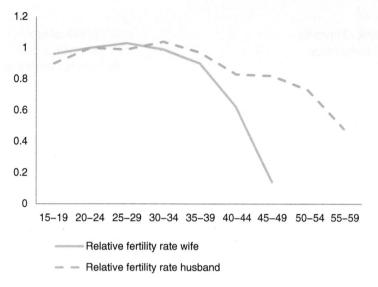

Figure 5.15 Graph showing the variation in relative fertility rate for wives and husbands, who are not using contraceptive measures, with age where the wives were born between the years 1840–1859 (data taken from Menken et al. 1986).

Table 5.4 Advanced maternal age: definitions

Classification terminology	Definition (age in years)	Authors
Advanced maternal age	≥35	Delbaere et al. (2007)
Delayed childbearing	≥35	SOGC Genetics Committee (2012)
High maternal age	≥40	Delbaere et al. (2007)
Advanced maternal age	≥35 modified to ≥40 to better reflect a cut-off in terms of identifying high-risk pregnancies in contemporary maternity care	Chan and Lao (2008)
Very advanced maternal age Mature gravida Extremely elderly gravida	≥44 or ≥45 at delivery reflecting the use of assisted reproductive technologies to achieve older age conceptions	Callaway et al. (2005); SOGC Genetics Committee (2012)

Heffner (2004; Table 5.5) reports the relative risks of conception of babies who have chromosomal abnormalities being born to women, according to maternal age. However, these figures may be negated, in individual women, by the use of pre-implantation genetic diagnosis and or donor gametes.

A predominantly biophysical approach to older parenthood tends to focus on the idea that later conception is both more difficult to achieve and attendant with poorer outcomes. This does not always reflect other confounding factors, such as the differing health statuses of a population of women who are considered older. Demonstrable benefits of older motherhood include a significant reduction in childhood unintentional injuries and hospital admissions for children by the age of three and a significant decline in hospital admissions for children up to

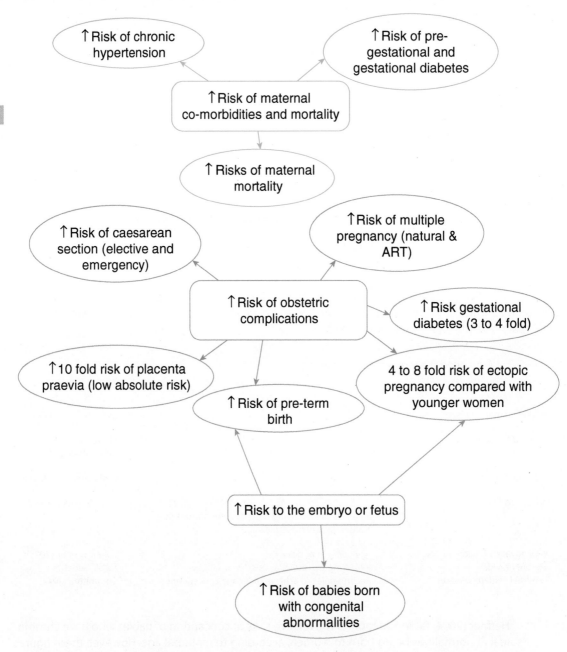

Figure 5.16   Risks attendant with older age conception (Didly et al. 1996; Callaway et al. 2005; Chan and Lao 2008; Mbuga Gitau et al. 2009; CMACE 2011; SOGC Genetics Committee 2012).

Table 5.5 Relative risk of babies with chromosomal abnormalities according to maternal age (Heffner, 2004)

Maternal age at birth (years)	Risk of Down's syndrome	Risk of any chromosomal abnormality
20	1/1667	1/526
25	1/1200	1/476
30	1/952	1/385
35	1/378	1/192
40	1/106	1/66
45	1/30	1/21

the same age (Sutcliffe et al. 2012). Midwives, obstetricians, practice nurses and General Practitioners (GPs) need to be aware of the influence of societal trends, personal and cultural factors, on the timing of parenthood. Partly due to the liberty afforded by availability of safe and effective contraceptive methods and also the provision of effective assisted reproductive technology, women are able to delay childbearing for a number of reasons (Velde and Pearson 2002). They may wish to pursue higher education, achieve career goals, become financially stable, obtain secure marriages, or intimate partnerships. Women may also wish to start second or subsequent families with new partners (Shaw and Giles 2009; Society of Obstetricians & Gynaecologists of Canada (SOGC) Genetics Committee 2012; Dabrowski 2013). Midwives should, therefore, be prepared to offer compassionate and sensitive support for older mothers. As with teenage mothers, care should not be based on assumptions, but rather evidence-based; it should respect the dignity of the woman and her family using effective communication to develop a positive partnership (NICE 2010; Commissioning Board Chief Nursing Officer and DH Chief Nursing Adviser 2012).

Disability and parenting

New mothers across the childbearing age spectrum may also have pre-existing disabilities. A person with a disability:

> …has a physical or mental impairment…which has…a substantial and long-term adverse effect on a person's ability to carry out normal day-to-day activities…
>
> (Equality Act 2010, p. 3)

More broadly speaking disability is 'an umbrella term, covering impairments, activity limitations, and participation restrictions' (WHO 2013). The White Paper, 'Valuing People' (DH 2001), found that parents with disabilities; including learning disabilities (intellectual and social disabilities affecting people's ability to learn and cope independently) received patchy and underdeveloped support. Walsh-Gallagher et al. (2013) found that disabled pregnant women were often impeded from experiencing a positive pregnancy. Disabled mothers may face stigma and prejudice from society, including health professionals: they may be perceived as being totally dependent on others, and therefore incapable of effective parenting. Disabled mothers may face assumptions about their suitability for parenthood, and distaste at the evidence of their being sexually active; they may also face heightened scrutiny due to concerns over their parenting adequacy (Malacrida 2007; MacDonald 2009; Rosqvist and Lövgren 2013; Walsh-Gallagher et al. 2013). Some of these objections may not be dissimilar to those faced by adolescent or older mothers. One of the key policy objectives from 'Valuing People Now' (DH 2009, p. 20) was to ensure that people with learning disabilities would '… *have the choice to have relationships, become parents and continue to be parents …*,' with the expectation of their being supported in doing so. Therefore, midwives should use their skills to coordinate the care of these mothers in partnership with them recognising their dignity, their abilities and love for their children (DH/Partnerships for Children, Families & Maternity 2007; Commissioning Board Chief Nursing Officer & DH Chief Nursing Adviser 2012). This care should be supportive rather than judgemental, or paternalistic, assessing the needs of women, their babies and the wider family and acting to achieve their best interests.

Parenting styles and expert advice

All new parents are faced with multiple decisions about how to care for their newborn babies from abundant information and advice from multiple sources (see Figure 5.17). Until relatively recently parenting was the preserve of parents and their families, involving close friends, colleagues and peers (Fatherhood Institute 2008; Smith 2010). Kinship networks and peers exert influence based on geographical, practical and personal considerations. Parenting expectations

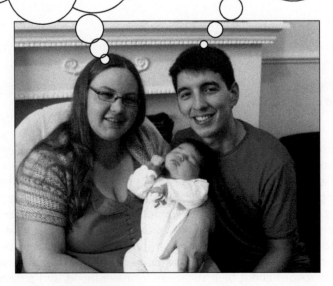

Figure 5.17   Examples of choices faced by new parents.

are shaped by culture (e.g. the tradition among Chinese women 'Tso-Yueh-Tzu' or 'doing-the-month') involving a range of practices in the first month after childbirth to restore women's strength. This is characterised by 'confinement and convalescence' leading to acknowledgment and compensation for childbearing (Chien et al. 2006; Liu et al. 2014). Midwives may encounter other customs such as the circumcision of male infants (Ingram et al. 2003) and must approach these sensitively, ensuring that their advice is evidence-based, with the welfare of the mothers and infants uppermost.

Information and advice also flows from statutory health professionals such as midwives, GPs, health visitors and obstetricians (NICE 2010). There are now many *'expert'* voices from which parents may choose, either through direct contact, or numerous media formats. These include traditional print media, broadcast media (such as radio and television) and electronic media including blogs, podcasts, social media and mobile phone applications (Robinson and Jones 2014). Parents may perceive any of these as authoritative voices, influencing their parenting styles.

Routine/schedule based style

Some parents highly value structure and certainty and are keen to establish schedules and routines for their babies. Well-intentioned medical experts such as 18th century physician, Dr William Cadogan and early 20th century public health specialist, Frederick Truby-King contributed such advice (Palmer 2009). Both men promoted breastfeeding of babies by their mothers; however, greatly fearing the danger of overfeeding, they advocated very restrictive feeding schedules, forbidding overnight feeding (Palmer 2009). One modern day counterpart, ex-maternity nurse Gina Ford, in her 'Contented Baby with Toddler book,' dictates a schedule for babies (and by extraction for their parents) incorporating the timing of nappy changes, the frequency, duration and time-of-day for infant feeding and sleeping (Ford 2009). Prescriptive schedules may provide a sense of security for parents who value predictability in their postnatal lives, but may rely on rather paternalistic and anecdotal premises rather than sound research evidence. For example Cadogan believed that the care and preservation of children should be in the hands of *men* of good sense, since:

> …this business has been too long fatally left to the management of women, who cannot be supposed to have proper knowledge to fit them for such a task…
>
> (Cadogan 1748, p. 2)

Strict, non-evidence-based routines may also negate maternal–infant physiological and psychosocial interactions, blunting parental responses to distressed infants (see Chapter 4: 'Psychology applied to maternity care'). Indeed, Ford (2009) does not warn of potential harm to maternal milk supply and infant immune sensitisation, by introducing formula feeds (see Chapter 10: 'Infant feeding'). Midwives working with parents wishing to adopt routine approaches should only reinforce positive aspects which may be gleaned, such as creating a distinction between day and night through managing the environment (e.g. venue, lighting, and noise) (NHS Choices 2012). However, they should clearly explain where strict adherence to routine conflicts with sound evidence, in order to allow parents to make an informed choice and to ensure the baby's wellbeing.

Attachment parenting

Another approach to parenting is attachment parenting, which includes granting the baby unlimited access to his or her parents, is characterised by closeness of proximity between the baby and his or her mother (in the main) and breastfeeding in response to infant cues. Devices such as slings or baby carriers are used and the baby is held frequently in his or her parents' arms. Aspects of this approach have some support in studies in relation to lactation physiology, infant immunology and maternal and infant bonding (Klaus and Kennell 1982; Colson et al. 2003; 2008; Chiu et al. 2005: see Chapters 4 and 10). However, it may sometimes be difficult for parents to fully accommodate this approach, due to lifestyle constraints. Potential problems occur with such aspects as co-sleeping. Co-sleeping is considered to be an independent risk factor for increase in the incidence of Sudden Infant Death Syndrome (SIDS) for all babies (Blair et al. 2009; Carpenter et al. 2013), but this is disputed and contextualised by others (Ball 2009; UNICEF UK 2013). Some aspects of bonding and attachment theory have been incorporated into contemporary UK maternity care. Women are supported to have their babies placed in skin-to-skin contact with them, soon after birth; babies room-in with their mothers throughout the day and night in maternity units, enabling mothers to respond to their babies' cues (NICE 2006). Additionally, a measure for the prevention of SIDS is for the baby to sleep in his or her parents' bedroom for the first six months of life (NHS Choices 2012) (see Chapter 8: 'Postnatal midwifery care', where the prevention of SIDS is also discussed).

Pragmatic parenting

A different approach to parenting was advocated by psychoanalyst Winnicott who spoke of 'good enough' parenting:

> ... The good enough 'mother' (not necessarily the infant's own mother) is one who makes active adaptation to the infant's needs, an active adaptation that gradually lessens, according to the infant's growing ability to account for failure of adaptation and to tolerate the results of frustration ...

(Winnicott 1953, p. 94)

Good enough parenting is a more pragmatic approach to parenting seen in parents who, prioritise and meet their children's needs, providing consistent care and routine, whilst engaging help from relevant services when problems are identified (Kellett and Apps 2009). This approach contains flexibility and allows parents to incorporate positive and evidence-based, aspects from a range of parenting styles.

Key points

- Parents are diverse.
- Midwives mainly support and care for childbearing women and their infants but also fathers and the wider family.
- Midwives must provide appropriate care and accurate information to and for all women and their babies, to facilitate good enough parenting.

Conclusion

Midwives have a duty to provide accurate information and advice to new parents, applying current research findings and other evidence into practice, ensuring that evidence-based advice and support is presented to childbearing women and their families, regarding the baby and self-care (NMC 2008). It is important that clinicians are not authoritarian, inaccurate or unhelpful, in their advice. They must show kindness, responsiveness and reassurance to help new parents nurture their infants. The midwife's role could be considered to facilitate good enough parenting.

End of chapter activities
Crossword

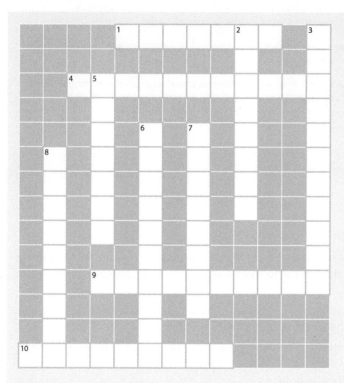

Across

1. When a married or cohabiting couple live together with children from previous relationships the family has become. ...
4. Midwives have a role in teaching this for parenthood
9. Pregnancy which occurs in a female aged between 10 to 19 years, according to the World Health Organization
10. The ability to produce offspring

Down

2. A family structure where a household is composed of one person and some other kin, in addition to a spouse or child
3. The Chinese tradition of 'doing-the-month' is characterised by a period of this
5. Parents who value structure and predictability may be likely to use this style of parenting
6. A mother who performs genetic, gestational and social roles as a parent
7. The age of a woman who conceives at the age of 35 years or above may be considered this
8. A woman who acts as the gestational carrier for a baby on behalf of commissioning parents, in an arrangement made prior to conception

Find out more

Below is a list of things you can find out about to enhance your knowledge of the issues and topics covered in this chapter. Make notes using the chapter content, the references and further reading identified, local policies and guidelines and discussions with colleagues.

- What is parenthood?

- On which people should midwifery care be primarily focussed, given their sphere of practice? http://www.internationalmidwives.org/assets/uploads/documents/Definition%20of%20the%20Midwife%20-%202011.pdf.

- Discuss how midwives can be involved in the care of teenage parents https://www.gov.uk/government/publications/teenage-pregnancy-past-successes-future-challenges

- To which kind of biological mother does the midwife have accountability for providing physical and emotional care? http://www.nmc-uk.org/Documents/NMC-Publications/Midwives%20Rules%20and%20Standards%202012.pdf

Glossary of terms

Amenorrhea   The absence of menstruation.

Conception   The start of pregnancy, at the fusion of the male germ call (sperm), with the female germ cell (ovum) – fertilization – resulting in the formation of a zygote, a single cell containing its own unique genetic code.

Consanguinity   A reproductive relationship between blood relations who share at least one common ancestor no more remote than a great grandparent.

Ethnic group   A group of people with social cohesion, sharing distinctive and common features. These include physical appearance, religious affiliation, language or dialect, culture, customs, values, geographical location and ancestral origins.

Fertility/fecundity   The innate ability to conceive offspring.

Illegitimacy   The status of children born out of wedlock (historically).

Kinship   A network of relatives (kin) connected by common ancestry or marriage.

Parity   Term indicating the number of pregnancies a woman has had, resulting in the birth of an infant capable of survival.

Paternalistic   An attitude of protecting people, over whom one has authority, in a way which restricts their freedom or responsibilities.

Progeny   Offspring.

Reproductive cloning   The creation of a genetically identical whole organism, which could be a plant, animal or human being.

Stepchild   Child of a person's husband or wife from a prior marriage or prior relationship.

(Henley & Schott 1999; Bhopal 2006; Soanes et al. 2005; Fulcher & Scott 2007; Tiran 2008; Martin 2010.)

References

Allen, E., Bonnell, C., Strange. V., Copas, A., Stephenson, A., Johnson, A., Oakley (2007) Does the UK government's teenage pregnancy strategy deal with the correct risk factors? Findings from a secondary analysis of data from a randomised trial of sex education and their implications for policy. *Journal of Epidemiology and Community Health* 61, pp. 20–27.

American Society for Reproductive Medicine (2012) *Age and Fertility* [Online]. Available: https://www.asrm.org/uploadedFiles/ASRM_Content/Resources/Patient_Resources/Fact_Sheets_and_Info_Booklets/agefertility.pdf [12 July 2013].

Aspinall, P.J., Hashem, F. (2010) Is our data on teenage pregnancy across ethnic groups fit for the purpose of policy formulation, implementation, and monitoring? *Critical Public Health* 20 (1), pp. 47–70.

Barter, C., McCarry, M., Berridge, D., Evans, K. (2009) *Partner exploitation and violence in teenage intimate relationships*, [Online], Available: http://www.nspcc.org.uk/inform/research/findings/partner_exploitation_and_violence_wda68092.html [17 July 2013].

Ball, H. (2009) Bed-sharing and co-sleeping. *New Digest* 48, pp. 22–27.

Benagiano, G., Carrara, S, Filippi, V. (2010) Sex and reproduction: an evolving relationship. *Human Reproduction Update* 16 (1), pp. 96–107.

Ber, R. (2000) Ethical Issues in Gestational Surrogacy. *Theoretical Medicine and Bioethics* 21, pp. 153–169.

Bhopal, R. (2006) Race and Ethnicity: Responsible Use from Epidemiological and Public Health Perspectives. *Journal of Law, Medicine, Ethics* (Fall), pp. 500–507.

Birkbeck, University of London (2012) *Issues Emerging from the First 10 Pilot Sites Implementing the Nurse Family Partnership Home Visiting Programme in England*, [Online], Available: http://www.iscfsi.bbk.ac.uk/projects/files/Issues%20arising%20from%20FNP%20-Evaluation-July-2012.pdf [16 July 2013].

Blackburn, S. (2013) *Maternal, Fetal, Neonatal Physiology*. 4th edn. Maryland: Elsevier Saunders.

Blair, P.S., Sidebotham, P., Evason-Coombe, C., Edmonds, M., Heckstall-Smith, E., Fleming, P. (2009) Hazardous co-sleeping environments and risk factors amenable to change: case-control study of SIDS in south west England. *British Medical Journal* 339, p. b3666.

Bottero, W. (2011) Personal life in the past. In: *Sociology of Personal Life*. (ed V. May), 1st edn. pp. 22–34. New York: Palgrave Macmillan.

Bradley, B.P., Mendels, F. (1978) Can the hypothesis of a nuclear family organization be tested statistically? *Population Studies* 32, pp. 381–394.

Brazier, M., Campbell, A., Golombok, S. (1998) *Surrogacy: Review for health ministers of current arrangements for payments and regulation: Report of the review team*. [Online]. Available: http://webarchive.nationalarchives.gov.uk/20130107105354/http://www.dh.gov.uk/prod_consum_dh/groups/dh_digitalassets/@dh/@en/documents/digitalasset/dh_4014373.pdf [10 February 2013].

Byrne, B., Campbell, A., Harrison, E., McKinley, B, Shah, P.S. (2011) *The impact of the global economic downturn on communities and poverty in the UK*, [Online], Available: http://www.abaco-project.eu/documents/experiences-of-economic-downturn-full.pdf. [30 Oct 2013].

Cadogan, W. (1748) *An essay on nursing and the management of children, from birth to three years of age* 1st edn. London: John Knapton.

Callaway, K., Lust, K, Mcintyre, H.D. (2005) Pregnancy outcomes in women of very advanced maternal age. *Australian and New Zealand Journal of Obstetrics and Gynaecology* 45, pp. 12–16.

Carolan, M., Davey, M.-A., Biro, M.A., Kealy, M. (2011) Older maternal age and intervention in labor: a population-based study comparing older and younger first-time mothers in Victoria, Australia. *Birth* 38 (1), pp. 24–29.

Carpenter, R., McGarvey, C., Mitchell, E.A., Tappin, D.M., Vennemann, M.M., Smuk, M., Carpenter, J.R. (2013) Bed sharing when parents do not smoke: is there a risk of SIDS? An individual level analysis of five major case–control studies. *British Medical Journal Open; BMJ Open* 3, p. e002299.

Centre for Maternal and Child Enquiries (CMACE) (2011) Saving Mothers' Lives: reviewing maternal deaths to make motherhood safer: 2006–08. The Eighth Report on Confidential Enquiries into Maternal Deaths in the United Kingdom. *British Journal of Obstetrics and Gynaecology* 118 (S.1), 1–203.

Chambers, D. (2012) *A Sociology of Family Life*. Basingstoke: Palgrave.

Chan, B.C-P, Lao, T.T-H (2008) Effect of parity and advanced maternal age on obstetric outcome. *International Journal of Gynecology & Obstetrics* 102 (3), pp. 237–241.

Cheal, D. (2002) *Sociology of Family Life*. Basingstoke: Palgrave.

Chen, Xi-Kuan., Wen, Shi Wu., Fleming, N., Yang, Q & Walker, M. C. (2007). Teenage pregnancy and congenital anomalies: which system is vulnerable? *Human Reproduction* 22 (6), pp. 1730–1735.

Chien, L-Y., Tai, C-J., Ko, Y-L., Huang, C-H and Sheu, S-J. (2006) Adherence to 'doing-the-month' practices is associated with fewer physical and depressive symptoms among postpartum women in Taiwan. *Research in Nursing, Health* 29, pp. 374–383.

Chiu, S-H., Anderson, G.C., Burkhammer, M.D. (2005) Newborn temperature during skin-to-skin breastfeeding in couples having breastfeeding difficulties. *Birth* 32 (2), pp. 115–121.

Christian Institute (n.d). *Civil Partnerships*, [Online]. Available: http://www.christian.org.uk/briefingpapers/civilpartnerships.htm#_edn7 [5 Aug 2013].

Church of England (2014) *Book of Common Prayer* Church House. [Online], Available: http://www.churchofengland.org/prayer-worship/worship/book-of-common-prayer.aspx. [20 Jan 2014].

Coates, M. (2010) Tides in breastfeeding practice. In: *Breastfeeding and Human Lactation.* (eds J. Riordan & K. Wambach), 4th edn, pp 117–161. Sudbury, MA: Jones and Bartlett.

Colson, S.D., Meek, J., Hawdon, J.M. (2008) Optimal Positions triggering primitive neonatal reflexes stimulating breastfeeding. *Early Human Development* 84 (7), pp. 441–449.

Colson, S., DeRooy, L., Hawdon, J. (2003) Biological nurturing increases duration of breastfeeding for a vulnerable cohort. *MIDIRS Midwifery Digest.* 13 (1), pp. 92–97.

Commissioning Board Chief Nursing Officer, DH Chief Nursing Adviser (2012) *Compassion in Practice*, [Online], Available: http://www.england.nhs.uk/wp-content/uploads/2012/12/compassion-in-practice.pdf [23 July 2013].

Dabrowski, R. (2013) The rise of the middle aged mother. *Midwives Magazine* 2, pp. 38–40.

Delbaere, I., Verstraelen, H., Gotgeluk, S., Martens, G., De Backer, G., Temmerman, M. (2007) Pregnancy outcome in primiparae of advanced maternal age. *European Journal of Obstetrics and Gynecology* 135, pp. 41–46.

Department for Children Families and Schools/Department of Health (2009) *Getting maternity services right for pregnant teenagers and young fathers: Revised edition (2009).* [Online]. Available: http://webarchive.nationalarchives.gov.uk/20130401151715/https://www.education.gov.uk/publications/standard/publicationdetail/page1/DCSF-00673-2009 [13 July 2013].

Department for Education (nd) *Family Nurse Partnership*, [Online], Available: https://www.education.gov.uk/commissioning-toolkit/Programme/Detail/7 [20 June 2013].

Department of Health/Office for National Statistics (2013) *Abortion Statistics, England and Wales: 2012: Summary information from the abortion notification forms returned to the Chief Medical Officers of England and Wales., [Online], Available:* https://www.gov.uk/government/uploads/system/uploads/attachment_data/file/211790/2012_Abortion_Statistics.pdf. [10 Oct 2013].

Department of Health (2009) *Valuing People Now: a new three-year strategy for learning disabilities*, [Online], Available: http://webarchive.nationalarchives.gov.uk/20130107105354/http://www.dh.gov.uk/prod_consum_dh/groups/dh_digitalassets/documents/digitalasset/dh_093375.pdf [22 Jan 2014].

Department of Health (2001) *Valuing People: A New Strategy for Learning Disability for the 21st Century. A White Paper*, [Online]. Available: http://www.archive.official-documents.co.uk/document/cm50/5086/5086.pdf. [24 Jan 2014].

Dewan, N., Brabin, B., Wood, L., Dramond, S. & Cooper, C. (2003) The effects of smoking on birthweight-for-gestational-age curves in teenage and adult primigravidae. *Public Health* 117, pp. 31–35.

Didly, G., Jackson, M., Fowers, G.K., Oshiro, B.T., Varner, M., Clark, S.L. (1996) Very advanced maternal age: Pregnancy after age 45. *American Journal of Obstetrics and Gynecology* 175 (3), pp. 668–674.

Department of Health/Partnerships for Children, Families and Maternity (2007) *Maternity Matters: Choice, access and continuity of care in a safe service.* London: DH.

Draper, J. (2002a) 'It's the first scientific evidence': Men's experience of pregnancy confirmation – some findings from a longitudinal ethnographic study of transition to fatherhood. *Journal of Advanced Nursing* 39 (6), pp. 563–570.

Draper, J. (2002b) 'It was a real good show': the ultrasound scan, fathers and the power of visual knowledge. *Sociology of Health and Illness* 24 (6), pp. 771–795.

Equality Act (2010) ch.10. London: The Stationary Office.

Fatherhood Institute (2008) *The Dad Deficit: The Missing Piece in the Maternity Jigsaw*, [Online], Available: http://www.fatherhoodinstitute.org/wp-content/uploads/2011/02/the-dad-deficit-the-missing-piece-in-the-maternity-jigsaw.pdf [10 Feb 2013].

FIGO Committee for the Ethical Aspects of Human Reproduction and Women's Health (2008) Surrogacy. *International Journal of Gynecology and Obstetrics* 102, pp. 312–313.

Ford, G. (2009) *The Contented Baby with Toddler Book.* London: Random House.

Fulcher, J., Scott, J. (2007) *Sociology*, 3rd edn. Oxford: Oxford University Press.

Giddens, A. (2009). *Sociology*, 6th edn. Cambridge: Polity Press.

Gilbert, W. M., Jandial, D., Field, N. T., Bigelow, P., Danielsen, B. (2004) Birth outcomes in teenage pregnancy. *The Journal of Maternal–Fetal and Neonatal Medicine* 16, pp. 265–270.

Gillespie, R. (2003) Childfree and feminine: understanding the gender identity of voluntarily childless women. *Gender and Society* 17 (1), pp. 122–136.

Ginther, D.K., Pollak, R.A. (2004) Family structure and children's educational outcomes: blended families, stylized facts, and descriptive regressions. *Demography* 41 (4), pp. 671–696.

Griffith, R. (2010) Assisted conception: recognizing the correct parents. *British Journal of Midwifery* 18 (10), pp. 660–661.

Gutteridge, K. (2010). Transition into parenthood: ideology and reality. In: *Essential Midwifery Practice: Postnatal Care*. (eds S. Byrom, G. Edwards, D. Bick), pp. 79–93. Chichester: Wiley-Blackwell.

Heffner, L. (2004) Advanced maternal age – how old is too old? *New England Journal of Medicine* 351, pp. 1927–1929.

Henley, A., Schott, J .(1999) *Culture, religion and patient care in a multi-ethnic society: a handbook for professionals*. London: Age Concern Books.

Higginbottom, G., Owen, J. M., Mathers, N., Marsh, P., Kirkham, M. (2006) Early parenthood among young people of minority ethnic origin in England. *British Journal of Midwifery*, 6 (3), pp. 142–146.

Human Fertilisation and Embryology Act (1990), ch 22. London: The Stationary Office.

Human Fertilisation and Embryology Act (1990), ch 37. London: The Stationary Office.

Human Fertilisation and Embryology Act (2008), ch. 22. London: The Stationary Office.

Human Fertilisation and Embryology Authority (2013). *Mitochondria replacement consultation: Advice to Government*, [Online]. Available: http://www.hfea.gov.uk/docs/Mitochondria_replacement _consultation_-_advice_for_Government.pdf [10 Feb 2014].

Human Reproductive Cloning Act, 2001, ch 23. London: The Stationary Office.

Ingram, J., Johnson, D., Hamid, N. (2003) South Asian grandmothers' influence on breast feeding in Bristol. *Midwifery* 19, pp. 318–327.

International Confederation of Midwives (ICM) (2011) *ICM International Definition of the Midwife*. [Online]. Available: http://www.internationalmidwives.org/assets/uploads/documents/Definition%20of%20 the%20Midwife%20-%202011.pdf. [7 July 2013].

Jayaweera, H., Hockley, C.A., Redshaw, M.E., Quigley, M.A. (2007) *Millennium Cohort Study First Survey Demographic and socio-economic characteristics of ethnic minority mothers in England*. [Online]. Available: http://www.cls.ioe.ac.uk/library-media%5Cdocuments%5CMCSTechnical%20Paper%20 March%2007.pdf [24 January 2014].

Kellett, J., Apps, J. (2009) *Assessments of parenting and parenting support need: A study of four professional groups*. York: Joseph Rowntree Foundation.

Klaus, M., Kennell, J.H. (1982) Labor, birth and bonding. In *Parent-Infant Bonding* (eds M. Klaus, J.H. Kennell), 2nd edn. St. Louis: The C. V. Mosby Company.

Lawrence, R.A, Lawrence, R.M. (2011) *Breastfeeding: A Guide for the Medical Profession*, 7th edn. Missouri: Elsevier Mosby.

Ledger, W, Cheong, Y. (2011) *Reproductive Ageing*. [Online]. Available: http://www.rcog.org.uk/files/rcog -corp/uploaded-files/SIP_No_24.pdf [16 June 2013].

Liu, Y.Q., Maloni, J.A., Petrini, M.A. (2014) Effect of postpartum practices of doing the month on Chinese women's physical and psychological health. *Biological Research for Nursing* 15 (1), pp. 55–63.

MacDonald, L. (2009) Do parents with learning disabilities have adequate parenting skills to safeguard their children? *Journal of Neonatal Nursing* 16 (6), pp. 212–217.

MacVarish, J. (2010) The effect of 'risk-thinking' on the contemporary construction of teenage motherhood. *Health, Risk and Society.* 12 (4), pp. 313–322.

Malacrida, C. (2007) Negotiating the dependency/nurturance tightrope: dilemmas of motherhood and disability. *Canadian Review of Sociology* 44 (4), pp. 469–493.

Marriage (Same Sex) Couple's Act 2013, ch. 30. London: The Stationary Office.

Martin, E.A. (2010) *Concise Oxford Colour Medical Dictionary*. Oxford: Oxford University Press.

Mbuga Gitau, G., Liversedge, H., Goffey, D., Hawthorn, A., Liversedge, N., Taylor, M. (2009) The influences of maternal age on the outcomes of pregnancies complicated by bleeding at less than 12 weeks. *Acta Obstetricia et Gynecologica* 88, pp. 116–118.

McCulloch, A. (2001) Teenage childbearing in Great Britain and the spatial concentration of poverty households. *Journal of Epidemiology and Community Health* 55, pp. 16–23.

Menken, J., Trussell, J., Larson, U. (1986) Age and Infertility. *Science* 223 (4771), pp. 1389–1394.

Murray, I., Hassall, J. (2009) Change and adaptation in pregnancy. In: *Myles Textbook for Midwives* (eds D.M. Fraser, M.A. Cooper), 15th edn, pp. 189–225. Edinburgh: Churchill Livingstone.

NHS Choices (2012) *Getting your baby to sleep* [Online], Available: http://www.nhs.uk/conditions/pregnancy-and-baby/pages/getting-baby-to-sleep.aspx#close [29 January 2013].

National Institute for Health and Clinical Excellence (2010) *CG62 Antenatal care: NICE guideline*, [Online], Available: http://www.nice.org.uk/nicemedia/live/11947/40115/40115.pdf. [10 Jan 2014].

National Institute for Health and Clinical Excellence (2006) *Routine postnatal care of women and their babies*, [Online], Available: http://www.nice.org.uk/nicemedia/pdf/CG37NICEguideline.pdf. [14 June 2013].

Nursing and Midwifery Council (NMC) (2012) *Midwives Rules and Standards 2012*. [Online]. Available: http://www.nmc-uk.org/Documents/NMC-Publications/Midwives%20Rules%20and%20Standards%202012.pdf. [5 June 2013].

Nursing and Midwifery Council (NMC) (2008) *The Code: Standards of conduct, performance and ethics for nurses and midwives*, [Online], Available: http://www.nmc-uk.org/Publications/Standards/The-code/Introduction/ [24 Mar 2013].

O'Donavan, O. (1984) *Begotten or Made?* Oxford: Oxford University Press.

Office for National Statistics (2013a) *Chapter 5 – Marriage and cohabitation (General Lifestyle Survey Overview -a report on the 2011 General Lifestyle Survey)* [Online], Available: http://www.ons.gov.uk/ons/dcp171776_302512.pdf [31 Oct 2013].

Office for National Statistics (2013b) *Trends in civil and religious marriages, 1966–2011*. [Online], Available: http://www.ons.gov.uk/ons/rel/vsob1/marriages-in-england-and-wales-provisional-/2011/sty-marriages.html. [10 Feb 2014].

Office for National Statistics (2013c) *Livebirths in England and Wales by Characteristics of Mother 1: 2011* [Online], Available: http//www.ons.gov.uk/ons/dcp171778_296157.pdf [10 Feb 2014].

Office for National Statistics (2013d) *Conceptions in England and Wales 2011*. [Online]. Available: http://www.ons.gov.uk/ons/dcp171778_301080.pdf [14 Feb 2014].

Ofsted (2009) The Schoolgirl Mum's Unit, [Online]. Available: http://www.ofsted.gov.uk/filedownloading/?id=928297&type=1&refer=0 [13 October 2013].

Palmer, G. (2009) *The Politics of Breastfeeding: When breasts are bad for business*, 3rd edn, London: Pinter and Martin.

Public Health England (2013) Sexually transmitted infections and chlamydia screening in England, 2012. *Health Protection Report* 23 (7), pp. 8–21.

Robinson, F., Jones, C. (2014) Women's engagement with mobile device applications in pregnancy and childbirth. *Practising Midwife* 17 (1), pp. 17–25.

Rosqvist, H., Lövgren, V. (2013) Doing adulthood through parenthood: Notions of parenthood among people with cognitive disabilities. *European Journal of Disability Research* 7 (1), pp. 56–68.

Royal College of Obstetricians and Gynaecologists (RCOG) (2011) *RCOG Statement on later maternal age*. [Online], Available: http://www.rcog.org.uk/what-we-do/campaigning-and-opinions/statement/rcog-statement-later-maternal-age [6th June 2013].

Sandall, J., Homer, C., Sadler, E., et al. (2011) *Staffing in Maternity Units*, [Online]. Available: http://www.kingsfund.org.uk/sites/files/kf/staffing-maternity-units-kings-fund-march2011.pdf [13 June 2013].

Sawyer, M. (2012) *The Teenage Pregnancy Myth*, BBC Radio 4 Broadcast, [Online]. Available: http://www.bbc.co.uk/radio/player/b01dhhpq [12 Feb 2013].

Shaw, R.L., Giles, D.C. (2009) Motherhood on ice? A media framing analysis of older mothers in the UK news. *Psychology and Health* 24 (2), pp. 221–236.

Sloggett, A., Joshi, H. (1998) Deprivation indicators as predictors of life events 1981–1992 based on the UK ONS longitudinal study. *Journal of Epidemiology and Community Health* 52, pp. 228–233.

Smith, M. (2010) Good parenting: Making a difference. *Early Human Development* 86, pp. 689–693.

Soanes, C., Hawker, S., Elliott, J. (2005) *Pocket Oxford English Dictionary*, 10th edn, Oxford: Oxford University Press.

Social Exclusion Unit (1999) *Teenage Pregnancy: Report by the Social Exclusion Unit*. London: The Stationary Office.

Society of Obstetricians and Gynaecologists of Canada Genetics Committee (2012) Delayed Child-Bearing. *Journal of Obstetrics and Gynaecology Canada* 34 (1), pp. 80–93.

Surrogacy Arrangements Act 1985, Ch 49. London: HMSO.

Sutcliffe, A.G., Barnes, J., Belsky, J., Gardiner, J., Melhuish, E. (2012) The health and development of children born to older mothers in the United Kingdom: observational study using longitudinal cohort data.

British Medical Journal, [Online]. Available. doi: http://dx.doi.org/10.1136/bmj.e5116 [24 January 2014].

Teenage Pregnancy Independent Advisory Group (2010) *Past successes – future challenges*. [Online], Available: https://www.gov.uk/government/uploads/system/uploads/attachment_data/file/181078/TPIAG-FINAL-REPORT.pdf [11 Nov 2013].

The Boulevard Centre (n.d) *About Us*, [Online]. Available: http://www.boulevardcentre.co.uk/public/mums004.html.nc [10 October 2013].

Thain, M. (ed.) (2009) *Penguin Dictionary of Human Biology*. London: Penguin.

Tiran, D. (2008) *Baillière's Midwives' Dictionary*, 11th edn. Edinburgh: Baillière Tindall,

The UK Collaborative Group for HIV and STI Surveillance (2006) *A Complex Picture: HIV, other Sexually Transmitted Infections in the United Kingdom*, [Online], Available: http://www.hpa.org.uk/webc/HPAwebFile/HPAweb_C/1194947365435 [19 June 2013].

UNICEF UK (2013) UNICEF UK Baby Friendly Initiative statement on Bed-sharing when parents do not smoke: is there a risk of SIDS? An individual level analysis of five major case-control studies, [Online], Available: http://www.unicef.org.uk/BabyFriendly/News-and-Research/News/UNICEF-UK -Baby-Friendly-Initiative-statement-on-new-bed-sharing-research/ [28 January 2013].

Velde, E., Pearson, P.L. (2002) The variability of female reproductive ageing. *Human Reproduction Update* 8 (2), pp. 141–154.

Walsh-Gallagher, D., McConkey, R., Sinclair, M., Clark, R. (2013) Normalising birth for women with a disability: The challenges facing practitioners. *Midwifery* 29 (4), pp. 294–299.

World Health Organization (WHO) (2004) *Adolescent Pregnancy: Issues in Adolescent Health and Development*. Geneva: WHO.

World Health Organization (2013) *Disabilities*. [Online], Available: http://www.who.int/topics/disabilities/en/ [9 November 2013].

Winnicott, D. (1953) The theory of the parent–infant relationship. *International Journal of Psychoanalysis* 41, pp. 585–595. Available: http://nonoedipal.files.wordpress.com/2009/09/transitional-objects-and -transitional-phenomenae28094a-study-of-the-first-not-me-possession.pdf.

Wyatt, J. (2009) *Matters of Life and Death*, 2nd edn. Nottingham: Intervarsity Press.

119

Chapter 6

Antenatal midwifery care

Julie Flint
University of Hull, Hull, UK

Carol Lambert
City University, London, UK

Learning outcomes

By the end of this chapter the reader will be able to:

* explain service provision for childbearing women experiencing normal pregnancy
* discuss choices open to women in relation to planning and preparing for the birth
* monitor the wellbeing of the woman and fetus throughout pregnancy
* determine when deviations in normal pregnancy may occur requiring support of the interprofessional team
* provide evidence based care in pregnancy.

Introduction

For the majority of women the childbirth journey should be a normal process that can be enjoyed and celebrated. Midwifery care is at the heart, supporting and educating a woman throughout the antenatal period. This ensures the woman is both physically and psychologically ready for giving birth and becoming a mother. Some women may begin with a normal pregnancy then develop complications along the way and some women begin with complicating factors, meaning they require medical care in addition to that fundamental midwifery care. This chapter will explore the provision and content of antenatal care for normal pregnancies, applying knowledge of anatomy and physiology of pregnancy, including maternal screening and examining the potential influence of birth preparation education. It will examine influences on women's decision-making and outcomes of birth, as well as highlighting some of the professional, legal and ethical responsibilities of the midwife and interprofessional team.

Fundamentals of Midwifery: A Textbook for Students, First Edition. Edited by Louise Lewis.
© 2015 John Wiley & Sons, Ltd. Published 2015 by John Wiley & Sons, Ltd.
Companion website: www.wileyfundamentalseries.com/midwifery

National policy on care provision in the United Kingdom

Activity 6.1

A woman has just taken a pregnancy test and it is positive; what thoughts and emotions do you think different women have?

The National Health Service (NHS) is available in the United Kingdom for all childbearing women to improve health and wellbeing of mothers and their infants. Through this statutory mechanism, NHS hospital Trusts are most commonly the providers of maternity services, although some independent and third sector providers are emerging. Clinical Commissioning Groups (CCGs) currently are tasked by Government to commission maternity services to provide maternity care. This procurement part of the commissioning system is undertaken through a tendering process determining who would be the best provider of a particular service. In effect a CCG receives a budget from the Government to advertise a required service for service users and invites businesses, from both the public (government financed) and private sectors, to apply to deliver that service for the NHS. The CCG will then 'buy in', procure those services from whichever they consider to be the most appropriate bidder in the process. The quality of the service provided should remain uppermost to any service provision regardless of provider. Quality of the service provision is monitored by the CCG alongside with other bodies such as Healthwatch England, Care Quality Commission (CQC) and The Kings Fund (Care Quality Commission 2014; Healthwatch 2014; The King's Fund 2014).

Some independent midwives (IMs) have historically provided care for individuals and groups of women, however, since October 2013 they are legally obliged to only practise midwifery with indemnity insurance. The cost of this is prohibitive for individual midwives or small group practices. Nonetheless, midwifery initiatives are emerging in cooperation with insurance underwriters to develop indemnity insurance for IMs work collectively, separate from NHS Trusts. One such scheme 'One to One' (no date) was developed in the Wirral; another is the 'Neighbourhood Midwives' in London (Neighbourhood Midwives 2013). They focus on women-centred care from a caseload holding operation, rather than a hospital set up, and it is organised to be economically efficient. The traditional NHS Trust way of working navigates women around different departments and professionals, referring them for consultations.

**All women need a midwife –
Some women need a doctor**

Although Department of Health policy determines provision of care, the woman's pregnancy and birth experience can be highly influenced by the support, care and education she and her birth partner receives. There is potential for individuals and cultural aspects to influence and alter birth outcomes, to both positive and negative degrees. For example, a woman may feel emancipated and in control at any given point and enjoy her experience, or she may be passive or fearful, possibly giving rise to an increased risk of potential intervention. Providing maternity care through an evidence-based approach ensures guidance and recommendations on clinical care which are developed from research, and have the woman at the centre of that care.

Changing Childbirth (DH 1993) symbolised the beginning of change in English maternity care policy. It recognised that services needed to change and put women at the centre of care. This was to enable for the first time, women to take part in decision-making about their own care. In the UK the government's agenda and current maternity policy, promotes the importance of services that are both flexible and individualised and fit with the needs of women (DH 2004). It values and guarantees their views, and what they value will be acknowledged and respected (National Institute for Health and Care Excellence (NICE) 2008). The Maternity Matters policy document (DH 2007) recommends that women should be given choice within maternity services; with guarantees of being able to make informed choices throughout pregnancy, birth and the postnatal period.

Choice of birth place for women has become a central focus for service providers. A major research project has been undertaken into the place of birth in England; the results support a policy of offering healthy women with low-risk pregnancies a choice of birth setting. Women who plan to give birth in a midwifery unit and multiparous women planning birth at home, experience fewer interventions than those planning birth in an obstetric unit with no impact on perinatal outcomes (Brocklehurst et al. 2011). Nulliparous women with planned home births also have fewer interventions, but do have some poorer perinatal outcomes.

Women are encouraged to access maternity services as early as possible; the Maternity Matters report (DH 2007) suggests that self-referral into a local midwifery service would speed up and enable that early access. Direct access pathways such as these could benefit women on multiple levels; however the anticipated beneficial outcomes of this have not yet been researched.

How women and partners view their care provision is highly influential; direct access to midwives can help to normalise the concept of childbirth. Previously, women went to their General Practitioners (GPs) to begin their childbirth journeys, which implied that a doctor was required in all pregnancies. This may instil a belief that things can go wrong and that medical assistance is required in all cases, thus perpetuating a perception that childbirth is risky and that pregnant women need rescuing by medicine (Wagner 1994). Midwives must protect the midwifery relationship and the underpinning concept of birth being normal, to prevent future erosion of that tentative midwifery lead in maternity care. Returning to a system where women are referred to a named consultant in all instances would be a threat to this fundamental aspect of care.

The Vision and Strategy from the Department of Health (DH), Public Health England, NHS England and the Royal College of Midwives (RCM) is clear in its support of midwifery led services for improved health and wellbeing, with women being screened and risk-assessed at the initial booking interview and throughout childbearing to determine the need for referral to other appropriate health professionals (DH, Public Health England 2013).

Further reading activity

Read this information in more detail:

[Available online] https://www.gov.uk/government/uploads/system/uploads/attachment_data/file/208815/midwifery_strategy_visual_A.pdf

Highlights:

- Midwives will be the first point of contact within accessible maternity services for women.
- Midwives will deliver innovative, evidence based, cost effective, quality care across integrated health and social care settings.
- Midwives will offer support as the lead professional for maternity care to all healthy women with uncomplicated pregnancies.

For women with complex pregnancies, it is suggested that midwives will still be the key coordinators of care within the interprofessional team, while working closely with obstetricians, GPs, health visitors, maternity support workers, breastfeeding support workers and social workers to enable women and families to access the care and support they require.

Activity 6.2

Read this information in more detail:

[Available online] www.gov.uk/government/publications/midwifery-services-for-improved -health-and-wellbeing Highlights

From a woman's perspective identify what you think a woman would want to know when she goes for her first booking appointment with the midwife.

Individualised care of a woman

It is understood that women accessing maternity services in England have choices and are required to make decisions within the antenatal period, about who cares for them and where to give birth. These decisions are influenced by their circumstances, level of ill health and potential risk of adverse outcomes.

Women and their partners are able to choose between Midwifery-Led-Care (MLC) and Consultant-Led-Care (CLC) (DH 2007). MLC is when all care is provided solely by midwives, who are fully accountable for all care provided; women remain within parameters of normality, without any cause to consult with an obstetrician (NMC 2012). CLC is when care is overseen by an obstetrician from the very beginning of a woman's pregnancy, or at any point where a deviation from the normal occurs. Obstetricians are accountable for the advice and decision-making in relation to birth complexities; whilst the wellbeing of the mother and fetus is still monitored by midwives throughout the pregnancy. Midwives continue to practise within their professional accountability for their individual practice, whilst referring back to consultant obstetricians for advice on any developing ill health and decision-making. If a GP continues to provide some of the antenatal surveillance, this would be termed 'shared care', with the care being shared between the primary healthcare providers (GPs) and secondary care hospital provision, often called the acute services (DH 2007). The team approach goes further to include other health professionals and practitioners such as managers, sonographers, phlebotomists, Children's Centre organisations and smoking cessation teams. Individual specialist midwives also exist in some areas, focusing on specific needs such as, for example, healthy lifestyle, infant feeding, substance misuse, mental health and supporting specialist medical disorders. All serve to provide a service that can provide seamless care for all women and their families.

These different models of care currently reflect different philosophies of care in pregnancy. The biomedical model, which has historically decreed the traditional model of pregnancy, is one that holds a medicalised approach to pregnancy, where technology holds supremacy, promotes observation of physical characteristics of pregnancy and measurement of wellbeing (Jomeen 2010). This medical model observes the pregnant body as a mechanical device where wellbeing can only be ensured by a process of monitoring and examination to avoid any fetal or maternal problems (Davis-Floyd 2001). This is in contrast to the holistic model of midwifery where care is women-centred and reflects the concept of being 'with women'; where there is a partnership between a woman and her midwife (Hunter et al. 2008). Care naturally focuses on not only the physical aspects of wellbeing, but her emotional and social wellbeing, recognising the individuality and uniqueness of each woman. How NHS Trusts operationalise the links between the professions still needs to be determined.

The determinants for the model of a woman's care are her parameters of 'normality' and therefore should be the case for the majority of women. A systematic review undertaken by Sandall et al. (2013) compared midwife-led continuity models and determined that women should be offered and encouraged to ask for this model of care. Some women within the midwife-led system require medical review; after review they may then be determined as satisfactory and go back to MLC. Some women are complex and so do not meet the strict MLC criteria; however obstetricians still require midwives to monitor care in the community, being ready to refer to them when a deviation is noted. Improvements could be made in the operational processes of this system to support midwives in monitoring care of complexity. This demonstrates how the midwife's role straddles normality and complexity, supporting the medical role for caring for ill-health with an opportunity to appropriately normalise some aspects and be woman-focused.

A review into the socioeconomic value of the midwife by Devane et al. (2010, p. 16) illustrated that when women were randomised into MLC, they were less likely than women randomised to other models of care, to have:

> …amniotomy, augmentation/artificial oxytocin during labour, regional analgesia (epidural/spinal), opiate analgesia, instrumental vaginal birth and an episiotomy…

Furthermore, women receiving MLC had more antenatal visits; were less likely to have analgesia as well as anaesthesia during labour; were more likely to be attended by a midwife they knew and had higher perceptions of control in labour and birth (Devane et al. 2010). This illustrates how MLC can be cost effective through a philosophy that works to reduce the intervention culture, promotes relationships and ensures continuity of care and carer.

This chapter continues by examining clinical care provision from a woman-centred perspective; highlighting her needs through the woman's journey and demonstrating how she might present. Further discussion and depth of thought about clinical issues can be found in publications elsewhere. Evidence based practice ensures some standardisation to the best way of conducting care and guides professionals in their advice and decision-making. Consulting national and local guidelines as well as up to date research, on an ongoing basis will ensure sound knowledge on which to determine best practice. Keeping abreast of changes made to policies such as screening and care recommendations is vital to maintain a professional status. This section sets the scene and highlights an ethos of care provision acknowledging that guidelines are guidance and might not always be pertinent or agreeable to individual women. Midwifery craftsmanship is celebrated and put forward as a platform of normality from which individual women may differ.

Being pregnant

Women have individual views and experiences of being pregnant; they need to accept many physical and emotional changes that evolve throughout the three trimesters of pregnancy.

Many women become aware of being pregnant very early on in their pregnancy. They can utilise accurate testing systems available commercially over the counter in any pharmacy to diagnosis their pregnancy. They often still seek confirmation and reinforcement of the pregnancy from professionals (Lambert 2013). This may give rise to various individualised feelings about the situation, she may feel happy or sad; the pregnancy may have been planned or unplanned. It may have occurred easily or after a long process of assisted reproduction treatment the most common being: In Vitro Fertilisation (IVF), including intracytoplasmic sperm injection (ICSI), gamete intrafallopian transfer (GIFT), zygote intrafallopian transfer (ZIFT), intrauterine insemination (IUI).

A normal gestation period for pregnancy is calculated from the last menstrual period of the woman and is estimated to last until approximately 40 completed weeks, which is regarded as being full term. However pregnancy length is considered normal if birth occurs anywhere between the weeks of 37–42 completed weeks' gestation.

Booking for care

A woman will meet her midwife at the booking interview where her medical, social and psychological history will be taken and advice will be offered in relation to screening and wellbeing for the woman and the growing fetus. This initial booking appointment is time-consuming within the midwife's day-to-day workload, although an extremely valuable opportunity to begin the woman's relationship with maternity services. Box 6.1 highlights some of the issues often discussed; the list is not exhaustive and needs to be in relation to the individual needs of the woman.

Risk assessment based on physical assessment and screening
Maternal physiological conditions

At the initial booking appointment the midwife assesses the wellbeing of the mother and the fetus (or multiples) which can be determined through a physical assessment, and this will continue at various points in the pregnancy. The midwife will assess the risk of:

- pre-existing medical conditions/relevant surgical procedures or trauma (e.g. cardiac anomalies, uterine surgery or fractured pelvis)
- obesity (over $30 \, \text{kg/m}^2$)
- diabetes (pre-existing or gestational relating to pregnancy)
- pre-eclampsia (new hypertension presenting after 20 weeks with significant proteinuria) (NICE 2010)
- venous thromboembolic disorder.

Box 6.1   Factors to discuss at the midwifery booking appointment

- Lifestyle
- Exercise, travel, sexual intercourse
- Healthy nutrition/supplements – Vitamin D as insufficiency thought to be common in pregnancy (WHO 2012); folic acid
- Employment and safe working
- Food acquired infections: Listeria/Toxoplasmosis
- Toxoplasmosis from animal faeces
- Potential exposure to hazardous substances
- Smoking, alcohol and other substance misuse

Infections
- Rubella, human Immunodeficiency virus (HIV), syphilis, hepatitis B (Hep B), Hep C, urinary tract infections (UTIs) and other sexually transmitted infections (STIs), for example, chlamydia.

Social, psychological and cultural aspects

The midwife will ask whether the woman is experiencing any of the following (see Chapters 4, 11 and 13 where these public health issues are discussed in greater depth).

1. Domestic abuse: routine enquiry should occur at any opportunity the woman is on her own.
2. Mental health problems: Whooley questions have been developed to screen for any potential mental health issues (NICE 2007).
3. Female genital mutilation (FGM): considerations for women of ethnic origin from countries where FGM practise is prevalent (Sub-Saharan Africa some SE Asian countries).
4. Lifestyle issues: such as diet, smoking, alcohol intake and/or other substance misuse (NICE 2010).

Fetal health screening and monitoring

Women need to be informed of the differences between screening tests that determine a statistical possibility of a disorder occurring (for example Down syndrome) and diagnostic tests that provide definitive evidence of a condition (for example Rubella). Further information about screening tests for childbearing women and their babies can be accessed using the online UK National Screening Committee (NSC) (2014). Screening is offered to all women; however it is not mandatory that a woman accepts the screening offered. Women need to understand the implications of undertaking screening tests, in that, the end-point decision could be for her to consider termination of the fetus. She needs to understand these consequences if she already knows that she would ultimately not want to terminate her pregnancy; she may go ahead with screening tests as she may still want to know the risk potential, even if they carry on with the pregnancy.

Fetal anomalies

Fetal anomaly screening aims to determine the potential for various inherited chromosomal disorders. The testing is most commonly known to screen for a 'likelihood' of the presence of Down syndrome. Screening provides a risk ratio of the condition; it does not diagnose the presence of the syndrome (NSC 2014).

The national performance standard for Down syndrome screening is offered in the form of a combined test which includes ultrasound scanning for nuchal translucency and biochemical serum screening for hCG (human chorionic gonadotrophin) and PAPP-A, (pregnancy-associated plasma protein A). The optimal time for undertaking this screening is between 11 weeks to 13 weeks +6 days pregnant. The diagnostic tests for detecting a fetus with Down syndrome are chorionic villus sampling (CVS) where a small amount of placental tissue is removed under ultrasound guidance from 10 weeks of pregnancy, or amniocentesis where a small amount of amniotic fluid is removed under ultrasound guidance. If a woman reports later in pregnancy (between 15–20 weeks) the quadruple test, a blood test, will be performed to assess serum markers, namely hCG, inhibin A, AFP (alpha fetoprotein) and uE3 (oestriol).

Ultrasound scanning

Ideally, an initial scan takes place between 10 weeks 0 days and 13 weeks 6 days to provide accurate dating for the pregnancy; followed by a fetal anomaly scan for structural anomalies, normally between 18 weeks 0 days and 20 weeks 6 days (NICE 2008). Ultrasound scanning has been used for over 30 years and is not thought to do any harm to a fetus; however Marinac-Dabic et al. (2002) suggest that more research is required to evaluate potential risks of ultrasound on the fetus. An ultrasound scan may identify a placenta praevia which could have serious implications for mother and baby. Therefore, closer surveillance and consultant guidance would be sought (see Chapter 16: 'Emergencies in Midwifery' where this is discussed in greater depth).

Inherited factors and disorders
Haematological elements

The midwife will have discussions with the woman who can access leaflets relating to the various screening tests – taking bloods for full blood count (FBC), blood group and Rhesus status, Hep B, HIV and Rubella. Sickle cell anaemia and thalassaemia screening takes place following completion of the Family Origin Questionnaire which determines whether they are at risk. People of certain ethnic origins (e.g. Black African, Black Caribbean, and Black British are screened for sickle cell anaemia or if from high prevalence areas such as the Mediterranean and malaria areas). There is some suggestion of a genetic link in malarial areas providing a protective factor against sickle cell and thalassaemia). For more information visit the UK National Screening Committee website.

- **Blood group** – Information relating to A, B or O grouping is important if the woman becomes ill and requires a blood transfusion, so should be considered at any point of care where the maternal or fetal condition becomes compromised.
- **Rhesus factor** – for detecting potential for isoimmunisation. This would occur if a sensitising incident occurred in pregnancy, for example a placental bleed, where there is the risk of fetal blood from a rhesus positive baby mixing with the maternal blood of a rhesus negative mother. This will stimulate the production of antibodies against rhesus D antigens, from the rhesus D positive blood of the baby, in the mother. If these antibodies then cross the placental barrier to the fetus, haemolysis can occur which begins to destroy the baby's red blood cells, resulting in haemolytic disease of the newborn (HDN). This can result in severe neonatal jaundice and anaemia, which may result in the newborn baby requiring a blood transfusion.
  - Anti-D is recommended as a treatment option for all pregnant women who are rhesus D negative and who are not known to be sensitised to the rhesus D antigen (NICE 2008). In addition, the risk of sensitisation can be reduced by offering anti-D immunoglobulin if there is any risk of feto-maternal haemorrhage (FMH) during the pregnancy, e.g. termination, abdominal trauma, antepartum haemorrhage, miscarriage or invasive procedures (NICE 2008). After birth the baby's cord blood is tested to determine blood group and rhesus status. Postnatal prophylaxis of anti-D immunoglobulin is recommended to the woman if her baby is rhesus positive. This prevents sensitisation of the woman following birth to protect any subsequent pregnancies. As anti-D is a blood product, the woman should be informed to enable her to consider her choice about blood products and potential transmission of blood-borne infections.
- **Full blood count** – primarily focuses on the haemoglobin (Hb) concentration, measured in g/dL, measuring the amount of oxygen-carrying protein. Alongside other features such as

mean corpuscular volume (MCV), red blood cell (RBC) count can give indications of different kinds of anaemias such as iron deficiency (microcytic, low haemoglobin concentration), or vitamin B12 deficiency (macrocytic) (Lab Tests Online UK 2013). The platelet count gives the number of platelets, per given volume of blood. Increases and decreases in platelets can indicate disorders of blood coagulation.

- Developing a disorder – iron deficiency anaemia may be caused by malnutrition or poor general wellbeing (or sometimes secondary to exposure to diseases such as malaria).

Routine care for all pregnant women

The elements described above continue to be part of an ongoing assessment and review, forming the basis for midwifery antenatal care.

Table 6.1 outlines the schedule of appointments for routine antenatal care for women. In addition the ongoing growth and wellbeing of the fetus requires monitoring.

Table 6.1   The schedule of appointments for routine antenatal care for women (adapted from NICE 2008; 2010 Guidelines)

Booking first trimester	Physical and psychological assessment; consider both history and current findings Discuss and offer maternal and fetal screening and begin baseline monitoring to assess wellbeing	Maternal baseline observations – Temperature, pulse, respirations, blood pressure, body mass index, urinalysis and screening for asymptomatic bacteriuria Assess previous history, general health and lifestyle issues. Offer haematologic screening Determine risk factors Advise on nutritional supplements vitamin D and folic acid Routine enquiry – For domestic abuse Whooley questions – To assess perinatal mental health status
Antenatal appointments 25–34 weeks, second trimester	Physical and psychological assessment; consider both history and current findings Discuss and offer maternal and fetal screening and monitor for deviations in the wellbeing of mother and baby	Maternal observations – At each antenatal appointment, blood pressure measurement and urinalysis for protein, to screen for pre-eclampsia At each antenatal appointment, woman to be informed of the need to seek immediate advice from a healthcare professional if she experiences symptoms of pre-eclampsia At each antenatal appointment, raise awareness of fetal wellbeing by discussing fetal movements At each antenatal appointment, from 25 weeks – Symphysis fundal height should be measured and recorded At 28 weeks – Offer repeat full blood count, blood group and antibodies It is recommended that routine antenatal anti-D prophylaxis is offered to pregnant women who are rhesus D-negative.
Antenatal appointments 34–42 weeks third trimester	Physical and psychological assessment; consider both history and current findings Discuss and offer maternal and fetal screening and monitor for deviations in the wellbeing of mother and baby Prepare for birth and motherhood	Maternal observations – Screening and monitoring (indicated above) at each antenatal appointment, including review of the screening undertaken at 28 weeks Plan impending birth – parental education From 36 weeks, check presentation and position of the fetus, engagement in the pelvis of the presenting part Discuss care of the newborn and the postnatal period From 38 weeks – Discuss management of prolonged pregnancy From 41 weeks – Support woman's decisions for induction of labour

Serial measurement of symphysis–fundal height and plotting on customised growth charts is recommended (Royal College of Obstetricians and Obstetricians [RCOG] 2013). There has been a recent drive to train midwives to ensure consistency in this skill.

Body changes

Changes in anatomy and physiology occur, and the nurturing of the fetus begins (Figure 6.1).

Activity 6.3

From your own clinical practice placements; discuss with colleagues and or clinical mentors some of the common changes of pregnancy you have observed in women for whom you have cared for during the first, second and third trimesters of pregnancy.

Seek to understand the causes and reasons for the anatomical and physiological changes by further reading. Read: Section 3, Pregnancy, in: (eds) Marshall, J., Raynor, M. (2014) *Myles Textbook for Midwives*, 16th edn. Edinburgh: Elsevier.

Deviations from normality

Antenatal surveillance aims to detect deviations from normality such as pre-eclampsia, Haemolysis, Elevated Liver enzymes and Low Platelets (HELLP) syndrome, and previously unknown medical conditions (see Chapter 16: 'Emergencies in midwifery' where pregnancy-related conditions are discussed in greater depth). Whilst the previous content reflects care for women who fall within the parameters of normality, demographics are changing in relation to the number of women in that category. Increasing maternal age and increasing levels of obesity are now major contributing factors that impact on the perception of wellbeing and parameters of normality (Bonar 2013). These issues can impact on the medicalisation of pregnancy and the opportunity to adequately monitor the pregnancy along with the woman's ability to give birth.

The midwife must be able to recognise physiological and psychological deviations throughout the pregnancy; refer to an obstetrician and provide seamless care, still aiming to normalise aspects despite variables to level of normality. The woman should feel in control of her situation and able to make informed decisions and choices to empower her sense of wellbeing and respecting her emotional perspective.

Wellbeing

The concept of wellbeing is about a mind–body–health relationship. Stacey (2011) describes how in the 1970s, science identified the link between the brain and immune system. In 1985 the discovery of signalling neuropeptides triggered the discipline of psychoneuroimmunology (PNI). Although acknowledging that the biomedical approach to health still dominates, exploring the PNI influences for childbirth can highlight the potential health impact and possible effect on the birth process. An emotional feeling will trigger the limbic system in the brain (thalamus, hypothalamus, hippocampus and amygdala) and transforms that feeling into the

(a)

- Tiredness

Emotional considerations:
- Potential depression and anxiety or ambivalence - particularly if the pregnancy was not planned.

Change of lifestyle considerations:
- Career
- Social lifestyle – smoking/alcohol/exercise

Breasts:
- Lactogenesis 1 begins - Stimulating Infant feeding decisions

Gastro-intestinal changes:
- Increased appetite
- Nausea and Vomiting
- Constipation
- Heartburn
- Haemorrhoid development

(b)

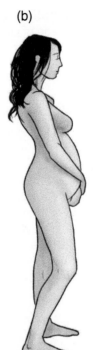

- Growing: Uterus, breasts and adipose tissue around the body
- Often enjoy this phase: "blooming"
- Acknowleging the pregnancy or not, sometimes women deny and do not plan until they are confident about viability of the fetus
- More connection with the baby, nurturing may become evident and protective instincts may emerge
- Becoming real for partner

(c)

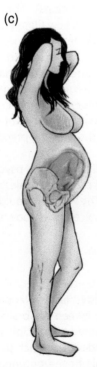

- Carpal tunnel syndrome
- Varicose veins
- Tiredness returns
- Frequency of micturition/vaginal discharge
- Back ache/pelvic girdle discomfort/pain
- Connection with the baby stronger, may talk to and dream of baby and protective instincts may emerge
- Planning for the birth and parenting, attending birth preparation classes
- Partners and others may become nurturing or anxious
- Possible maternity leave if working
- Shopping and preparing for caring for baby

Figure 6.1   (a) First trimester of pregnancy: a hidden but dramatic influence; (b) second trimester of pregnancy: body shape changing; (c) third trimester of pregnancy: now obviously pregnant. Source: Reproduced with permission from J. Green.

chemical cascade that prepares the body for fight or fright, or equally when the response is resulting from a sexual interaction. If arousal (which can be fear) continues and the hypothalamic–pituitary–adrenal (HPA) axis is stimulated for a sustained length of time, cortisol is secreted. Although this has clear implications for acutely affecting the optimal hormonal balance, low level secretion also needs to be considered, particularly as Jomeen and Martin (2005) highlight that women can be at risk of anxiety in pregnancy anyway.

Having looked at the influences of policy and pregnancy screening on maternal choices throughout antenatal care, women's ability to make choices should be considered, particularly about their intentions for coping with the discomforts of pregnancy, labour and birth and how this can be influenced by the culture of birth around them. Women often share their experiences of pregnancy and birth; these stories contribute to influencing the culture, knowledge and confidence in the birthing process of subsequent childbearing women. Therefore, potentially if more women share good experiences they may generate more confidence and potentially less intervention in the women who follow them into the childbirth journey. This, in turn, re-informs women, service providers, the wider community and general culture of birth. Figure 6.2 highlights the influences on a woman's decision making.

As previously stated, initiatives have called for service providers to promote choice and empowered decision-making (DH 2007). It has long been apparent that an effective interface between users and service providers is crucial to ensure women are confident and prepared for their birth experience (Green et al. 2003). Increased use of birth technologies and interventions over recent years has alarmed experts and women (Johanson et al. 2002).

Women's self-identity and decision-making about care

Women are consumers in maternity services and therefore active decision-makers about their care and as such should be valued. Their self-identity influences how they will interact with health professionals and their self-perception throughout childbirth. Pregnant women are exposed to new situations and dilemmas and may feel potentially vulnerable as they navigate choices about care (Edwards 2005). For some women, this vulnerability in making decisions about themselves and their unborn babies may be overwhelming (Santalahti et al. 1998). Van de Vusse (1999) demonstrated that more positive birth experiences occur when women are involved in decision-making and more negative experiences are experienced when they are not. Even though women are encouraged to take part in decision-making, some might be actively involved (Harrison et al. 2003) and some may refrain, assuming a passive role (Moffat et al. 2007). This does not mean they are any less satisfied with the decisions made (Blix-Lindstrom et al. 2004), but as women experience increased feelings of responsibility for their own and their babies' health, they differ in the level of involvement they want to have in the decision-making process. Therefore, some women seem satisfied with passive involvement; women with pregnancy complications seem to have less opportunity for involvement in decision-making and are often content to rely on the expertise of the practitioner. For some women it might be enough that they are consulted about decisions even if they do not want to take an active role in decisions about their care. This does not mean they are excluded from, or not offered opportunities to participate in decisions regarding their bodies. Midwives should remain mindful of different women's situations, so opportunities for women to remain active in decision-making about their care are offered throughout the childbearing journey. The most

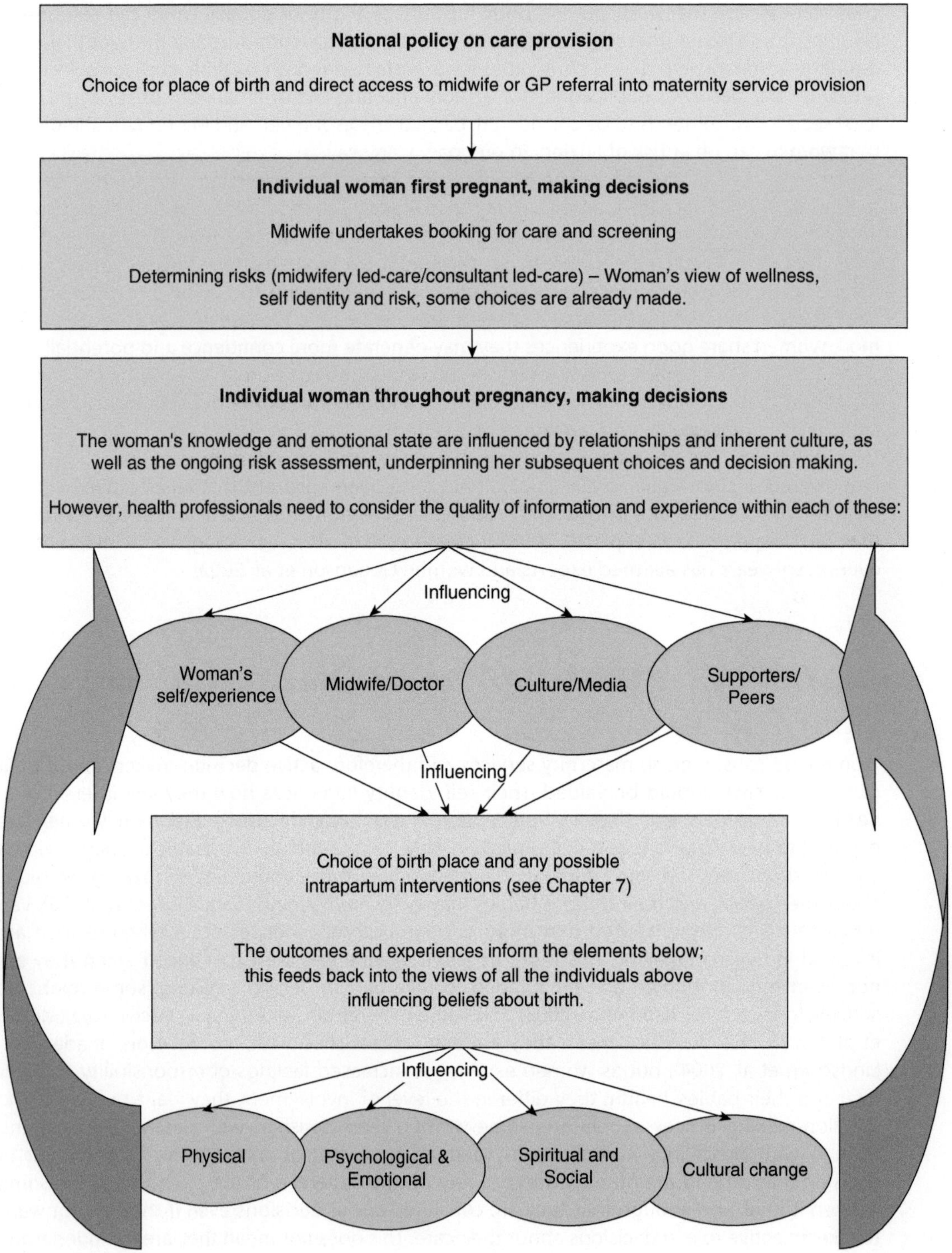

National policy on care provision

Choice for place of birth and direct access to midwife or GP referral into maternity service provision

Individual woman first pregnant, making decisions

Midwife undertakes booking for care and screening

Determining risks (midwifery led-care/consultant led-care) – Woman's view of wellness, self identity and risk, some choices are already made.

Individual woman throughout pregnancy, making decisions

The woman's knowledge and emotional state are influenced by relationships and inherent culture, as well as the ongoing risk assessment, underpinning her subsequent choices and decision making.

However, health professionals need to consider the quality of information and experience within each of these:

Influencing

Woman's self/experience

Midwife/Doctor

Culture/Media

Supporters/Peers

Influencing

Choice of birth place and any possible intrapartum interventions (see Chapter 7)

The outcomes and experiences inform the elements below; this feeds back into the views of all the individuals above influencing beliefs about birth.

Influencing

Physical

Psychological & Emotional

Spiritual and Social

Cultural change

Figure 6.2 Factors influencing maternal choices in pregnancy.

important factor seems to be the ability of the professional to support them in their preferred role in the decision-making process (Harrison et al. 2003).

Midwife–woman relationship for decision-making

Midwives and women have a relationship that is fundamental to midwifery and one that is the foundation to midwifery care (Kirkham 2010). Hunter et al. (2008) describes maternity care as a tapestry; weft threads represent clinical outcomes, policies, protocols and technologies and the interwoven warp threads represent the relationships between midwives and woman that hold it all together. Women trust and use the expertise of health professionals and feel more satisfied if care from them is harmonious with what they want (Harrison et al. 2003). For some time now that trust has been recognised; Tinkler and Quinney (1998) demonstrated that trust is just one factor that affects satisfaction. They consider how the midwife–woman relationship influences experiences and perceptions of care, and re-affirm the midwife–women relationship as an important aspect of satisfaction. Others who have written on this subject found that women implicitly trust the midwives who care for them and even when their own wishes were disregarded, trust is maintained (Bluff and Holloway 1994). Such implicit trust must be handled professionally in open dialogue so that midwives do not simply dictate what will happen.

Influencing women in their decision-making

There is limited literature that illuminates understanding about what truly influences women's decision-making for birth. Barber and Rogers (2006) illustrated how midwives have great influence over women with regard to choice of birth places and they found that women are often left with limited information on which to base their choice options on. The influence midwives have on women is also highlighted by Levy (1999), who was first to research how midwives facilitate the process of informed choice to women in pregnancy and aimed to identify the processes midwives engage in for assisting women to make informed choices. Levy identified ways midwives communicated with women about their choices, steering them towards a safer course of care, which she termed 'protective gate keeping'. Midwives would both provide information to women, but also guard it and release it at the time to suit the midwife. Levy highlighted how midwives 'walked a tightrope' when facilitating informed choice in an attempt to meet the wishes of women. Midwives would steer themselves through a number of dilemmas, anxious to meet the desires of women and appear impartial in their advice, while acknowledging their own sentiments about certain issues (Levy 1999).

So the implication of this influence on women's decision-making is that women might simply comply with the professionals who care for them. Women's decisions are guided by the professionals because women see them as experts. Women accept suggestions because they feel listened to, but this means women comply with midwives, rather than actually choosing how they want to give birth (Kirkham 2010; Van de Vusse 1999; Freeman et al. 2006). These notions of professional gate keeping and influential practitioner beliefs could lead to manipulation of women in the decision-making process, where women comply with professional judgement because they do not want to be seen in a bad light.

Further reading activity

Human rights in childbirth (http://www.birthrights.org.uk/) is a UK organisation dedicated to improving women's experiences of pregnancy and childbirth.

Birth preparation and parent education

More than cultural awareness, women seek specific information about pregnancy and birth. It is suggested in the United States of America, that a third of women seek information from popular childbirth education books. Information however is variable, with inaccuracies in the presentation of scientific evidence and recommendations (Powell et al. 2009). Women may attend classes in the antenatal period wanting the opportunity to understand the process of childbirth and develop confidence in becoming a parent. Part of that process can be learning how to communicate with caregivers to make the choices and decisions discussed earlier, rather than them merely conforming to practitioner preferences and prescriptive policy guidance. Such learning could enhance that empowerment and personal control within the childbearing domain for women, their families and the wider community.

Birth preparation and the traditionally known 'Parent Education' classes have been part of UK maternity service provision for some time. During the 1960s and 1970s, a focus on active birth developed and aimed to give women information about labour that included birthing positions and breathing techniques (Walsh 2012). Such classes are provided through NHS midwifery services, and private and charitable organisations across the country, the National Childbirth Trust (NCT) being the largest non-NHS organisation that is paid for by individuals. Research has predominantly focused on birth outcomes, such as mode of birth or use of analgesia, as a measure of the effectiveness of antenatal classes, finding their merits to be consistently inconclusive (Gagnon and Sandall 2011). There is some evidence that women's experience of birth and parenting may be improved if they attend participant-led classes compared with more traditional classes (NICE 2008). Nolan (2009) also highlights that studies have universally failed to take into account the quality of the education provided. Recent research on the provision of birth preparation classes identifies consensus across stakeholders, that current provision is seriously inadequate and that midwives are inadequately prepared and supported in this role; also identifying that an expanded focus is needed on relationships and the transition to parenthood (Barlow et al. 2009).

The 'Birth and Beyond' package developed by McMillan et al. (2009) provides practitioners with a framework and content for delivering a quality programme of learning to women and families. However, this work did not explain how facilitators were meant to deliver it. Midwives are expected to deliver classes within their clinical role (NMC 2012) and traditionally within their working hours, despite their increased pressures and reduction in staffing levels more recently. Provision of birth preparation/parent education classes can therefore be a challenge for NHS Trusts. Midwives or health visitors receive little or no training on how best to facilitate them and there is no obvious quality assurance on the content and delivery of the sessions. Robust facilitation by experts trained in adult education, more than just curriculum planning, along with satisfaction evaluation would demonstrate quality and urgently needs to be developed nationally.

Barlow et al. (2009) conducted research into the provision of birth preparation classes; at the time of the review an outgoing NHS Primary Care Trust (PCT) in a Northern city in England was becoming an example of an organisation looking to do things differently. The PCT contracted out these services to be delivered outside the conventional midwifery contracted time (Reports to the PCT 2010–13) by a small social enterprise organisation rooted in midwifery to pioneer and develop the service. Social enterprise business models are able to sit within the NHS framework working alongside other providers (DH 2008; DH 2010). Ethically and morally, not for profit organisations complement the NHS promoting organisational autonomy and staff engagement (Addicott 2011). This commissioned service in the North of England, was highly successful in improving parent attendance and quality of class provision. However, the venture was not re-commissioned despite excellent satisfaction scores from attendees. The state of antenatal education provision is therefore, somewhat precarious and subject to market forces.

Activity 6.4

- Write a birth plan for a woman who is pregnant for the first time, has experienced a normal pregnancy and is intending to give birth in a hospital labour ward staffed by midwives and obstetricians.
- Write a birth plan for a woman for the second time after an instrumentally assisted first birth, who intends to have a baby at home with a community midwife attending.

Think about the differences each woman will have. What might influence each of these women and who might have the greatest risk of a medically assisted outcome?

Key points

- Women should be offered a choice for their birth place.
- Screening and surveillance of the mother and fetus monitors for abnormalities.
- Good midwife–woman relationships and education assists a woman in her decision making.
- Care must always be woman-centred and individualised.

Conclusion

This chapter highlights how pregnancy can be a normal process for women to enjoy and celebrate. National policy guides the journey for women in relation to choices about where to give birth and utilising information for the wellbeing of herself and her baby. Midwifery care is at the heart of service provision, supporting and educating women throughout the antenatal period. This ensures the woman is both physically and psychologically prepared for giving birth and becoming a mother. However, variables and complexities of pregnancy do exist and a good midwife–mother relationship, based on individualised woman-centred care, will ensure best outcomes and satisfaction.

End of chapter activities
Crossword

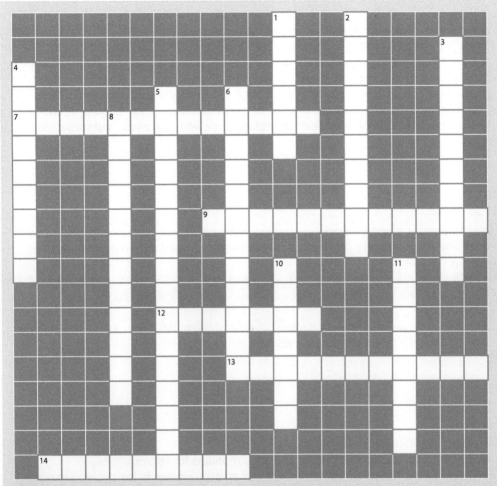

Across

7. Infection from animal faeces
9. Care without Doctor involvement
12. To observe for
13. Having not yet given birth to any viable infants
14. One of the three periods of pregnancy

Down

1. Leading to the opening of the uterus
2. Reflects the evidence base and recommends practice
3. The presenting part descending into the pelvis
4. Before labour
5. Recommends women should be offered choice of place of birth
6. Caused by hormonal influence on the bowels
8. Extracts blood
10. Screening questions for mental health issues
11. A deviation from the normal

Find out more

Below is a list of things you can find out about to enhance your knowledge of the issues and topics covered in this chapter. Make notes using the chapter content, the references and further reading identified, local policies and guidelines and discussions with colleagues.

1. Read the Antenatal Care Guidelines: Routine care for the healthy pregnant woman (NICE 2008; 2010).

2. Read the Hospital Trust Guideline/Policy which identifies reasons for pregnant women needing additional care and referral to consultant-led care.

3. Read the Hospital Trust Guideline/Policy which identifies reasons for referral to the paediatrician.

4. Make a list of some of the commonly used abbreviations in antenatal care and find out the meanings.

Glossary of terms

AFP (alpha fetoprotein)   Protein that is produced by the yolk sac and liver during fetal development.

Body Mass Index   The weight of a person (in kilograms) divided by the square of their height (in metres), the units are therefore kg/m^2.

Carpal tunnel syndrome   A combination of parasthesia (pins and needles), numbness, and pain in the fingers and hands. Often worse at night. Caused by pressure on the median nerve as it passes through the wrist.

Cervix   Relating to the 'neck' of the uterus. The area below and inclusive of the cervical OS.

Chorionic villus sampling (CVS)   An invasive procedure in which a sample of placental tissue is aspirated through the cervix or abdomen under ultrasound visualization.

Chromosomal disorders   Problems within the structure of the cell nucleus that carries the genetic information.

Down syndrome   A condition resulting from a chromosomal abnormality most commonly due to the presence of three copies of chromosome 21; most likely to occur with advanced maternal age.

Fracture   Breakage of a bone.

Fundus   The part furthest from the opening of an organ.

Gamete intrafallopian transfer (GIFT)   A procedure for assisting conception, suitable only for women with healthy Fallopian tubes.

Gestation   The period during which a fertilized egg cell develops into a baby that is ready to be delivered; averages 266 days in humans.

Haemolysis   The destruction of red blood cells.

Haemorrhoid   Enlargement of the normal spongy blood-filled cushions in the wall of the anus.

hCG (human chorionic gonadotrophin)   A hormone produced by the placenta during pregnancy. Maintains the secretion of progesterone by the corpus luteum of the ovary.

Hepatitis B or C   Inflammation of the liver caused by viruses, toxic substances or immunological abnormalities.

HIV   Human immunodeficiency virus.

Immunisation   The production of immunity by artificial means through administration of a vaccine.

Intracytoplasmic sperm injection (ICSI)   A technique of assisted conception. Spermatazoa are extracted and injected into the cytoplasm of the egg and implanted into the uterus.

Intrauterine insemination (IUI)   Carefully washed spermatozoa are injected into the uterus through the vagina at the time of ovulation.

Iso-immunisation   The development of antibodies within an individual against antigens form another individual of the same species.

Listeria   Bacteria that are parasites of warm-blooded animals. Affecting many domestic and wild animals. Can be transmitted to humans by eating infected animals or their products.

Macrocytic   Larger than normal cells.

Microcytic   Smaller than normal cells.

Micturition   Act of passing urine.

Nuchal translucency scanning   Ultrasound screening test to measure the maximum thickness of the translucency between the skin and the soft tissue overlying the cervical (neck) region of the spine of the fetus.

Nulliparous (woman)   Having not yet given birth to any viable infants.

Oedema   Excessive accumulation of fluid in the body tissues. It can be local because of injury or inflammation, or more general, as in heart or kidney failure which can include pre-eclampsia in pregnancy.

Os   Cervical opening (internal: to the uterus/ external: to the vagina).

PAPP-A   Pregnancy-associated plasma protein A: a marker for Down syndrome.

Placental   Relating to the placenta. An organ within the uterus by which the embryo is attached to the wall of the uterus. It links between the fetal and maternal blood systems to transfer nutrients and waste products.

Prophylaxis   Any means taken to prevent disease.

Rhesus (Rh) factor   Antigens that may or may not be present on the surface of red blood cells; people who lack the factor are Rh negative. Incompatibility between Rh negative and positive is the cause of haemolytic disease of the newborn.

Rubella   German Measles – a mild highly contagious viral infection, mainly of childhood. It can cause malformations in the fetus in early pregnancy.

Sickle cell anaemia   A hereditary blood disease. Production of an abnormal type of haemoglobin (red blood cells) leading to episodes of anaemia and jaundice and has no cure only able to treat symptoms.

Symphysis pubis   Joint between the pubic bones of the pelvis.

Syphilis   Sexually transmitted disease caused by bacteria entering the body through mucous membranes during sexual intercourse, resulting in the formation of lesions throughout the body.

Thalassaemia   A hereditary blood disease. Red blood cells cannot function normally leading to anaemia and enlargement of the spleen and abnormalities of the bone marrow.

Toxoplasmosis   A disease in mammals and birds caused by a protozoan. Transmitted to humans through ingesting undercooked meat or contaminated by faeces of infected cats.

Urinary tract   The entire system of ducts and channels that conduct urine from the kidneys to the exterior. It can be susceptible to infections in pregnancy.

Varicose veins   Veins that are distended, lengthened and tortuous. Superficial veins in the legs are most commonly affected.

Venous thrombo-embolic (VTE)   The formation of a blood clot in a vein, which may become detached and lodged else-where. In pregnancy the risk of VTE is more common and can result in death.

139

Zygote intrafallopian transfer (ZIFT)   Following in-vitro fertilisation the zygote is introduced into the fallopian tube. Commonly used when tubes block the normal binding of the sperm and egg.

(Adapted from Martin 2010.)

References

Addicott, R. (2011) *Social Enterprise in healthcare.* Kingsfund Available at: http://www.kingsfund.org.uk/sites/files/kf/field/field_publication_file/social-enterprise-in-health-care-kings-fund-report-august-2011.pdf

Barlow, J., Coe, C., Redshaw, M., Underwood, A. (2009) *Birth and Beyond: Stakeholder perceptions of current antenatal education provision in England.* Department of Health: London [Available online] www.chimat.org.uk/resource/item.aspx?RID=82144

Barber, T., Rogers, J. and Marsh, S. (2006) The Birth Place Choices Project: Phase one. *British Journal of Midwifery* 14 (10), pp. 609–613.

Birth & Beyond (2010–13) Reports to the PCT: Available direct from the chapter author.

Bonar S. (2013) *State of Maternity Services report 2013.* London: The Royal College of Midwives.

Blix-Lindström, S., Christensson, K., Johansson, E. (2004). Women's satisfaction with decision-making related to augmentation of labour. *Midwifery* 20, pp. 104–112.

Bluff, R. and Holloway, I. (1994) 'They know best': women's perceptions of midwifery care during labour and childbirth. *Midwifery* 10, pp. 157–164.

Brocklehurst, P., Hollowell, P., Hardy, J., et al. (2011) Perinatal and maternal outcomes by planned place of birth for healthy women with low risk pregnancies: the Birthplace in England national study. *British Medical Journal* 343, p. d7400 doi: 10. 1136/bmj.d7400

Care Quality Commission (2014) *About us.* [Online], Available: http://www.cqc.org.uk/about-us [13 Mar 2014].

Davis-Floyd, R. (2001) The technocratic, humanistic and holistic paradigms of childbirth. *International Journal of Gynaecology and Obstetrics* 75, pp. S5–S23.

Department of Health (2010) *Equity and excellence: Liberating the NHS.* Gateway reference 14385. London: Crown.

Department of Health (2008) *High Quality Care for All: NHS Next Stage Review Final Report (Darzi).* London: Department of Health.

Department of Health (2007) *Maternity Matters: Choice, access and continuity of care in a safe service.* London: HMSO.

Department of Health (2004) *National Health Service Framework for children, young people and maternity services: Maternity Services.* London: HMSO.

Department of Health (1993) *Changing Childbirth Part 1: Report of the Expert Maternity Group.* London: HMSO.

Department of Health, Public Health England (2013) *Midwifery Services for improves health and well-being* [Available online] www.gov.uk/government/publications/midwifery-services-for-improved-health-and-wellbeing

Devane, D., Brennan, M., Begley, C., et al. (2010) A systematic review, meta-analysis, meta-synthesis, and economic analysis of midwife-led models of care. Royal College of Midwives: London.

Edwards, N. (2005) *Birthing Autonomy Women's Experiences of Planning Home Births*, 1st edn. Oxon: Routledge.

Freeman, L.M., Adair, V., Timperley, H., West, S.H. (2006) The influence of birthplace and models of care on midwifery practice for the management of women in labour. *Women and Birth* 19, pp. 97–105.

Gagnon, A.J., Sandall, J. (2011) Individual or group antenatal education for childbirth or parenthood, or both (Review). *The Cochrane Collaboration* Issue 10 Available at http://www.thecochranelibrary.com Wiley Ltd.

Green, J., Baston, H., Easton, S., McCormick, F. (2003) *Greater Expectations?* Summary report. Mother infant Research Unit (MIRU), University of Leeds.

Harrison, M.J., Kushner, K.E., Benzies, K., Rempel, G.K. (2003) Women's satisfaction with their involvement in health care decisions during a high-risk pregnancy. *Birth* 30 (2 June), pp. 109–115.

Healthwatch (2014) *About us*. [Online], Available: http://www.healthwatch.co.uk/about-us [16 Mar 2014].

Hunter, B., Berg, M., Lundgren, I., Olafsdottir, O.A., Kirkham, M. (2008) Relationships: The hidden threads in a tapestry of maternity care. *Midwifery* 24 (2), pp. 132–137.

Johanson, R., Newburn, M., MacFarlane, A. (2002) Has the medicalisation of childbirth gone too far? *British Medical Journal* 324, pp. 892–895.

Jomeen, J., Martin, C.R. (2005) Self-esteem and mental health during early pregnancy. *Clinical Effectiveness in Nursing* Mar–June 9 (1–2), pp. 92–95.

Jomeen, J. (2010) *Choice, control and contemporary childbirth understanding through women's stories*, 1st edn. United Kingdom: Radcliffe Publishing.

Kirkham, M. (ed.) (2010) *The Midwife-Mother Relationship*, 2nd edn. England: Palgrave Macmillan.

Lab tests online UK (2013) *Full Blood Count*. [Online]. Available: http://www.labtestsonline.org.uk/understanding/analytes/fbc/tab/test

Lambert, C. (2013) *The influence of self in women's decision-making about birthplace: An Interpretive Phenomenological Study*. Doctoral Thesis University of Hull. Hull.

Levy, V. (1999) Protective Steering: A grounded theory study of the processes by which midwives facilitate informed choices during pregnancy. *Journal of Advanced Nursing* 29 (1), pp. 104–112.

Marinac-Dabic, D., Krulewitch, C.J., Moore, R.M. Jr. (2002) The safety of prenatal ultrasound exposure in human studies. *Epidemiology* 13 (3), pp. 19–S22.

Marshall, J., Raynor, M. (2014) *Myles Textbook for Midwives*, 16th edn. Edinburgh: Elsevier.

Martin, E.A. (2010) *Concise Oxford Colour Medical Dictionary*. Oxford: Oxford University Press.

McMillan, A., Barlow, J., Redshaw, M. (2009) Preparation for birth and beyond. A resource pack for leaders of community groups and activities. Available at: http://www.yor-ok.org.uk/Downloads/Parenting/Preparation%20for%20Birth%20and%20Beyond.pdf

Moffat, M.A., Bell, J.S., Porter, M.A., Lawton, S., Hundley, V., Danielian, S., Bhattacharya, S. (2007) Decision making about mode of delivery among pregnant women who have previously had a caesarean section: a qualitative study. *MIDIRS Midwifery Digest* 17 (2), pp. 210–221.

National Institute for Clinical Excellence (2007) *Antenatal and Postnatal Mental Health; Clinical Management and Service Guidance*. London: Department of Health.

National Institute for Health and Clinical Excellence (2008) *Routine antenatal anti-D prophylaxis for women who are rhesus D negative Review of NICE technology appraisal guidance 41*. London: NICE.

National Institute for Health and Clinical Excellence (2008) *Antenatal Care: Routine care for healthy pregnant women*. Full Guideline. London: NICE.

National Institute for Health and Clinical Excellence (2010) *Antenatal Care: Routine care for the healthy pregnant woman NICE clinical guideline 62*. London: NICE.

National Institute for Health and Clinical Excellence (2010) *Quick reference guide Hypertension in pregnancy guideline 107*. London: NICE.

Neighbourhood Midwives (2013) *Our service*. [Online], Available: http://www.neighbourhoodmidwives.org.uk/midwifery-service.php [15 Mar 2014].

Nolan, M.L. (2009) Information Giving and Education in Pregnancy: A Review of Qualitative Studies. *Journal of Perinatal Education* 18 (4), pp. 21–30.

Nursing & Midwifery Council (2012) *Midwives rules and standards*. London Publications: NMC.

One to One (no date) *Our service*. [Online], Available: http://www.onetoonemidwives.org/our-service [15 June 2014].

Powell Kennedy, H., Nardini, K., Mc-Leod-Waldo, R., Ennis, L. (2009) Top-selling childbirth advice books: a discourse analysis. *Birth* 36 (4), pp. 318–324.

Royal College of Obstetrics and Gynaecologists (RCOG) (2013) *Green Top Guideline 31: The investigation and management of small for gestational age fetus*. London: Royal College of Obstetrics and Gynaecologists.

Sandall, J., Soltani, H., Gates Shennan, A., Devan, D. (2013) Midwife-led continuity models versus other models of care for childbearing women [Available on line] http://onlinelibrary.wiley.com/cochranelibrary/

Santalahti, P., Hemminki, E., Latikka, A., Ryynänen, M. (1998) Women's decision-making in prenatal screening. *Social Science & Medicine* 46 (8), pp. 1067–1076.

Stacey, C. (2011) Psychoneuroimmunology and wellbeing. In: Knight, A., McNaught, A. *Understanding Wellbeing: An Introduction for Students and Practitioners of Health and Social Care*. Banbury: Lantern.

The King's Fund (2014) *About us*. [Online], Available: http://www.kingsfund.org.uk/about-us [15 Mar 2014].

Tinkler, A., Quinney, D. (1998) Team Midwifery: the influence of the midwife-women relationship on women's experiences and perceptions of maternity care. *Journal of Advanced Nursing* 28 (1), pp. 30–35.

UK National Screening Committee (2014) *Screening Tests for You and Your Baby*. [Online], Available: http://www.screening.nhs.uk/getdata.php?id=17806

UK National Screening Committee (2014) [online] Available: http://www.screening.nhs.uk/uknsc.

Van de Vusse, L. (1999) Decision making in analyses of women's birth stories. *Birth* 26 (1), pp. 43–50.

Wagner, M. (1994) *Pursuing the Birth Machine; The Search for Appropriate Birth Technology*. Australia: Ace Graphics.

Walsh, D. (2012) *Evidence-based Care for normal Labour and Birth; A Guide for Midwives*, 2nd edn. London: Routledge.

World Health Organization (WHO) (2012) *Guideline: Vitamin D supplementation in pregnant women*. Switzerland: World Health Organization. [Available online] http://www.who.int

Chapter 7

Intrapartum midwifery care

Julie Flint

University of Hull, Hull, UK

Sue Townend

Calderdale and Huddersfield NHS Foundation Trust, West Yorkshire, UK

Learning outcomes

By the end of this chapter the reader will be able to:

- explain parameters of normality in labour
- discuss some of the challenges that midwives and women face in reducing the medicalisation of labour and birth
- monitor the wellbeing of mothers and their unborn children in normal labour
- determine when deviations from the norm may occur in the intrapartum period
- provide evidence based care in the intrapartum setting.

Introduction

The emphasis of the midwife's role in the provision of maternity care continues to lie within the boundaries of normal childbirth. The increasing rates of intervention in childbirth cause a great deal of debate, and the current medical model for childbirth is much criticised. It is paramount that student midwives base their knowledge and skills within the context of women centred care when pregnancy and birth are physiologically normal. Equally, as all women deserve the best care, all aspects of compassionate and competent care need to be applied to complex situations to give all women and their babies the best start to family life.

This chapter will focus on normal labour and birth and the role and responsibilities of the midwife, highlighting how an understanding of anatomy and physiology informs care provision and ensures a woman-centred approach. Place of birth and the influence of birth preparation education as a way to empower women are also included.

Fundamentals of Midwifery: A Textbook for Students, First Edition. Edited by Louise Lewis.
© 2015 John Wiley & Sons, Ltd. Published 2015 by John Wiley & Sons, Ltd.
Companion website: www.wileyfundamentalseries.com/midwifery

Facilitating and maintaining normality in childbirth

The birth of a baby is a time when a woman has an opportunity to develop as an individual and reach her full potential; the support and care she receives can influence her outlook and progress throughout that journey and for the rest of her life. It is evident that if she feels some sense of personal control of the situation, she may have a more positive experience and higher levels of satisfaction (Goodman et al. 2004). This can be achieved by having the ability to make choices about the place of birth that best suits her wherever possible; having some understanding of what is happening to her through the process of labour and planning some coping strategies both prior to and during labour, making decisions along with the professionals giving care at the time (see Chapter 6: 'Antenatal midwifery care' where decision making is explored in greater depth).

Those persons present at the time of labour and birth can influence the outcome both positively and negatively, through their actions and words, with the potential to increase or decrease intervention. Often, this person is someone unknown to the woman. It is therefore essential for midwives to develop and feel confident in practising midwifery that is reflexive and adaptable within that midwife–woman relationship as explained by Kirkham (2010), in a gentle supportive manner. The midwifery role is one of expert practitioner. Practising as a skilled birth attendant (World Health Organization (WHO) 2004) requires an absolute grounding in the fundamental skills of midwifery which encompass the softer, caring and nurturing nature, sound knowledge base and clinical skills. This is what makes a midwife different and unique. A woman needs assurance that the person – the midwife she is putting her trust in – has the knowledge, skills and expertise including intuition, to care for her appropriately.

It is during the intrapartum period that woman-centred care reaches the peak of importance for influencing the birthing experience. Women seek to have a carer who is 'on their side' one who discusses the benefits, risks and potential alternatives to any suggested interventions; allowing the women to make her own informed choice. This can help to support women to have personal control, rather than the carer assuming responsibility for knowing best and choosing options from a menu of actions to assist the woman (Kirkham 2004).

The more straightforward and uncomplicated the birth, the greater the likelihood for the mother of achieving skin-to-skin contact with her baby, enjoying that first meeting and encouraging the baby's pre-feeding behaviours (Porter and Winberg 1999). The woman is less likely to have untoward outcomes such as genital tract trauma, suffer exhaustion or have undergone surgery. If the woman feels she has had a satisfactory experience she may feel increased self-worth, self-esteem and self-confidence in the transition into parenthood, with perhaps less potential for postnatal depression (Thompson et al. 2002).

Armed with knowledge and compassion, the skill for the midwife is to provide safe, effective care for all women regardless of the level of complexity in the pregnancy or throughout the intrapartum period. Some women face challenges when they have hopes and choices that lie outside clinical guidance, or are hoping to prevent interventions they may feel are unnecessary when known medical conditions and situations become evident.

Figure 7.1 Demonstrates how different pathways of care and intervention can lead to different outcomes in birth experience. The flow chart represents how the lead carer for the woman may fluctuate between the midwife and the obstetrician. Confusion may occur when the woman remains within the parameters of normality, monitored by midwives, but with varying degrees of intervention to achieve a vaginal birth, for example; pharmacological methods of pain relief, amniotomy, intravenous infusion and cardiotocograph (CTG) monitoring. The woman may

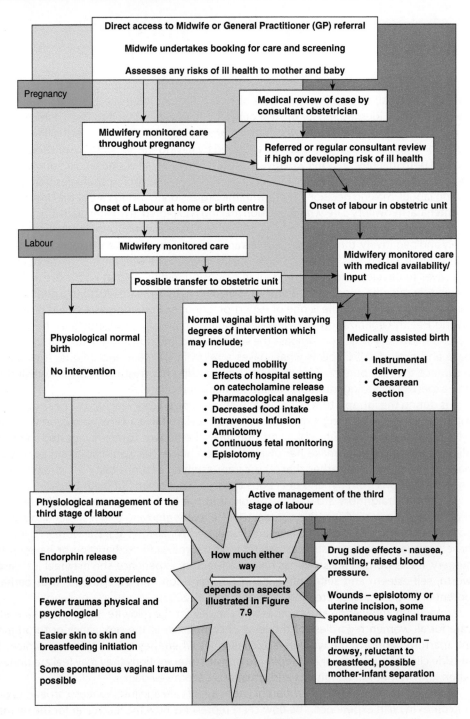

Figure 7.1 Pathways of care during the intrapartum period.

require the knowledge and skills provided by a medical practitioner and a transfer to consultant-led care, but the majority of care will still be monitored and provided by the midwife. It is the clinical decision making skills of the midwife to support appropriate referral to medical staff when there is recognition of normal processes being compromised (NMC 2009) that is crucial to the safety of woman and baby.

Place of birth

The evidence from the Birthplace in England study (Birthplace in England Collaborative Group 2011), highlights the effect of ownership of the environment and the authority stance that can result. A community midwife is the guest in the woman's home, whilst medical ownership exists in the hospital. A birth centre setting seems to be a woman-centred balanced ownership with a nurturing orientation (Walsh 2004). The environment debate to date has been focused on how the surroundings should be homely, improving the surroundings with wallpaper and pictures aimed at reducing anxiety, allowing the physiology of labour to unfold. However Lothian (2006) argues that women say they would just like it to be less medicalised and that they feel safe knowing things are at hand 'just in case'. Hospital birth centres have been associated with lower rates of intervention and higher rates of satisfaction (Hodnett et al. 2012). For those women choosing home birth, is it about feeling 'in control' in her own environment, or 'safe' cocooned by the familiar in the heart of her family?

Activity 7.1

Think about a woman who decided on a home birth; why did she want this? How confident was she about birthing? Did the staff support her decision? Were there any issues? What skills must the midwife employ to ensure that this is the best environment for the woman? What special skills will be needed if the woman's decision to have a home birth goes against medical advice?

Birth preparation for coping with labour

Some women may choose to prepare for giving birth by attending formal or informal group sessions. As discussed in Chapter 6, maternity services and other organisations provide antenatal classes in some form in most areas. Equally some women look to complementary and alternative therapies such as hypnotherapy and acupuncture, not provided for in mainstream health services (see Chapter 14: 'Complementary and alternative medicines' where these are explored in greater depth). The aim is to prepare women and partners for the birth experience and the early weeks of parenting; to discuss what to expect and develop coping strategies. This may follow the traditional maternity service provision or classes that women pay for individually. Some women choose not to undertake any preparation or antenatal education and recognise they have prepared themselves by their virtual presence at the labours of others by watching reality television programmes. Some women enter the intrapartum experience without preparation and appear to do very well, while others appear to have prepared well and have a desire to do birth without intervention, yet start to fear the pain of contractions and doubt their ability in being able to birth normally once in labour.

Table 7.1 The bio-physical mechanism by which the fetus undertakes the journey through the birth canal

1. Longitudinal lie of the fetus, an anterior fetal denominator (occiput for cephalic presentation) and an attitude of flexion.
2. The onset of strong regular contractions to enable the fetus to descend through the pelvis.
3. Following further descent through transition: the head rotates on the pelvic floor; the face sweeps the perineum and the head is born; internal rotation of the shoulders occurs and is demonstrated as restitution.
4. At the next contraction the shoulders are born and the body follows by lateral flexion.

Clinical consideration

Look out for women who seem to just believe they can do it and those who seem very scared. What are the interventions and outcomes of each of their birth experiences?

Onset, process and progress of labour

It is useful to consider three elements when assessing labour and the potential success of a vaginal birth – the power, passage and passenger. The power relates to the effectiveness of the uterine activity attempting to expel the fetus from the woman's body. The passage is through the pelvis and soft tissues, often called the birth canal. The passenger is the fetus undertaking the journey, playing an active part, in relation to its position and lie in the birth canal. The bio-physical mechanism by which this all happens is depicted in Table 7.1.

Labour has traditionally been identified and documented in a prescriptive way as 'stages' of labour. This suggests that a woman ends one stage, suddenly entering the next stage, highlighting different care approaches and requirements for each of the stages and any potential assistance that may be required. More recently, from a woman-centred approach for normal labour, phases or rhythms of labour have been described, highlighting the experience of each phase (Walsh 2011). Midwives are perfectly placed to watch and monitor women to know when the stability of maternal and fetal wellbeing is evident and when support, recommendations and actions are required to assist them. A deep understanding of labour progress and the signs of developing problems is therefore essential.

The latent phase of labour

For some time now the latent phase has been considered from a clinician's perspective rather than the lived experience of the woman, which Walsh (2011) highlights may be very different. This phase is determined as the time when the cervix is effacing (softening, shortening and becoming thin) in the presence of the hormone prostaglandin. A woman may or may not experience painful uterine activity during this time; at some point however uterine activity becomes evident. Deciding whether this is the process of effacement and labour preparation or an active labour that will progress is sometimes difficult for both the woman and the midwife. Diagnosing onset of labour is generally undertaken by performing a vaginal examination, assessing the findings and utilising the information gained to advise the woman and plan care. Effacement of the cervix and its application to the cephalic presenting part, along with good descent of the

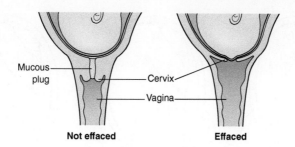

Not effaced   Effaced

Figure 7.2 Cervix not effaced and cervix effaced. Source: Cruickshank and Shetty 2009, Figure H, p. 11. Reproduced with permission of Cruickshank and Shetty.

presenting part, demonstrates the best indicator of good potential (Figure 7.2 illustrates the not effaced and effaced cervix). Effacement and dilatation of the cervix occurs during the latent phase and despite this being progress, it is not yet regarded as active labour. It can be quite normal for a woman to have an effaced and dilated cervix but not be in active labour. It is only the additional presence of painful and regular uterine contractions that determines the onset of active labour as determined by the National Institute for Health and Clinical Excellence (NICE, 2007).

The latent phase has long since been regarded as something the woman is responsible for coping with at home in a normal pregnancy, and does not require admission to a birthing environment. Recommendations are for maternity services to provide one-to-one care once the woman is in established labour (NICE 2007; Hodnett et al. 2013). This suggests that if the woman has a normal pregnancy she does not require midwifery or medical activities or support to assist her during that early phase. There is evidence to suggest that women are more at risk of intervention and subsequent assisted birth if admitted in the latent phase of labour, since diagnosing it is so subjective. Becoming more established in labour at home is therefore beneficial (Greulich and Tarrant 2010). However Barnett et al. (2008) reiterate that women have difficulty identifying the onset of labour and seek reassurance from the professionals. Their study concluded that for women, being sent home because they were not in labour only increased their anxiety.

If we are aiming to be woman-centred, then maternity service provision needs to consider the individual needs of women and ensure women who are in need during this time, have access to a midwife. As a profession midwifery must not throw the baby out with the bathwater and lose sight of how a midwife must care for the woman rather than her cervix!

Active phase

This active phase of labour is generally regarded as a time where there is no turning back and that labour will progress by further dilatation of the cervix and descent of the fetus through to the impending birth of the baby. Diagnosis of the established and progressive first 'stage' of labour is accepted as being from when the cervix of the uterus has dilated (during the latent phase) to four centimetres around the presenting part of the fetus (NICE 2007). Active labour then progresses until the cervix has fully dilated around the presenting part, often termed as being 10 centimetres dilated or 'fully', as illustrated in Figure 7.3.

Diagnosing dilatation of the cervix and the progress of labour is generally through the continued performance of vaginal examinations, to advise the plan of care, although how often this should be undertaken is open to debate (Downe et al. 2013). Effacement of the cervix and application to the descending part (pressure and stretch) is a most important aspect to consider, indicating good labouring potential, rather than the cervical dilatation measurement alone. A

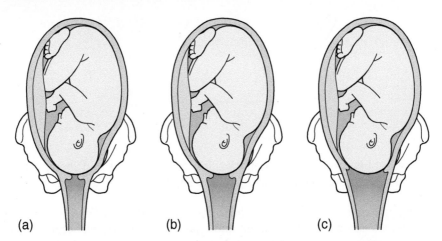

(a)   (b)   (c)

Figure 7.3   Progressive dilation of the cervix in the first stage of labour. Source: Cruickshank and Shetty 2009, Figure I, p. 11. Reproduced with permission of Cruickshank and Shetty.

woman could have a cervix dilated to 5 centimetres (cm), but if the presenting part is high and the cervix is not well applied, her contractions may not stimulate the production of oxytocin well. Equally, a woman with a well-effaced cervix at 3 cm dilatation and tightly applied to a low presenting part, has great potential to labour very efficiently, because of the effect the pressure and stretch has on the production of oxytocin (see 'Optimal hormonal balance' below). There are many ways of 'knowing' that labour is happening and progressing from the woman's behaviour (Walsh 2011). The clinical picture will commonly be described from the bio-physical parameters in relation to the mechanism of labour; Figure 7.9 illustrates how other factors can affect the progress in labour.

Monitoring progress of the active phase of labour

In common practice and recommended by WHO (1994) and NICE (2007) the pictorial record known as the Partogram is used. This tool is used to demonstrate labour progress, recommending the four-hour action line if 1 cm progress per hour is not achieved. However, a systematic review by Lavender et al. (2008) concluded that further evidence is required to determine the efficacy of its use in normal labour. In a randomised controlled trial conducted by Lavender et al. (2006), the evidence suggested that allowing for a slower rate does not necessarily increase caesarean sections and women can be just as satisfied with longer labours. Enkin et al. (2000) recommend 0.5 cm dilatation per hour as progress in primigravida women; this has been endorsed by the NICE (2007) intrapartum guideline.

Partogram use is underpinned by regular vaginal assessment. Recognising landmarks and interpreting the findings of a vaginal examination is a skill that students focus on and causes some anxiety. Vaginal assessment is a skill, which midwives must utilise as efficiently as possible. Midwives may shy away from performing such intimate examinations on occasion, stating it is not necessary if they feel labour is established and progressing. That may be the case in some situations, but midwives must understand the physiology along with safe parameters of progress and wellbeing to determine when such examinations are required. The skill of the midwife lies in knowing when to do and when not to do. Downe et al. (2013) have determined there is widespread use of vaginal examinations without good evidence of its effectiveness.

Therefore, every vaginal examination performed must be justified. Too frequently midwives fail to define position of the baby on vaginal examination or determine that descent through the pelvis is not occurring. This information is of crucial importance. If the examination is being done – make it count. The fewer examinations the better, but to ensure that is the case, as much information from that examination must be obtained as possible.

Clinical consideration

Notice next time medical assistance is requested because a woman has not progressed in her labour; note the first thing a doctor does. The doctor will palpate the abdomen to assess if the fetal head has moved down into the pelvis. The doctor is assessing whether the biparietal diameter (the widest part of the skull) has negotiated the pelvic inlet and whether it will go through with assistance or whether it is obstructed.

A reflexive, woman-centred midwife will actively find ways to encourage decent of the fetus and encourage good uterine activity through fundamental midwifery skills such as encouraging mobilisation and changing positions.

Mobilisation and positioning in labour

Applying anatomical knowledge of the pelvis and fetal skull to the birth process arms midwives with skills to help the birth process progress. The changing shape of the pelvis makes more space in the passage, while moulding of the fetal skull to reduce its diameter assists with travelling through the pelvis (Coad and Dunstall 2011). This pelvic change can be seen as the rhombus of Michaelis, and becomes evident on the mother's lower back (Wickham and Sutton 2002). As the sacrum flattens and moves to give space to the passing fetus, the outer skin stretches and flattens the cleft between the buttocks. This is shown as what has been described as a purple line, seen from the anal margin and extending between the buttocks (Hobbs 1998). A recent longitudinal study concludes there is a positive correlation between the length of the purple line, cervical dilation and station of the fetal head, and it may provide a useful guide of labour progress alongside other measurements (Shepherd et al. 2010).

Midwives are now seeing the benefits of birthing balls, making 'nests' and utilising a platform rather than a bed to assist mobilisation. There is clear evidence that walking and adopting upright positions (see Figure 7.4) shortens the duration of labour, reduces the risk of caesarean and the need for epidural. It is therefore recommended that women are encouraged to adopt positions and be mobile in labour that suit them (Laurence et al. 2013). Figure 7.5 illustrates different positions for labour.

Optimal hormonal balance

Assessment of uterine activity is crucial in determining the progress of labour along with assessment of the cervical dilatation. A midwife spending time with her hand gently resting on the fundus of the uterus throughout the contractions will gain invaluable knowledge of the effectiveness of the uterine activity. Good, powerful and effective contractions occur due to the presence of a rich mix of hormones influencing the labour process. Oxytocin production from the posterior pituitary gland is stimulated through the pressure and stretch of the cervix sending signals through the brain. Therefore the lower the presenting part is within the pelvis, pressing down on and stretching the cervix, the more oxytocin will be produced. This will continue to accumulate through the increased intensity and act as a bio-feedback mechanism know as the Ferguson reflex (Buckley 2011).

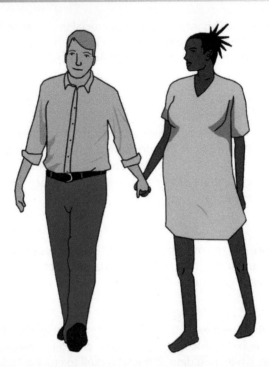

Figure 7.4   Mobilising in labour with support from partner. Source: Reproduced with permission from J. Green.

Although this description may sound daunting to women, her body compensates through endorphin release to support the woman's own ability. This status quo can remain if the woman is undisturbed and unstimulated, allowing her to progress through the labour phases unhindered. Fear however, can have a major influence on a delicately balanced cocktail of hormones. The influence of adrenaline and catecholamine can completely hinder the release of the beneficial hormones of oxytocin and endorphins (Buckley 2004).

Women in childbirth can be seen to become submissive when they recognise they are vulnerable; maintaining an optimal hormonal balance will ensure she submits to her own body's natural instincts.

Activity 7.2

Think of a woman who seemed to cope well in labour without much support from others. What emotional and behavioural characteristics did she display?

Transitional and pushing phases or 'second stage'

With a phases view, the behaviour of the women may vary between demonstrating a strong and uncontrollable urge to push her baby out, with or without full dilatation of the cervix, to a woman having no urge to push at all with a fully dilated cervix. Both can be in transition between the first and second stages. The second stage is recognised as being from when full dilatation has been diagnosed through vaginal examination, to the birth of the baby. Some women experience an early urge to push and this can sometimes be distressing for both the woman and the midwife, impacting on their birth experience. It is however an area with little evidence yet to demonstrate its implications and inform midwifery management (Downe et al. 2004).

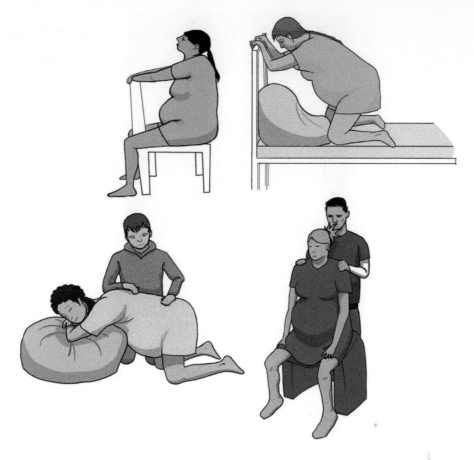

Figure 7.5   Different positions for labour. Source: Reproduced with permission from J. Green.

Women entering second stage without an urge to push are equally noteworthy. A passive delay in active pushing, if maternal and fetal wellbeing are evident can be acceptable (Frazer et al. 2000). The debate continues into how to support women in pushing out their babies. Yildirim and Beji (2008) found neonates fared better and women had shorter second stages when adopting spontaneous pushing. This is in contrast to the more traditional valsalva, closed glottis, breath-holding pushing which reduces oxygen availability at the point in labour when the fetus is most vulnerable. Hollins Martin (2009) confirms this, and the Royal College of Midwives (RCM) second stage guidelines (RCM 2012) also recommend encouraging women to push instinctively.

Monitoring maternal and fetal wellbeing in labour

Every interaction the midwife has with the woman must count. In other words, it is fine to body-watch, gleaning as much information about the woman from the woman without even touching her, but it is totally appropriate to ensure that clinical findings concur with observation. Baseline abdominal palpation is essential, particularly if the midwife has never met the woman previously, since this will give her and the woman vital information about the position and descent of the baby. These assessments will inform decision-making regarding positions for labour and pain relief.

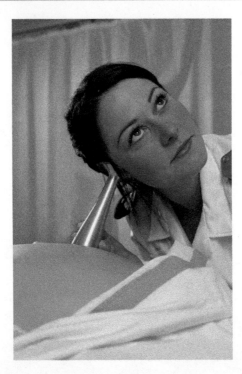

Figure 7.6   Use of a pinard to auscultate the fetal heart. Source: Copyright University of Hull.

The true skills of a midwife lie in the ability to interpret findings, predict potential in the woman's situation and to guide the suggested care; this is often viewed as instinctive midwifery. A midwife will utilise her hands, eyes, ears and nose translating those findings via her experience to inform her decision-making. She uses a pinard stethoscope to hear the fetal heart rate (Figure 7.6), undertakes maternal observations of temperature, pulse, respirations and blood pressure measurement to determine baselines and detect any changes.

Energy levels need to be maintained to enable a woman to labour efficiently. Singata et al. (2013) found inconclusive evidence and therefore no justification to restrict fluids and food intake during labour for low-risk women.

Care and compassion

The importance of good one-to-one support in labour from a midwife cannot be over-emphasised (DH 2007; NICE 2007). This does not mean that the midwife must be constantly at the woman's side, unless of course that is what the woman requires, but that the midwife is available whenever the woman feels she needs that midwifery support. Communication during this time is paramount – the midwife utilising all her skills and most importantly listening to the woman for she knows herself better than anyone else. It is important for a midwife to recognise those women who have confidence in themselves and support them. This may not always be comfortable for the midwife, since the woman may wish to make choices the midwife may not agree with. Conversely the midwife must be aware of the influence she may have over a woman who has no confidence. By communicating and explaining fully, the midwife has the best opportunity to allow the woman to understand a situation and work with it.

There are many examples of procedures and examinations, which often form part of the intrapartum care and which women find uncomfortable, embarrassing or intrusive. The compassionate midwife ensures that nothing is done without good reason and that if an intervention or procedure is performed, it is done with as much expertise as possible and always with informed consent.

Comfort and support to maintain maternal wellbeing and coping is overarching in the midwife's role. Helping her to wash, encouraging oral hygiene and changing sheets if in bed, are all actions that help the woman to feel cared for. General hygiene is important, particularly necessary for women having long or complex births as they may be at higher risk of developing infection.

A philanthropic attitude underpins all the care we give regardless of whoever is involved in providing care. Women in childbirth can be seen to submit when they recognise they are vulnerable. A woman must be allowed to submit to the most appropriate person for her – the doctor, the midwife, a lay support person or best of all herself.

Clinical consideration

When considering the options, interventions and care pathways for women in labour, think about the benefits and the risks to mother and fetus, and the alternatives.

Birth partners

The woman must have control over the choice of who is her birth partner, and whoever that is must be made to feel welcome and involved. There are recognised positive outcomes from the involvement of birth partners (RCM 2011a; Dellman 2004), as long as they are well-supported and informed. The RCM (2011a; 2011b) identify the challenges in involving fathers in a system which is so woman-focused and give top tips on how to facilitate their participation in the birth and other aspects of maternity care. When this is done well then it has a positive effect on the mother, father and their relationship, parenting and breastfeeding. Fathers and other birth partners can have a role in assisting with relaxation techniques and act as an advocate for the woman. It is important that the birth partner wants to be there; sometimes there can be negative effects on fathers who witness traumatic births or are at the birth because they feel pressured to be there. Dellman (2004) identifies how a man being present at the birth is beneficial for most women and also identifies circumstances when they may have a negative effect on outcomes. In addition, there are women who prefer men not to be present at the birth. Hollins Martin (2008) identifies the pressures from UK society for fathers to be present at the births. She cautions making assumptions about a father's willingness to participate at the birth. There are strategies to assist with the anxieties that fathers might have around attending the birth, which includes identifying and agreeing their role of what they do and do not want to see or participate in (Hollins Martin 2008). It is essential that the midwife is in tune to the needs of the father and other birth partners, but not to the detriment of the woman who must always be the focus of her care.

Further reading activity

Go to the link below which is listed on the Fathers Institute website, which is part of Warwick University study on experiences of childbirth. Go to Dad's stories and read their memories, which identify similarities and differences in each Dad's experience. Next time you observe or participate in a birth, think about the experience from the birth partner's perspective.

[Available online] http://www2.warwick.ac.uk/fac/arts/history/chm/outreach/hiding_in_the_pub/memories/

Assisting the normal physiological process

A midwife is part of an interprofessional team that works closely together to keep the woman and her baby safe. A midwife's role is to detect deviations from normal and call a health professional who is reasonably expected to have the necessary skills and experience to assist her in the provision of care (NMC 2012). As a midwife it is important to understand the appropriate use of interventions and how sometimes midwifery expertise can assist the process of labour prior to medical assistance being required. Labour is not a black and white situation with a clear-cut pathway from low to high-risk. For example, a woman may have an epidural and perhaps an intravenous infusion of oxytocin aiming to improve uterine function and propel the passenger through the passage with more power. She may require a lot of encouragement in the pushing phase and even an episiotomy; however she may still achieve a vaginal birth with the continued care and compassion from the midwife.

Outside the parameters of normality

In situations where the midwife is faced with factors not deemed to be normal, she must use her knowledge and clinical judgment about the most appropriate way forward. If she can justify what she is doing – keeping the woman and her baby the focus of providing safe effective care, then her clinical judgement should not be called to question. For example, in a situation where transfer to hospital from a birth centre or home birth is being considered, then the whole picture must be evaluated. This will include taking into consideration not only the facts presenting at the time, but also the background, the woman's obstetric history and whether there is time to safely transfer. As identified by the NMC (2012) midwives must seek help and support from appropriate professionals when there are deviations from the norm.

Artificial rupture of membranes

Artificially rupturing the membranes along with the use of intravenous oxytocin became common practice in 1969 after O'Driscoll pioneered the managed labour to speed up the process of birth to accommodate the move from birth at home to birth in hospital. His impression was that this intervention did not result in untoward outcomes with some suggestion that women were satisfied with such care (O'Driscoll et al. 1969). It is now seen as an intervention to be considered when other possibilities have been exhausted in a normal physiological labour (Walsh 2011). In midwifery-led care, the midwife would not rupture the membranes unless there was a clinical reason to do so. The cushion of amniotic fluid in front of the baby's head is protective and intact membranes allow the amniotic fluid to act as a shock absorber throughout contractions. If labour progress has stalled and the midwife and mother have done everything they can to help labour move forward, it may be appropriate to transfer care to the obstetricians. However, before this happens, since this will probably be the first intervention employed by the obstetricians, artificial rupture of membranes by the midwife at this point may be all that is required and the care can continue midwife-led, removing the need to transfer care.

Equally there may be occasions when the midwife detects an abnormality of the fetal heart. This may raise alarm to the potential for distress of the fetus. Detecting the presence of meconium by either artificially rupturing the membranes, or if it becomes evident on spontaneous rupture, gives the midwife more information on which to base her care and advice.

Pain management in labour

Women have a choice of different types of analgesia and other forms of pain management in labour. It is the midwife's responsibility to ensure the woman understands how each form of pain relief will affect them, their baby and the course of their labour.

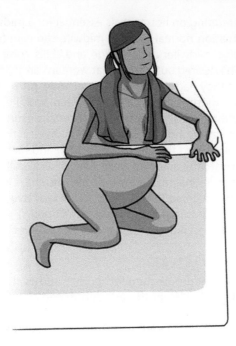

Figure 7.7   Woman using water for relaxation in labour. Source: Reproduced with permission from J. Green.

A summary of the evidence from Cochrane Systematic Reviews suggests that non-pharmacological methods such as: immersion in water (see Figure 7.7), relaxation, acupuncture and massage may improve management of labour pain, with few adverse effects, although their efficacy is unclear (Jones et al. 2012). Hypnotherapy and acupuncture have been acknowledged as having benefits to assisting women cope with labour (Smith et al. 2009). The popularity is increasing for considering water immersion for coping with labour and giving birth. Evidence suggests that its use in the first stage of labour reduces the need for epidural analgesia and the length of labour (Cluett and Burns 2009).

Pharmacological methods including local anaesthetic nerve blocks or non-opioid drugs also improve management with few adverse effects (Jones et al. 2012). There is evidence to suggest that epidurals relieve pain, but can increase the numbers of instrumental births and run the risk of causing hypotension, motor blocks (hindering leg movement), fever and urine retention (Jones et al. 2012). It could be argued there are pros and cons; at times an epidural can be a valuable part of modern medicine when complications occur or if requested by the woman as an option for managing pain in labour. If a woman is so anxious and tense in response to the pain of contractions the optimal hormonal balance may be hindered. By having an epidural the woman relaxes and the oxytocin release improves; it can often be seen at the next vaginal examination that the cervix is fully dilated with good descent of the presenting part.

Midwifery craftsmanship

A midwife learns her craft through experience; repeatedly noticing subtle patterns and commonalities in women's behaviour. This experiential knowledge forms the bedrock of an individual midwife's skill. Although we focus on normality, most midwives work in environments where the use of interventions can be common and routine. Having confidence in midwifery rather than just concentrating on normality is essential for a midwife; since it is not possible to make an abnormal situation normal, but the midwife can care for the woman with the same midwifery skill. Applying midwifery knowledge and skills complements the obstetric care a woman may require. The desired outcome is that women can still feel in control even if the birth experience is not what they had hoped (Fahy and Hastie 2008). The role of the woman within the team is discussed in more detail in Chapter 2: 'Team working'.

Judicious use of midwifery skills and knowledge is vital, ensuring that clinical skills have been appropriately employed throughout to support the midwife in her accountability; utilising what is known about physiology and the individual women and having confidence in the woman's ability to birth. Being a watchful guardian with honed clinical skills and the knowledge to be able to use all that information is what makes the midwife who she is. There is no place for routine and ritual, without justification. Doing things just because we have always done them is not good enough, but doing the right things with the woman's understanding and consent, even if that means something the woman may prefer to avoid, is good practice of an educated midwife.

Medical intervention

It is acknowledged that modern Western technology and evidence-based medicine has indisputably contributed to safer childbirth, reducing maternal and fetal mortality. However it is questionable whether the benevolent aspect of paternalism has gone too far and being at the detriment of women's autonomy in childbirth (Walsh et al. 2004). It is part of the midwives' role to keep elements of normality as part of the holistic care for women, for those also needing a doctor and medical intervention. Figure 7.8 illustrates a woman receiving some medical intervention, using different positions to help labour progress.

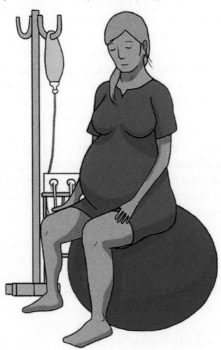

Figure 7.8   Woman on a birthing ball receiving medical intervention. Source: Reproduced with permission from J. Green.

Meeting the baby

The moment a mother meets her baby has been awaited with anticipation. Women's expectations will differ greatly, for some there may be fear and sense of responsibility; some may not be intending to be the social parent of the child and maybe facing some very difficult times. (See Chapter 5: 'Parenthood', where defining parents is discussed in greater depth). Whatever the situation, this is a moment in the lives of the parents and the newborn that will stay with them both forever. The midwife has an opportunity to assist in making this moment memorable and the most optimal physiologically.

Midwives must be alerted to the sudden change of environment for the newborn; a stimulating environment may potentially trigger stress responses in the baby. Very little evidence exists about the emotional status of a newborn, although it is known there is an increase in fetal catecholamines in labour in response to birth (Coad and Dunstall 2011). Providing a gentle transition for the newborn simply seems a logical approach. The benefits of skin-to-skin contact for mother and baby are well recognised (Anderson et al. 2006). Skin-to-skin and gentle handling may help to instil a calmness that will stay with the baby in the early weeks. The joy of birth and bonding potential is needed even more if labour has resulted in intervention and an assisted or traumatic birth, for example caesarean section or an instrumental birth.

Third stage management

When discussing the third stage of labour with a woman, it is really important to ensure that she understands this can be achieved without intervention as the natural conclusion of a normal uncomplicated labour (Soltani 2008), only separating the baby and the placenta and membranes once the baby has been born. Alternatively the third stage can be actively managed by the midwife with uterotonic drugs, clamping and cutting the cord and controlled cord traction. Giving information about the third stage of labour would form part of birth planning and should include discussion about both methods of delivery and the benefits and risks for mother and baby. However, the woman should be aware that this decision does not need to be made until the end of the second stage of labour, with full information of the clinical picture.

Where there is a risk of the uterus not contracting to expel the placenta and membranes and achieve haemostasis of the blood vessels at the placental site, or other risk factors for haemorrhage. The woman should be advised regarding active management of the third stage with uterotonic drugs and controlled cord traction (NICE 2007). By giving a simple explanation of the physiology of the third stage, the woman can make the most appropriate decision for her. Some women have no strong feeling regarding this part of labour, wishing to get it over with as soon as possible allowing them to concentrate on their baby, whilst for others it is extremely important.

Midwives should ensure they have the skills for both physiological and managed delivery of the placenta, avoiding mixing elements of the two methods since this may have implications on outcome (Begley et al. 2011). Skin-to-skin contact and breastfeeding at this point is a mother's well-deserved reward for her hard work. This helps the mother to be more relaxed and produce the hormonal response to encourage separation of the placenta. Soltani (2008) has shown that gravity too can play its part in helping the placenta to separate and expel from the body. It is suggested the woman should be in an upright position for this part of labour.

Birth in water may alter the timing of use of drugs if active management of the placenta is to be employed, with midwives waiting until the woman has exited the pool before starting the process for active management. The reality in practice is that midwives and doctors whilst broadly following the principles of active management do vary in their techniques, and as evidence has emerged to support delaying the clamping and cutting of the cord, to allow full transfusion of blood to the baby, this too has further complicated management (Farrar et al. 2009). Partners or women themselves may want to be involved in the cutting of the umbilical cord, seeing this as a symbolic moment where baby becomes truly independent.

Lotus birth involves physiological delivery of the placenta, but the cord and placenta remain intact until the cord separates naturally from the baby. The placenta may be treated with salt and herbs and is wrapped with the baby following birth. This practice whilst not common is increasingly requested.

Activity 7.3

Think about how third stage of labour is managed in your unit. What differing practices have you seen, and how does this relate to current evidence?

List the advantages and disadvantages of both physiological and active management of the third stage of labour for mother and baby.

Perineal care

Antenatal discussion with women around perineal trauma offers them the opportunity to be proactive in preparing themselves, both physically and emotionally, and the use of perineal massage has been found to be useful (Beckmann and Garrett 2006).

Over the last 30 years the incidence of episiotomy, which in some cases was routine, has significantly reduced. Research has shown this is not protective of further perineal damage. Indeed, episiotomy has been strongly associated with a higher frequency of anal sphincter trauma (Dudding et al. 2008). Since this has become a much more restricted practice, now mainly associated with instrumental birth or birth with intervention (Birthplace in England Collaborative Group 2011; Hatem et al. 2008) many student midwives will never have performed an episiotomy during their training. It is, however important for students to be familiar with how this procedure would be carried out, should the need arise. It is also important for midwives to have the skill to repair perineal trauma since perineal tearing and episiotomy is associated with 85% of births (Albers et al. 2005). A reduction in episiotomy does not mean that there is no indication for perineal repair.

Recently there seems to have been a trend towards leaving perineal trauma unsutured. It is unclear in the practice setting, whether this is because fewer women require or want suturing, or because midwives do not have the skills or do not want to suture because this is their preference. Whilst the evidence is limited regarding suturing or not suturing perineal tears, midwives are advised to be cautious of leaving trauma unsutured, unless the woman has expressly declined suturing (RCM 2012). Midwives must be aware of the way in which they impart information and the influence they have in their position as a trusted knowledgeable professional and must not abuse this in order to avoid carrying out a procedure they know women dislike and find uncomfortable. If midwives are not able to suture, then in the best interests of the woman, the midwife must seek assistance from either another midwife or a doctor to perform perineal repair.

Suturing is a skill all midwives need to develop and maintain through ongoing education and training. It is part of timely, holistic and continued care, which the midwife should provide, reducing unnecessary exposure to multiple professionals. The Royal College of Midwives has produced comprehensive, evidence-based guidelines for midwives to follow (RCM 2012), and readers are advised to access these.

Activity 7.4

Follow the link below to access this research article by Ismail et al. (2013).

Think about what this article says about perineal repair.

Perineal Assessment and Repair Longitudinal Study (PEARLS): a matched-pair cluster randomized trial [Available online] http://www.biomedcentral.com/1741-7015/11/209

159

Decision-making

Figure 7.9 depicts a nurturing and enclosing womb, demonstrating the best way to assist the decision-making process for birth, that is, to formulate a rationale based on the best evidence and guidance available. This is done while working through the experiential knowledge and intuitive views of both the woman and the midwife; discussing the benefits risks and alternatives and making collective decisions based on the woman's needs.

Being aware of the instinctive, innate, deeply emotional information the woman shows in her behaviour, such as being talkative, dependant, tearful, excited or fearful, will help to inform a midwife's decision-making. The midwife will consider how the environment is impacting on the hormonal balance and how these are linked with factors such as nourishment, fluids, position and movement in labour. Also assessing any impact of pharmacological and non-pharmacological pain management support e.g. water immersion, coupled with how the cognitive, knowledgeable aspects are helping or hindering progress. Together, women and carers can formulate a rationale that includes the expertise of the professional. Only then can the woman's decisions about her needs and birth experience be informed.

Key points

- Set a woman up with confidence in her capability to birth through providing compassionate woman-centred care.
- Support her by managing the environment to prevent unnecessary stimulation and anxiety for her, and encourage the optimal hormonal balance.
- Always palpate the abdomen to determine descent of the fetal head in determining progress of labour; do not rely on what can be seen at the vulva during slow pushing.
- Know what deviations may occur and be that watchful guardian, yet being adequately proactive when necessary.
- Watch, listen and feel the progress of a woman's labour, and your craftsmanship as a midwife will develop rapidly.

Conclusion

Caring for a birthing woman brings many midwives immense pleasure in their professional role. It is an emotive time, laced with hard work, assessing risks and monitoring signs of wellbeing. Within the parameters of normality a midwife has a great opportunity to minimise unnecessary interventions and protect the birthing environment. Observing birthing behaviour through its phases as well as the bio-physical observations ensures that compassionate, woman-centred

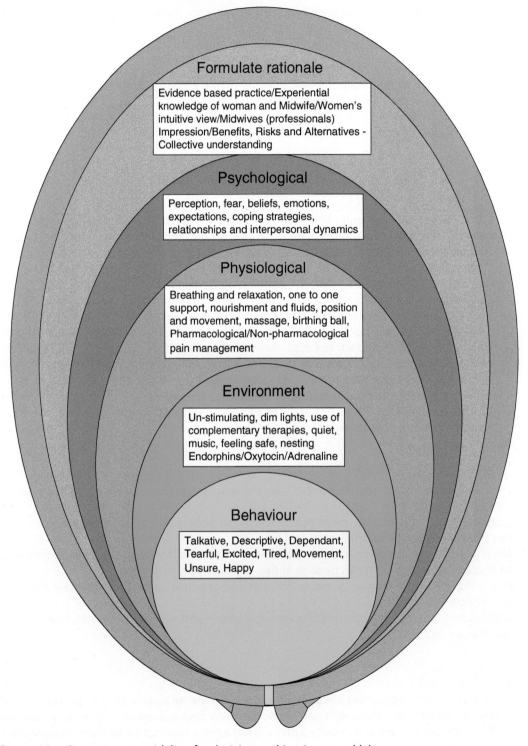

Formulate rationale

Evidence based practice/Experiential knowledge of woman and Midwife/Women's intuitive view/Midwives (professionals) Impression/Benefits, Risks and Alternatives - Collective understanding

Psychological

Perception, fear, beliefs, emotions, expectations, coping strategies, relationships and interpersonal dynamics

Physiological

Breathing and relaxation, one to one support, nourishment and fluids, position and movement, massage, birthing ball, Pharmacological/Non-pharmacological pain management

Environment

Un-stimulating, dim lights, use of complementary therapies, quiet, music, feeling safe, nesting Endorphins/Oxytocin/Adrenaline

Behaviour

Talkative, Descriptive, Dependant, Tearful, Excited, Tired, Movement, Unsure, Happy

Figure 7.9 Concept map guideline for decision-making in normal labour.

care is provided, leading to a better potential for women to feel they have had some control. A midwife, therefore, can help the woman to achieve an optimal hormonal balance, even when medical intervention is needed to assist the birthing process, ensuring the best outcomes for mother and baby and satisfaction with the experience.

End of chapter activities
Crossword

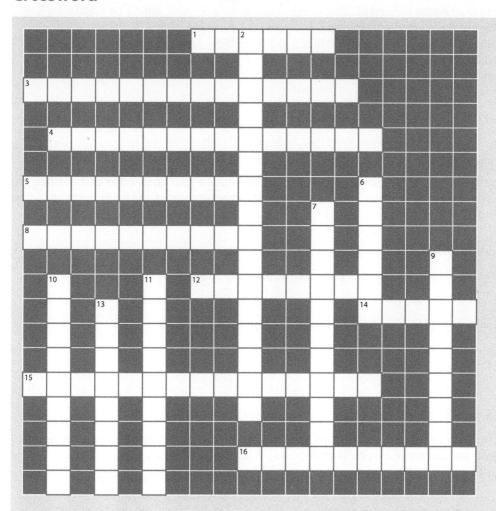

Across

1. Stage of labour when the cervix is fully dilated until the birth of the baby
3. Biofeedback mechanism
4. Chemicals which have roles in the central nervous system and sympathetic nervous system
5. Hormone which stimulates the sympathetic nervous system
8. Describing the phases between the stages of labour
12. Person in control during labour and birth

14. Stage of labour involving delivery of the placenta and membranes
15. Electronic monitoring of the fetal heart

16. Surgical incision to widen the vaginal orifice

Down

2. Surgical operation where the baby is delivered via an incision in the abdomen
6. The phase when the cervix is effacing in the presence of the hormone prostaglandin
7. The arrest of bleeding involving blood coagulation and contraction of blood vessels

9. Includes a graphical record of progress of labour
10. What midwives should be facilitating and maintaining
11. Artificial rupture of the amniotic sac
13. A regional anaesthetic

Find out more

Below is a list of things you can find out about to enhance your knowledge of the issues and topics covered in this chapter. Make notes using the chapter content, the references and further reading identified, local policies and guidelines and discussions with colleagues.

1. Read the Hospital Trust guideline/policy for midwifery-led care in labour.

2. Read the Royal College of Midwives (2012) Evidence-based guidelines for midwifery-led care in labour.

3. Find out what resources are available to facilitate an active birth in the area you are working.

4. Find out about the local provision for birth preparation for pregnant women and birth partners.

Glossary of terms

Acupuncture   Acupuncture is a form of ancient Chinese medicine in which fine needles are inserted into the skin at certain points on the body. It is a complementary therapy.

Adrenaline   Hormone secreted by adrenal gland, which stimulates the sympathetic nervous system.

Amniotomy   Artificial rupture of the amniotic sac.

Caesarean section   Surgical operation where the baby is delivered via an incision in the abdomen.

Cardiotocograph   Electronic monitoring of the fetal heart.

Catecholamines   Chemicals which have roles in the central nervous system and sympathetic nervous system.

Craftmanship   A person who is skilled.

Effacement   The cervix softening, shortening and becoming thin.

Endorphin   Natural pain relieving chemicals.

Epidural anaesthesia   A local anaesthetic is injected into the epidural space, which suppresses sensation in the lower part of the body.

Episiotomy   A surgical incision to widen the vaginal orifice.

Ferguson reflex   Bio feedback mechanism, caused by an increase in oxytocin due to stimulation of the cervix and lower vagina, leading to increased uterine contractions.

Haemostasis   Process which stops haemorrhage.

Hormone   A chemical substance which is has a specific effect on particular cells or organs, they travel around the body to the target cells or organs.

Instrumental delivery   When the birth is assisted with the use of forceps or ventouse.

Latent phase   The time when the cervix is effacing in the presence of the hormone prostaglandin.

Local anaesthetic   A reduction or removal of sensation in a particular area of the body.

Mechanism of labour   Manoeuvres which the fetus undertakes in order to move through the birth canal.

Meconium   The first stools of a newborn baby, which are sticky and dark green, composed of cellular debris, mucus and bile pigments.

Mortality   Death.

Oxytocin   A hormone released by the posterior pituitary gland, which causes uterine contraction and stimulates milk flow.

Partogram   A graphical record of the progress of labour.

Philanthropic   Benevolent, humane.

Purple line   A purple line, seen from the anal margin and extending between the buttocks.

Skin-to-skin   Baby being placed naked, skin-to-skin on mother or father immediately after birth.

Transitional phase   Moving between one phase of labour to another.

Uterotonic   Drugs that cause contraction of the uterine muscle.

References

Albers, L., Sedler, K., Bedrick, E., Teaf, D., Peralta, P. (2005) Midwifery care measures in the second stage of labour and reduction of genital tract trauma at birth: A randomised trial. *Journal of Midwifery and Women's Health* 50 (5), pp. 365–372.

Anderson, G.C., Moore, E., Hepworth, J., Bergman, N. (2006) Early skin to skin contact for mothers and their healthy newborn infants. *The Cochrane Database of systematic reviews Issue 3*.

Barnett, C., Hundley, V., Cheyne, H., Kane, F. (2008) 'Not in labour': impact of sending women home in the latent phase. *British Journal of Midwifery* 16 (3), pp. 144–153.

Beckmann, M., Garrett, A. (2006) Antenatal perineal massage for reducing perineal trauma. *Birth Issues in Perinatal Care* 33(2), p. 159.

Begley, C.M., Gyte, G.M.L., Murphy, D.J., et al. (2011) Active versus expectant management for women in the third stage of labour. *Cochrane Database of Systematic Reviews*, Issue 11. Chichester: John Wiley.

Birthplace in England Collaborative Group (2011) Perinatal and maternal outcomes by planned place of birth for healthy women with low risk pregnancies: The Birthplace in England National Prospective Cohort Study. *British Medical Journal* 343 d7400.

Buckley, S. (2011) Undisturbed birth. *AIMS Journal* 23 (4), pp. 4–7.

Buckley, S. (2004) Undisturbed birth: nature's hormonal blueprint for safety, ease and ecstasy. *MIDIRS* 14 (2), pp. 203–209.

Cluett, E.R., Burns, E. (2009) Immersion in water in labour and birth. *The Cochrane Library* Accessible at: http://onlinelibrary.wiley.com/doi/10.1002/14651858.CD000111.pub3/abstract

Coad, J., Dunstall, M. (2011) *Anatomy and Physiology for Midwives*. Edinburgh: Churchill Livingstone.

Cruickshank, M., Shetty, A. (2009) *Obstetrics and Gynaecology: Clinical Cases Uncovered*. Oxford: Wiley-Blackwell.

Department of Health (2007) *Maternity Matters*. London: DoH.

Dellman, T. (2004) The best moment of my life: a literature review of fathers' experience of birth. *Australian Midwifery Journal* 17 (3), pp. 20–26.

Downe, S., Gyte, G.M.L., Dahlen, H.G., Singata, M. (2013) Routine vaginal examinations for assessing progress of labour to improve outcomes for women and babies at term. *The Cochrane Collaboration* Accessed at: http://onlinelibrary.wiley.com/doi/10.1002/14651858.CD010088.pub2/abstract

Downe, S., Young, C., Hall Moran, V. (2004) The early pushing urge: practice and discourse. In: Downe, S. (ed.) (2004) *Normal Childbirth Evidence and Debate*. London: Churchill Livingstone.

Dudding, T.C., Vaizey, C.J., Kamm, M.A. (2008) Obstetric anal sphincter injury; risk factors, and management. *Annals of Surgery* 247 (2), pp. 224–237.

Enkin, M., Keirse, M.J., Neilson, J. (eds) (2000) *A Guide to Effective Care in Pregnancy and childbirth*, 3rd edn. Oxford: Oxford University Press.

Farrar, D., Airey, R., Tufnell, D., et al. (2009) Measuring placental transfusion for term births: weighing babies with the cord intact. *Archives of Disease in Childhood, Fetal Neonatal Edition* 94 (7).

Fahy, K., Hastie, C. (2008) Midwifery guardianship: reclaiming the sacred in birth. In: (eds) Fahy, K., Foureur M., Hastie, C. *Birth Territory and Midwifery Guardianship*. Philadelphia: Butterworth Heinemann Elsevier.

Frazer, W.D., Marcoux, S., Krauss, I., Douglas, J., Goulet C., Boulvain, M. (2000) Multicentre, randomised, controlled trial of delayed pushing for nulliparous women in the second stage of labour with continuous epidural analgesia. *American Journal of Obstetetrics and Gynaecology* 182, pp. 1165–1172.

Goodman, P., Mackey, M.C., Tavakoli, A.S. (2004) Factors related to childbirth satisfaction. *Journal of Advanced Nursing* 46 (2), pp. 212–219.

Greulich, B., Tarrant, B. (2010) The latent phase of labour: diagnosis and management. *Journal of Midwifery & Women's Health* 52 (3), pp. 190–198.

Hatem. M., Sandall, J., Devane, D., et al. (2008) Midwife-led versus other models of care for childbearing women. *Cochrane Database of Systematic Reviews* Issue 4. Chichester: John Wiley.

Hodnett, E., Downe, S., Walsh, D. (2012) Alternative versus conventional institutional settings for birth. *The Cochrane Library* Available at: http://onlinelibrary.wiley.com/doi/10.1002/14651858.CD000012.pub4/abstract;jsessionid=F4B19E07F65C4697EB611C2AEB7D71DF.f04t01

Hodnett, E.D., Gates, J.G., Hofmeyr, S., Sakala, C. (2013) Continuous support of women during childbirth. *The Cochrane Library* Accessible on: http://onlinelibrary.wiley.com/doi/10.1002/14651858.CD003766.pub5/abstract

Hollins Martin, C.J. (2009) Effects of valsalva manoeuvre on maternal and fetal wellbeing. *British Journal of Midwifery* 17 (5), pp. 279–285.

Hollins Martin, C. (2008) A tool to measure fathers' attitudes and needs in relation to birth. *British Journal of Midwifery* 16 (7), pp. 432–437.

Hobbs, L. (1998) Midwife to Midwife – Assessing cervical dilation without VE's: watching the purple line. *Practising Midwife* 1 (11), pp. 34–35.

Ismail, K.M.K., Kettle, C., Macdonald, S.E., Tohill, S., Thomas, P.W., Bick, D. (2013) Perineal Assessment and Repair Longitudinal Study (PEARLS): a matched-pair cluster randomized trial. *BioMed Central Medicine*, 11 (209) doi:10.1186/1741-7015-11-209.

Jones, L., Othman, M., Dowswell, T., et al. (2012) Pain management for women in labour: an overview of systematic reviews. *Cochrane Database of Systematic Reviews* 2012, Issue 3. Art. No.: CD009234. DOI: 10.1002/14651858.CD009234.pub2.

Kirkham, M. (2010) *The Midwife–Mother Relationship*. Basingstoke: Palgrave MacMillan.

Kirkham, M. (2004) *Informed Choice in Maternity Care*. Basingstoke, Palgrave MacMillan

Laurence, A., Lewis, L., Hofmeyr, J.G., Styles, C. (2013) Maternal positions and mobility during labour. *The Cochrane Library*. Accessible at: http://onlinelibrary.wiley.com/doi/10.1002/14651858.CD003934.pub4/abstract

Lavender, T., Hart, A., Smyth, R.M.D. (2008) Effect of partogram use on outcomes for women in spontaneous labour at term. *The Cochrane Library* Accessed at: http://onlinelibrary.wiley.com/doi/10.1002/14651858 .CD005461.pub4/abstract

Lavender, T., Alfirevic, Z., Walkinshaw, S. (2006) Effects of different partogram action lines on birth outcomes: a randomised controlled trial. *Obstetrics & Gynaecology* 108 (2), pp. 295–302.

Lothian, J. (2006) Birth plans: The good , the bad and the future. *Journal of Obstetrics, Gynaecologic and Neo-natal nursing* 35 (2), pp. 295–303.

NICE (2007) *CG55 Intrapartum Care: Care of healthy women and their babies during childbirth*. London: NICE.

Nursing & Midwifery Council (2009) *Standards for pre-registration midwifery education*. London: NMC.

Nursing & Midwifery Council (2012) *Midwives Rules and Standards*. London: NMC.

O'Driscoll, K., Gallagher, J.T. (1969) Prevention of prolonged labour. *British Medical Journal* 2 (5655), pp. 477–480.

Porter, R.H., Winberg, J. (1999) Unique salience of maternal breast odours for newborn infants. *Neuroscience and Biobehavioral Reviews* 23, pp. 439–449.

Royal College of Midwives (2011a) *Reaching Out: Involving Fathers in Maternity Care*. London: RCM.

Royal College of Midwives (2011b) *Top Tips for Involving Fathers in Maternity Care*. London: RCM.

Royal College of Midwives (2012) *Evidence Based Guidelines for Midwifery-Led Care in Labour. Second Stage of Labour Guidelines*. London: RCM.

Royal College of Midwives (2012) *Evidence Based Guidelines for Midwifery-Led Care in Labour. Suturing the perineum*. London: RCM.

Shepherd, A., Cheyne, H., Kennedy, S., McIntosh, C., Styles, M., Niven, C. (2010) The purple line as a measure of labour progress: a longitudinal study. *BMC Pregnancy Childbirth* 10 (54).

Singata, M., Tramna, J., Gyte, G.M.L. (2013) Restriction fluid and food in labour. *The Cochrane Library* Accessible at: http://onlinelibrary.wiley.com/doi/10.1002/14651858.CD003930.pub3/abstract

Smith, C.A., Collins, C.T., Cyna, A.M., Crowther, C.A. (2009) Complementary and alternative therapies for pain management in labour. (Review) *The Cochrane database of systematic reviews*. A reprint of a Cochrane review, prepared and maintained by The Cochrane Collaboration and published in The Cochrane Library, 2009, Issue 1.

Soltani, H. (2008) Global implications of evidence 'biased' practice: management of the third stage of labour. *Midwifery* 24 (2), 138–142.

Thompson, J.F., Roberts, C.L., Currie, M.C., Elwood, D.A. (2002) Prevalence and persistence of health problems after childbirth: Association with parity and method of birth. *Birth* 29 (2), pp. 83–94.

Walsh, D., El-Nemer A., Downie, S. (2004) Risk, safety and the study of physiological birth. In: *Normal Childbirth: Evidence and Debate*. Edinburgh: Churchill Livingstone.

Walsh, D. (2011) *Evidence-based Care for Normal Labour and Birth*. London: Routledge.

Walsh, D.J. (2004) 'Nesting' and matrescence as distinctive features of a free-standing birth centre in the UK. *Midwifery* 22 (3), pp. 228–239.

Wickham, S., Sutton, J. (2002) The rhombus of Michaelis: a key to normal birth, or the poor cousin of the RCT? *Practising Midwife* 5 (11), pp. 22–23.

World Health Organization (2004) *Making Pregnancy Safer: The Critical Role of the Skilled Attendant*. Geneva: WHO.

World Health Organization (1994) World Health Organization partograph in management of labour. *Lancet* 343 (8910), pp. 1399–1404.

Yildirim, G., Beji, N.K. (2008) effects of pushing techniques in birth on mother and fetus: a randomized study. *Birth* 35 (1), pp. 25–30.

165

Chapter 8

Postnatal midwifery care

Louise Lewis

University of Hull, Hull, UK

Lisa Lachanudis

Women and Children's Hospital, Hull, UK

Learning outcomes

By the end of this chapter the reader will be able to:

- understand the roles and responsibilities of the midwife in assessing, monitoring and evaluating the care of the mother and baby in the postnatal period
- explain the basic anatomy and physiology of the puerperium
- provide evidence-based information to promote health and well-being of the mother and baby
- explain the provision, organisation and content of postnatal care
- support involvement of fathers in the postnatal period
- understand the responsibilities of the midwife in safeguarding vulnerable adults and children.

Introduction

The postnatal period marks an important time of adaptation, encompassing many physical, emotional, socioeconomic and life changing experiences for the mother and partner. The Nursing and Midwifery Council (NMC) of the United Kingdom, in 'Midwives Rules and Standards' (2012, p. 6) define the postnatal period:

> ...as the period after the end of labour during which the attendance of a midwife upon a woman and baby is required, being not less than ten days and for such longer period as the midwife considers necessary...

The National Institute for Health and Care Excellence (NICE) (2013) suggest the postnatal period lasts six to eight weeks after the birth, concluding with a postnatal examination of mother and baby by an appropriately qualified practitioner, marking the end of the maternity care provision.

Fundamentals of Midwifery: A Textbook for Students, First Edition. Edited by Louise Lewis.
© 2015 John Wiley & Sons, Ltd. Published 2015 by John Wiley & Sons, Ltd.
Companion website: www.wileyfundamentalseries.com/midwifery

The aim of postnatal care is to facilitate a smooth transition to parenthood, promote a bio-psycho-social recovery in the mother, monitor the wellbeing of the newborn and provide evidence-based information to the parents. For many women and babies the postnatal period is uncomplicated; this chapter will provide an overview of the key aspects of midwifery care aiming to address the needs of the normal postnatal recovery of the healthy mother whilst offering an insight into recognition of deviations from the normal and the appropriate management (see Chapter 9: 'Care of the newborn', where the needs of the neonate are explored in more depth).

The history of postnatal care

During the 17th century, childbirth in England was inherently a social domestic event, firmly rooted in a female domain. Historically, women and infants were cared for by unqualified local women known as 'gossips' who were usually more mature, married and had themselves given birth. They provided support during labour and for up to six weeks after the birth, helping with domestic duties and supporting the mother to recuperate after the birth (Wilson 1995). Birth predominantly took place within the home and was followed by a 'lying in period' described by Calder in 1912 (cited in Marchant 2010, p. 17) as

> ... Rest in the horizontal position is essential to the lying in if the double results of involution are to be accomplished. The rest should continue for at least a month, the first two weeks in bed, then one week out of bed lying on the sofa, and the fourth week in the bedroom, lying down at intervals ...

The passing of the Midwives Act 1902 set the framework for the training and education of midwives along with provision of care for women and their families. Subsequent guidance and standards have regulated the profession, developing a family-centred, professional and safe service that women are afforded today.

Statistics show the number of births within England and Wales in 2012 to be 729,674 increasing by 0.8% from 723,913 in 2011 (Office of National Statistics 2013). With rising birth rates and increased pressures upon midwifery services to deliver a high quality service, traditional routine practices in the postnatal period have inevitably changed. The days of the 'lying in period' where women were advised to stay in bed in hospital, have now been superseded by early ambulation, early discharge and the promotion of maternal independence. Even for women having undergone caesarean sections, NICE (2011) suggest women who wish to be discharged may be discharged after 24 hours, with follow-up care at home, providing there are no other complications. It should be acknowledged, however that this applies to England and Wales and that international practice along with cultural beliefs will differ. For example, Greece and India continue to follow a traditional 40-day confinement period of recuperation, whilst China follows a 30-day confinement period after the birth.

Activity 8.1

What are the potential complications associated with the 'lying in period' where women were often kept in bed for in excess of ten days?
How are these issues addressed by current evidence-based guidelines?

Anatomy and physiology of the puerperium

The puerperium is traditionally defined as the period of time from immediately after the birth of the baby and placenta and membranes, until the reproductive organs have returned to their non-pregnant state. It is estimated to last six to eight weeks, although the evidence base to support this duration is lacking and health problems are known to exist beyond this period (Coad and Dunstall 2011). The puerperium is characterised by anatomic and physiological changes which relate to involution and lactation. It is also a time of major psychological, emotional and social change as the new mother emerges into the world with the new infant.

Involution of the uterus

Involution of the uterus is the physiological process of the uterus returning to be a pelvic organ. It is a process of contraction, autolysis and epithelial regeneration and proliferation (Azulay Chertok 2013). Oxytocin is released from the posterior pituitary gland inducing strong intermittent myometrial contractions, which may be further increased by the infant suckling at the breast. Immediately following birth of the fetus, myometrial spiral fibres occlude compressing the blood vessels supplying the placental site, causing haemostasis and separation of the placenta from the uterine wall. Haemostasis is achieved by ischemia, pressure from the uterine walls becoming realigned in opposition to each other and the blood clotting mechanism (Coad and Dunstall 2011). The initial postpartum contractions known as 'afterpains' may be strong, particularly in multiparous women which gradually reduce in intensity within the first week (Azulay Chertok 2013). The breakdown of excess myometrial muscle fibres is influenced by proteolytic enzymes within the cells; a process known as autolysis (Jackson 2011). The end products of autolysis are disposed of by phagocytosis. Following birth, the uterus lies about halfway between the umbilicus and the symphysis pubis and over the next 12 hours after birth, the fundus of the uterus rises to the level of the umbilicus. According to Azulay Chertok (2013), the height of the fundus continues to decrease by about 1 cm per day and by 2 weeks, the uterus has descended into the pelvis and the fundus can no longer be palpated abdominally; it gradually decreases in size over the next month to six weeks. Involution is checked by abdominal palpation, after a woman has been asked to empty her bladder.

Subinvolution of the uterus

Slow, delayed or incomplete involution of the uterus can be caused by ineffective uterine contractility, retained placental products, membrane fragments and infection (Azulay Chertok 2013), predisposing the patient to postpartum haemorrhage. The signs and symptoms of infection can include fever, abdominal tenderness, and offensive and excessive vaginal blood loss, although, pyrexia is no longer favoured as a diagnostic category because it is not always present in the presence of infection (Sinha and Otify 2012). The signs and symptoms of postpartum haemorrhage can include tachycardia, hypotension and on palpation of the fundus, the uterus can feel soft described as 'boggy' and may palpate above the umbilicous (Azulay Chertok 2013). Postpartum haemorrhage is discussed in greater depth in Chapter 16: 'Emergencies in midwifery'. If subinvolution is suspected immediate medical treatment is required. The presence of uterine fibroids can also distort the size and shape of the uterus, and requires medical assessment.

Lochia

The decidual lining of the uterus degenerates and is shed in the postpartum blood loss; known as the lochia. The process of involution and restoration of the endometrium is reflected in the characteristics of the lochia which varies in amount and colour as healing occurs. This varies between individuals and generally starts as a red to brown vaginal loss (rubra) lasting the first few days, changing to pinkish-brown discharge (serosa), becoming whitish-yellow (alba) which can last until 6 weeks postpartum (Azulay Chertok 2013).

Regeneration of the endometrium

Regeneration of the uterine epithelial lining rapidly grows, reforming a new epithelium layer over most of the surface within 10 days (Coad and Dunstall 2011). By 2–3 weeks, the endometrial lining is regenerated, reflecting the proliferative stage of the menstrual cycle, except the placental site which takes around 6 weeks (Azulay Chertok 2013).

Cervix and vagina

Following birth the vaginal walls are decreased in tone and oedematous. The vagina gradually reduces in size and regains tone, although following a vaginal birth it does not return to its pre-pregnant state (Azulay Chertok 2013). Over the next 3–4 weeks, the cervix and vagina decrease in vascularity and oedema is reabsorbed.

The perineum

Women are likely to feel some degree of bruising around the vaginal and perineal tissues irrespective of whether the birth resulted in actual laceration or trauma. The effects of perineal pain can impact on the first experiences of motherhood. It is the responsibility of the midwife to minimize morbidity caused by perineal trauma, promote healing and effectively manage pain.

Hormones

Following delivery of the placenta, oestrogen and progesterone fall to non-pregnant levels within 72 hours of birth (Coad and Dunstall 2011). Oxytocin and prolactin levels are dependent upon lactational demands. Increased prolactin levels during breastfeeding, inhibit follicle stimulating hormone (FSH) and luteinizing hormone (LH) release, resulting in lactational amenorrhoea (see Chapter 12: 'Contraception and family planning', for more detail on lactational amenorrhoea).

Haematologic and haemostatic systems

The increased blood and plasma volume during pregnancy results in a physiological hypervolaemia that allows the woman to tolerate some blood loss after birth, normally 300–500 millilitres (Coad and Dunstall 2011). Clotting factors increase after delivery due to the removal of the placenta, resulting in a hypercoaguable state in the postpartum period. This predisposes women to the increased the risk of thromboembolic disorders, being the major cause of maternal death identified in previous Confidential Enquiries into Maternal Deaths (2007). Figure 8.1 highlights the risk factors for thromboembolic disorders in women.

Cardiovascular system

The birth of the baby, placenta and membranes, amniotic fluid and loss of blood; results in dramatic maternal haemodynamic changes rendering the cardiovascular system transiently unstable during the immediate postpartum period (Coad and Dunstall 2011). During the first week after the birth, body fluid is mobilised and excreted leading to a decrease in circulating blood volume as haemoconcentration occurs and the components of blood return to normal (Jackson 2011).

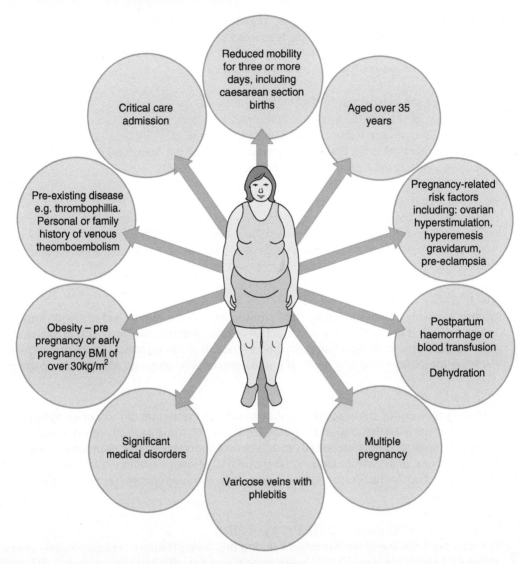

Figure 8.1   Women at risk of venous thromboembolism.

Renal system

Rapid diuresis occurs particularly during days 2–5 postpartum as the sodium and water reten-tion of pregnancy is reversed (Azulay Chertok 2013). Fluid and electrolyte balance is generally restored to non-pregnant homeostasis by 21 days (Coad and Dunstall 2011). It is important the midwife ensures the woman passes an adequate amount of urine within 6 hours following birth (NICE 2006).

Respiratory system

There is immediate reduction in intra-abdominal pressure when the baby is born, allowing expansion of the diaphragm. Respiratory rate returns to normal within 1–3 weeks (Coad and Dunstall 2011).

Gastrointestinal system

The effect of progesterone reduces gastrointestinal muscle tone and relaxes the abdomen, increasing the likelihood of constipation following birth. The first bowel movement usually occurs within 2–3 days postpartum, but may be complicated by the presence of haemorrhoids (Coad and Dunstall 2011).

Thermoregulation

Transient maternal temperature elevations due to the stress of labour and dehydration can occur following a normal birth which may resolve spontaneously and can be non-infectious. However, women should be monitored closely in the postpartum period, because deviations from the normal may indicate infection (Coad and Dunstall 2011).

Immediate postnatal period

In the United Kingdom (UK) the day of birth is always classified as Day 0, and is important in relation to the timing for the newborn blood spot screening (see Chapter 9: 'Care of the newborn', where neonatal screening is discussed in greater depth). The definition of the day of birth varies internationally; some areas define the day of birth as day 0 and in other countries it depends on the time of the day the baby is born. In terms of assessing the health of the newborn in relation to establishing feeding, monitoring sufficient milk intake or jaundice levels, it is advisable to consider how many hours old the baby is.

Either in the home, midwifery-led unit or hospital environment, immediate postnatal care is guided by an evidence-based approach to care (NICE 2006; 2013). The immediate postnatal period is defined as the first one to two hours after birth; the aim during this period is to support the physiological recovery of the mother, transition to motherhood and support the newborn's transition to extra uterine life (Dixon 2013). Assessment of the woman's physiological wellbeing is a crucial part of this period and includes the following assessment; any deviations from the normal would require urgent, immediate medical review.

Postnatal examination of the WOMAN by the midwife

W Wound assessment – Observe and evaluate for infection and adequate wound healing of the perineum and caesarean section wounds.

O Observations – Temperature, pulse, respirations and blood pressure.

M Measure and record first void of urine (should be within 6 hours of birth: NICE 2006).

A Assessment of the uterus – In the absence of abnormal vaginal loss, or signs of endometritis, assessment of the uterus by abdominal palpation as a routine observation is unnecessary (NICE 2006). Abdominal palpation should be undertaken if a woman has abnormal, excessive or offensive vaginal loss, abdominal tenderness, or fever. Any abnormalities detected, including in the size, tone and position of the uterus, must be evaluated urgently by a medical practitioner.

N Note the colour and circumference of the lower limbs and presence of any calf pain – observe and assess for deep vein thrombosis (DVT), although more than 50% of DVTs can be asymptomatic (Day 2003; Meetoo 2010).

Monitoring the baby's health and wellbeing is also a fundamental role of the midwife in the postnatal period (see Chapter 9: 'Care of the newborn', where examination of the newborn baby is discussed in greater depth).

Postnatal examination of the NEWBORN by the midwife

N Note the baby's skin colour – should be pink and warm or normal colour for their ethnicity. Any jaundice within the first 24 hours is pathological, and requires immediate review by paediatrician (see Chapter 9: 'Care of the newborn', where neonatal jaundice is discussed in greater depth).

E Elimination – assess adequate passing of urine and stools. Babies who have failed to pass either urine or meconium within the first 24 hours need immediate review by the paediatrician. Evaluation of normal elimination patterns is part of the ongoing infant feeding assessment and baby's general wellbeing.

W Weight loss – within normal parameters within the first few days (not more than 10% of birth weight)

B Behaviour – the baby should have periods of alertness, normal sleep patterns, waking for regular feeds, normal muscle tone, should lustily cry and be responsive to handling.

O Observations – should fall within normal ranges; respiratory rate 30–60 breaths per minute, heart rate 100–160 beats per minute, temperature of around 37°C (NICE 2006). Oral mucus membranes should be moist and pink with no evidence of oral *Candida albicans* (thrush), ankyloglossia (tongue tie) or abnormalities with the palate.

R Rashes – assess for any skin rashes, lesions, birth marks or spots. Attention should also be given to mother's previous medical history for risk factors such as group B streptococcus.

N Note the frequency, duration of breastfeeding and effective milk transfer. If formula feeding note the frequency, amount taken and type of formula milk used. Ensure parents are fully informed about the safe preparation of formula milk. (see Chapter 10: 'Infant feeding'; where feeding is explored in greater depth).

Further reading activity

Read the sections on wellbeing of the mother and baby in National Institute for Health and Clinical Excellence guidelines for postnatal care of women and their babies (NICE 2006) [Available online] http://www.nice.org.uk/nicemedia/live/10988/30143/30143.pdf

Additional information:

England, C. (2014) Recognizing the healthy baby at term through examination of the newborn screening. In: (eds) Marshall, J., Raynor, M. *Myles Textbook for Midwives*, 16th edn. Edinburgh: Elsevier.

Venous thromboembolism

Following on from The House of Commons Health Committee (2005), who reported an estimated 25,000 people in the UK to have died from preventable hospital-acquired deep vein thrombosis (more than the combined total of deaths from breast cancer, AIDS-related diseases and traffic accidents), the NHS has made prevention of deep vein thrombosis a priority (NICE 2010).

Despite falling to third place as a leading cause of death in the latest confidential enquiries into maternal deaths (Centre for Maternal and Child Enquiries (CMACE) 2011), thromboembolism still claimed the lives of 18 women between 2006 and 2008. This was a marked reduction from 41 between 2003 and 2005 and was largely attributed to the introduction of guidelines (RCOG 2004) superseded in 2009.

One of the main causative factors associated with venous thromboembolism (VTE) is obesity; NICE recommend all women to have assessment of their body mass index (BMI) at the first antenatal appointment, with any women who have a BMI above $30\,kg/m^2$ being referred for additional care. Women should be assessed at the booking interview, during any hospital admissions, reassessed if further risk factors occur and assessed again during the postnatal period. It is the midwives' responsibility to ensure risks are identified and appropriate referral for treatment is made – Figure 8.1 highlights the women who are at most risk for VTE.

When looking at the risk factors identified in Figure 8.1, it is important to consider how many women may be at increased risk due to the rising age of childbearing women, the rising rate of obesity, and the number of women undergoing instrumental and surgical deliveries. Maternity care providers therefore need to be confident and competent to teach women, their partners or family members to administer anticoagulant medication to ensure compliance is achieved. For many women this may be the first time they have held a medical syringe, let alone self-injected and some may feel less confident in being able to self-administer. It may be necessary to teach their partners or significant others how to administer the anticoagulant. With hospital stays becoming increasingly shorter, women may only experience one demonstration before being discharged to community care. Some units may therefore provide a supporting digital versatile disc (DVD).

Changes to postnatal care

Demands upon midwives to deliver high quality effective care have evolved over time: a shift in public health priorities, increasingly higher risk vulnerable families, pressures to balance heavy workloads with early hospital discharge, and increased clerical work may have contributed to midwives becoming disillusioned with the quality of care they are realistically able to provide in the postnatal period (Cattrell et al. 2005; Dykes 2005). A recent Royal College of Midwives (RCM) (2013) survey identified that over half of the midwives in the study said they would like to offer a lot more in terms of the standard of care in the postnatal period. Since the 1990s, the demand for postnatal care in the community within the UK has increased due to shorter hospital stays and an increasing number of mothers choosing to initially breastfeed, requiring support to establish effective lactation and ensure optimal infant nutrition (Walsh 2011). The responsibility and care does not always lie with the midwife alone. More commonly, midwives are seeking support offered by maternity support workers, Children's Centre staff and peer supporters, although the midwife still remains the main provider of care in an uncomplicated postnatal recovery of mother and baby.

The effects of global migration to the UK have contributed to the changing health needs of the population. Increasingly, midwives are working supported by interpreters and engagement with other services, increasing the demands upon the role of the midwife in the postnatal period. With increasing numbers of births to women aged 30 and over as a result of delayed marriage, increased participation in education and establishing a career (ONS 2013) this has also contributed to the increase in women with potentially complex needs, particularly for those women over 40 years. The number of live births to mothers aged 40 and over has more than quadrupled over the past three decades from 6519 in 1982 to 29,994 in 2012 (ONS 2013). Mills and Lavender (2011) cite risks associated with increased maternal age to include: hypertensive disorders; diabetes; chromosomal conditions, particularly trisomy 21 (Down syndrome) trisomy 13 (Patau syndrome) and trisomy 18 (Edwards syndrome); increased risk of multiple pregnancy; and increased risk of stillbirth. Women of this age group may also have co-existing morbidities, with some having conceived through assisted reproduction, both of which could lead to the woman being considered higher risk. With the ever-changing needs of the population and increasing pressure to provide effective postnatal care within a reduced timeframe, midwives

173

need to ensure they are skilled in being able to optimise the care and support they provide. Every postnatal contact with a mother and baby counts and should be afforded appropriate assessment, planning, implementation and evaluation of care. The RCM (2014) have launched a new initiate 'Pressure Points' to push for improved funding and additional resource to improve postnatal care services.

Physiological maternal morbidity

Evidence of postnatal morbidity has been an area of research and focus of maternity policy for many years. As early as the 1990s, research has highlighted the psychological and physical health problems women experience postpartum. The most common health problems include: back pain, urinary incontinence, perineal pain, intercourse problems, constipation and headaches (Bick and MacArthur 1995; Glazener et al. 1995). Practical suggestions to address the common areas of morbidity have been recommended by Bick and colleagues and readers are encouraged to access the latest recommendations to assist them in providing appropriate care (Bick et al. 2009).

Sepsis has become the most common cause for direct maternal death in the UK, with an increase in deaths relating to genital tract sepsis, particularly from community-acquired Group A streptococcal disease, which mirrors the increased incidence of streptococcus A in the general population (CMACE 2011). One of the ten recommendations in the CMACE report highlights the need for health professionals to go 'back to basics', recommending healthcare providers are competent in recognising basic signs and symptoms of ill health. In some of the women described in the CMACE report, earlier recognition of the severity of the illness, recording and appropriate evaluation of vital signs may have prompted earlier action and possibly an improved outcome (CMACE 2011). Sepsis may have an insidious onset, whereby young, previously healthy women can maintain normal vital signs until the late stages of acute disease. Readers are encouraged to look at the latest CMACE 2011 report (Chapter 7: Sepsis) to raise awareness in the prevention and ability to recognise and respond quickly to antenatal, intrapartum and postpartum sepsis. The results of a recent prospective case-control study (Acosta et al. 2014), are consistent with the trend in maternal sepsis deaths in the UK identified in the CMACE 2011 report. The case-control study emphasises that all health care practitioners should remain aware that pregnant or recently pregnant women with suspected infection need closer attention than women who are not pregnant and that signs of severe sepsis in peripartum women particularly those with confirmed or suspected Group A streptococcal infection should be treated as an obstetric emergency (Acosta et al. 2014).

The recent survey by the RCM (2013) identified that a third of women are rarely or never advised of the signs and symptoms of potentially life-threatening conditions in the postnatal period that should prompt urgent referral and treatment. The importance of undertaking, interpreting and acting appropriately on basic observations, understanding normality and improving the exchange of information to women and families about the signs and symptoms of life threatening complications are highlighted by CMACE (2011). In addition, appropriate use of Modified Early Obstetric Warning Scoring Systems (MEOWS) is recommended to help reduce deaths through early detection of serious illness. All health professionals who care for pregnant and recently delivered women are expected to follow local infection control protocols, to inform women about the signs and symptoms of sepsis, and to explain the importance of regular hand hygiene, particularly if the woman has a perineal, or caesarean wound, or is in contact with those that have a respiratory tract infection or a sore throat. This is particularly pertinent to community midwives, who may be the first to recognise potentially abnormal signs during the postnatal observations for all women, not just those who have had caesarean sections. If puerperal infection is suspected, the woman must be referred back to the obstetric services urgently (CMACE 2011).

Further reading activity

Read the signs and symptoms of life-threatening conditions in a woman, requiring Emergency Action in National Institute for Health and Clinical Excellence guidelines for postnatal care of women and their babies (NICE 2006) [Available online] http://www.nice.org.uk/nicemedia/live/10988/30143/30143.pdf

Quality standards influencing postnatal care provision

The National Service Framework for Children, Young People and Maternity Services (Department of Health 2004) recommended all women to receive coordinated postnatal care according to relevant guidelines responsive to the physical, emotional and social needs of the mother and baby. The policy also supported longer duration of midwifery contact for women and families in the postnatal period of up to three months. Maternity Matters (Department of Health 2007) promoted a high quality, accessible maternity service proposing four national choice guarantees which included the choice of how and where to access postnatal care. The introduction of the routine postnatal care of women and their babies (NICE 2006) in England and Wales was developed to standardise care and improve outcomes in the postnatal period. The guideline identified the importance of healthcare professionals caring for women and their babies being able to demonstrate relevant core competences. The value of ritualistic intervention that has no proven benefit was revised and a problem-based, systematic approach with emphasis on early detection of physical and psychological health problems and timely, appropriate intervention has been endorsed (NICE 2013).

Further reading activity

Read the latest quality standard for postnatal care published by NICE 2013 Information for people who use NHS postnatal care services [Available online] http://www.nice.org.uk/nicemedia/live/14217/64473/64473.pdf

A time-honoured tradition or a dying art?

Despite revision to the content and timing of postnatal care, government policy and national standards to support evidence-based care, there is evidence to suggest postnatal provision remains the Cinderella of maternity services (Bick 2012). Recent surveys have demonstrated that postnatal care is an area where women still report negative experiences (Bhavnani et al. 2010; Care Quality Commission (CQC) 2013), both in the UK and internationally (Schmied et al. 2008). Consequently, there is an ever increasing demand to provide quality postnatal care. Caring for women with more complex health needs contributes to the pressures in being able to provide woman focused care in the postnatal period. Shorter stays in hospital, a move away from the 'lying-in' period and reduced contact with maternity services in the postnatal period has changed the emphasis of care. The responsibilities lie more with the mother to self-care and monitor her own recovery from birth (Walsh 2011; Wray and Bick 2012). The changes in the organisation of postnatal care in England have resulted in a gradual shift from the longevity of postnatal home visiting to the introduction of postnatal clinics and reduced number of home visits. Compared to the CQC report of 2010, more women wanted to see a midwife more often and fewer felt they saw a midwife as much as they wanted in the postnatal period (Care Quality Commission 2013).

Postnatal clinics have challenged traditional relationships between women and midwives, albeit implemented in many areas to improve choice and continuity for women and increase the daily efficiency of midwives. The findings of a study designed to illicit the views and experiences of women and midwives using postnatal clinics, highlighted that women felt positive about having the choice to access care in a clinic. Many of the women viewed the clinics as being more convenient and flexible; associated with positive feelings of being able to 'get out' creating independence and motivation, easing the transition to motherhood (Lewis 2009). The community midwives viewed the clinics with optimism due to the efficiency achieved though reduced time spent travelling and parking. The availability of handwashing facilities and the privacy of the clinic environment was also favoured by the midwives (Lewis 2009). Research has indicated that women would prefer to see the midwife for a longer postnatal period (Hunter 2004; Jomeen 2010; CQC 2013). Perhaps the time saved through travelling and increasing daily efficiency of appointments will enable midwives to offer continued care beyond the existing 10–14 days. Currently the system of postnatal provision in England is based on an undefined number of home visits and postnatal contacts; NICE (2006) guidance has not specified the number of postnatal contacts to be offered to women and families.

The number of contacts from the midwife is influenced by a combination of the health professional's clinical judgement, the women's choice and anecdotally workload pressures encouraging midwives to limit postnatal contact to 10–14 days. Only a quarter of midwives have said postnatal visits were determined most significantly by women's needs. Nearly two-thirds of the sample of midwives recently surveyed said that the main reason determining the number of postnatal visits was organisational pressures (RCM 2013), implying women and babies are not at the centre of postnatal care provision. Figure 8.2 illustrates a community midwife performing a postnatal home visit.

Activity 8.2

Find out how postnatal care is organised in your area of clinical practice. Think about the different models of care provided and how effective you think they are at meeting the needs of women and families.

Care and compassion: promoting a healthy psychological adaptation to motherhood

The transition to parenthood can have profound effects on the mother and family both physically and psychologically (Gutteridge 2010; Bastos and McCourt 2010). Providing effective postnatal care can enhance the women's experiences and health outcomes (MacArthur et al. 2002) and is viewed by mothers as a fundamental aspect of care provision known to increase their satisfaction with childbearing (Jomeen 2010). It is important that midwives demonstrate

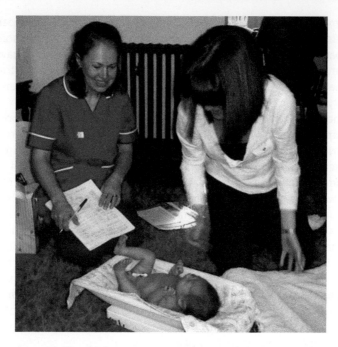

Figure 8.2   Community midwife visiting a woman at home in the postnatal period.

effective communication skills by listening to women and treating families with kindness, aimed at helping them adapt to their new roles confidently. Giving consistent information that validates the mother and partner's role, providing care that is culturally sensitive, respecting individuality, choice and additional needs, are also fundamental skills of the midwife. Giving positive verbal feedback to parents about infant care, involving fathers, significant others and providing opportunities for appropriate peer support can enhance maternal self-efficacy and improve the experience and transition to parenthood (Warren and McCarthy 2011). However, Jones et al. (2013) highlighted that peer support may not be of value for all women, particularly for those who feel they cannot talk openly about how they are really feeling, leading to feelings of isolation. The midwife can help to build a mother's confidence in her mothering abilities, promote the development of the mother–infant relationship, parenting competence and self-efficacy (Rowe et al. 2013). However, with reduced midwifery contact in the postnatal period, perhaps there is a danger of pushing mothers too quickly into fostering their own independence rather than allowing them time for replenishing and healing following birth. Midwifery-led units can offer the ideal postnatal environment promoting calmness; a place for the mother to feel nurtured, the opportunity to restore vitality, learn and gain confidence in her new role supported by the midwives (Smythe et al. 2013). The transfer of care from midwives and effective communication with the health visitor and General Practitioner (GP) is a crucial part of the ongoing continuum of postnatal care for the mother and baby.

Engaging fathers

During the provision of postnatal care, maternity care workers need to be sensitive to the families' needs; whilst much focus is on the woman and baby it is important to acknowledge the fathers' needs and emotions; to include them in the care. Whilst maternity care providers may perceive women to have had a routine normal labour and birth, some partners may find the birth distressing and may manifest symptoms of post-traumatic stress disorder following negative emotional experiences from the birth (White 2007). Partners who have witnessed a traumatic birth may require de-briefing by maternity care providers whilst in the hospital. It is important that the discussions with the family are reflected in the woman's maternity records so community staff can offer further support in the postnatal period.

Active fathering, particularly in the early years, has shown to have a positive impact on the child's development (RCM 2011a). It has been identified that young fathers in particular are less likely to be involved in the care of their children (Fisher 2007) and some fathers experience their place in maternity care as being a 'non-patient' and a 'non-visitor' with the consequence of feeling excluded and fearful (Steen et al. 2012). A man's own experience of being fathered can impact on how he develops relationships with his own children; society's expectations of being a good dad can add to the challenges for fathers adapting to their new role (Raynor and England 2010). Fathers may worry about the financial implications that arrive with a new baby and how they will manage to provide. However, the demography of families have changed dramatically over the past 50 years and it is more common for mothers and fathers to both be working, and sharing earnings and caring responsibilities for the children (Fatherhood Institute Annual Report 2012–13). In the UK, fathers may be entitled to one or two weeks ordinary statutory paternity pay and up to 26 weeks paid additional paternity leave (but only if the mother returns to work); further details can be found online at GOV.UK. For those families requiring additional financial support, maternity care providers may need to signpost families to other appropriate agencies. Some Children's Centres provide specialist sessions for fathers which allow them to share their experiences; details of these can be found within the local area of maternity service provision.

Embedding father-inclusive practices and listening to fathers is a crucial part of the provision of postnatal care, promoting a smooth transition to parenthood. The RCM have published guidelines to help health professionals facilitate the involvement of fathers in maternity care (RCM 2011b). Figure 8.3 illustrates some of the positive and challenging elements of fatherhood.

Safeguarding vulnerable adults and babies

Safeguarding means '*protecting people's health, wellbeing and human rights, enabling them to live free from harm, abuse and neglect*' (Care Quality Commission 2014). The groups identified as particularly requiring this protection are children, young people and vulnerable adults, but anyone can find themselves in circumstances in which they need safeguarding.

Midwives are seen as key workers in relation to safeguarding both adults and children (NMC 2009). Community midwives in particular, have the opportunity to meet with families and visit them in their homes, and therefore can assist in the prevention, identification, monitoring and reporting of concerns about the welfare of family members. Midwives are also important elements of the safeguarding team as it is known that pregnancy and the postnatal period are times when abuse can start or become worse (NICE 2014). Midwives can assist in the support of families in order to facilitate an environment within the family which will reduce the risk of abuse of both children and adults. Focus should not just be on the woman and her baby, but also any other children or family members they meet. Health professionals need to be up to date and vigilant in identifying the signs of abuse and know the systems in place to report abuse (NICE 2014). This involves asking appropriate questions to all pregnant women about domestic abuse (Hardacre 2005), examining babies for signs of physical abuse (NICE 2009) and observing the interactions between women, partners and their babies (Williams et al. 2013). The recently

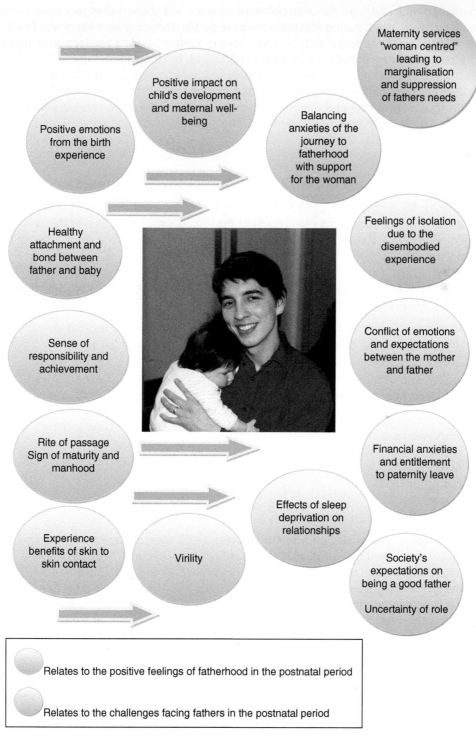

Figure 8.3   The positive elements and challenges of fatherhood.

published NICE (2014) guidance on domestic violence and abuse makes specific recommendations on these issues, stating that there needs to be *'the creation of an environment for disclosing domestic violence and abuse' and that questions about this should be a 'routine part of good clinical practice, even where there are no indicators'* (NICE 2014, p. 11, p. 12).

This is an opportunity for interprofessional and interagency working; it is important to keep accurate and contemporaneous records and to communicate effectively with all those involved in the families care. Lack of communication and effective team working are key features in many serious case reviews, which examine the deaths of women and children (Saunders 2004).

Activity 8.3

Go to the NSPCC website and look at the serious care reviews listed below:

1. Oxfordshire, December 2013, Child Y. This demonstrates how poor communication can affect the protection of children and also identifies other lost opportunities to save the child.
2. York, October 2013, Baby A. Again poor communication between professionals was identified as an issue.
3. Coventry, September 2013, Daniel Pelka. The issues of culture, race, language and domestic abuse are relevant in this case. As well as the fact that the mother was manipulative and deceptive. What implications does this have for midwives?

. As part of midwifery education programmes, students attend specific sessions on safeguarding children and adults. These will continue throughout a midwive's career.

The Department of Education (2011a, p. 5) set out six principles of adult safeguarding which are:

- empowerment
- prevention
- proportionality
- protection
- partnership
- accountability.

These are further explained within the document focused on the role of healthcare professionals (Department of Education 2011b). Readers are encouraged to access the document. An example of a relevant case is given on page 16; look at the case related to Susan, which will give some further insight as to how this system should work. Within the first principle of empowerment is embedded the ideal that a person has the capacity to give or refuse consent unless proven otherwise. This is related to the Mental Capacity Act 2005; all student midwives and midwives should be fully aware of the implications of this Act.

Activity 8.4

The five key principles of the Mental Capacity Act 2005 are outlined and explained on the NMC website. [Available online] http://www.nmc-uk.org/Nurses-and-midwives/Regulation-in-practice/Regulation-in-Practice-Topics/consent/

Go to the site and read these principles; think about their implications for midwifery practice.

Where to get help

There are identified workers within all Trusts and working environments who play a key role in the safeguarding of children and adults. They can be contacted to ask for advice and to seek support when there are concerns. Supervisors of Midwives can assist in this process and student midwives and midwives should use the supervisory framework in order to safeguard those in their care (see Chapter 1:'To be a midwife', where supervision of midwives is discussed in greater depth). Student midwives should also seek advice from their mentors.

Activity 8.5

Find out who are the key workers for safeguarding children and adults in the placement areas.
   Access specific safeguarding information on the relevant Trust and Council websites, where the process for reporting concerns will be set out. This will include safeguarding boards for both children and adults.
   Speak to a Supervisor of Midwives from the placement area and discuss with them the process for seeking advice about and reporting suspected abuse of both children and adults.

One of the key principles of all safeguarding whether that be children or adults is that it is everybody's business, not just healthcare workers such as midwives but society as a whole.

Reducing the risk of sudden infant death syndrome

One of the biggest challenges for new parents is adjusting to a new routine at night. UNICEF Baby Friendly Initiative offers practical suggestions for parents and recommendations to promote safety with the aim of reducing the risks of sudden infant death syndrome (SIDS). A guide has been written to help health professionals who will be using the *Caring for Your Baby at Night* guide with new parents. It highlights the evidence underpinning the recommendations in the leaflet and offers guidance on discussing these issues; it is available to download or can be accessed online.

The current body of evidence overwhelmingly supports the following key messages, which should be conveyed to all parents when discussing bed-sharing (UNICEF UK 2013):

*   The safest place for your baby to sleep is in a cot by your bed for the first 6 months.
*   Sleeping with your baby on a sofa puts your baby at greatest risk.
*   Your baby should not share a bed with anyone who is a smoker.

Further reading activity

Read the guidelines midwives need to discuss with parents to reduce the risk of SIDS, from the UNICEF Baby Friendly Initiative website.
   [Available online] http://www.unicef.org.uk/Documents/Baby_Friendly/Leaflets/HPs_Guide _to_Coping_AtNight_Final.pdf and http://www.unicef.org.uk/Documents/Baby_Friendly/Leaflets/ caringatnight_web.pdf
   Read the following article [Available online] http://bmjopen.bmj.com/content/3/5/e002299.full
   Carpenter, R., et al. (2013) Bed sharing when parents do not smoke: is there a risk of SIDS? An individual level analysis of five major case-control studies. BMJ Open. doi:10.1136/bmjopen-2012-002299

Postnatal exercise advice for new mothers

It is part of the midwife's role and responsibilities to ensure the new mother is provided with relevant information and advice regarding safe exercise in the postnatal period. Physiotherapists working in maternity units are available for specialist advice to women; information is also available for health professionals and women from the Association of Chartered Physiotherapists in Women's Health. Readers are encouraged to access the recommendations and guidelines available on the website.

Activity 8.6

Access the information about postnatal exercise for women in the postnatal period [Available online] http://acpwh.csp.org.uk/publications/fit-safe-exercise-childbearing-year.

Other responsibilities of the midwife in the postnatal period

The midwife also needs to assess if the woman is rhesus negative and whether she requires the administration of anti-D immunoglobulin in the postnatal period; it is imperative that this is administered within 72 hours of birth, if required. Appropriate blood samples from the mother and the baby's cord will have been taken immediately after the birth to identify the blood groups and any potential antibody transfer (see Chapter 6: 'Antenatal midwifery care', where isoimmunisation is discussed in greater depth).

The midwife will also need to evaluate whether the woman requires the MMR vaccine to prevent against measles, mumps, and rubella in the future.

Methods and timing of resumption of contraception should be discussed within the first week of birth as recommended by (NICE 2006). Healthcare professionals advising women about contraceptive choices should be competent to discuss the methods available, the benefits and risks of different methods (see Chapter 12: 'Contraception', where methods are discussed in greater depth).

Key points

- The postnatal period is a time of adaptation, encompassing many physical, emotional, socioeconomic and life changing experiences for the mother and partner.
- In the UK postnatal care provision is a fundamental part of maternity services.
- Effective postnatal care is known to increase woman's satisfaction and health outcomes.
- Changing demographics and health needs have led to an increase on the pressures of postnatal services.
- The demise in postnatal provision in the UK is concerning, with the potential to affect health outcomes for women and their babies.
- The midwife has a key role in being able to support a healthy adaptation to parenthood for mother and partner.

Conclusion

The postnatal period is a time of immense change for women and families. Midwives have a pivotal role in promoting confidence in parenting abilities and supporting a healthy physiological, psychological and social transition to parenthood. With the demise in postnatal care provision, it is vital that every contact with the woman and baby is optimised in terms of assessing health risks, shared decision-making, giving information, planning and evaluating care that is safe and meets the needs of women and babies. The introduction of collaborative working will hopefully increase daily efficiency and the provision of postnatal care will continue to be supported as an essential aspect of the childbearing experience for women and families.

183

End of chapter activities
Wordsearch

L	W	A	F	S	I	A	R	B	U	R	U	O	X	K	V	U	J	J	R
F	S	D	B	O	U	R	J	O	V	E	J	Y	G	L	V	W	M	D	E
V	G	I	X	A	U	F	R	U	H	H	A	O	V	A	K	G	H	E	T
K	A	I	S	J	B	R	C	S	Z	Y	R	L	D	Q	N	R	C	H	A
X	U	H	M	O	Y	Y	C	C	D	Y	P	R	B	P	A	Y	V	I	I
A	F	W	I	E	R	P	B	X	Z	X	X	B	T	A	N	E	M	S	N
I	M	W	O	T	O	B	E	L	C	F	K	U	N	N	K	M	A	C	E
S	D	E	G	C	T	S	I	M	U	U	E	T	V	U	Y	M	S	E	D
P	X	T	I	C	Z	X	G	F	T	E	T	P	F	P	L	E	T	N	P
M	B	N	N	N	T	L	L	I	C	V	S	S	R	K	O	L	I	C	R
A	S	S	V	V	D	I	S	G	K	I	N	I	N	D	G	T	T	E	O
L	Y	B	O	H	I	U	C	K	X	I	T	I	H	T	L	S	I	O	D
C	Z	R	L	X	R	S	F	N	A	Z	M	S	A	S	O	I	S	M	U
E	Z	V	U	E	L	B	K	P	I	A	E	T	Y	X	S	N	J	G	C
E	C	V	T	G	Z	G	R	E	T	C	Q	B	N	C	S	B	B	Y	T
R	X	U	I	T	A	E	X	I	A	S	O	R	E	S	I	L	D	G	S
P	J	P	O	V	T	G	V	Y	G	V	H	T	R	G	A	D	K	G	J
H	X	V	N	F	R	T	Y	V	K	R	U	L	Y	X	W	O	I	J	G
I	T	G	A	A	R	G	P	H	S	K	W	Y	U	X	K	Q	V	P	P
V	E	G	S	F	K	Z	X	A	V	B	J	H	Y	I	O	Z	V	Q	Z

1. Physiological process of the uterus returning to be a pelvic organ.
2. Often detected within the antenatal period but may occur postnatally.
3. May manifest with a pyrexia, inflammation and painful breasts.
4. The hormone secreted by the posterior pituitary gland at the initiation of the baby sucking at the breast.
5. Three words used to describe the stages and colour of lochia.
6. May be detected from newborn bloodspot screening.
7. May present clinically as; a tender uterus on abdominal palpation, excessive and or offensive lochia and or pyrexia.
8. Mother feeling emotional and tearful around the third day postnatally, referred to as..........
9. Returns to a pelvic organ after approximately 10–14 days.
10. Name used to describe the breakdown and separation of caesarean section wound site.
11. Postpartum contractions, often stronger in multiparous women.
12. Recommended for newborns as a prophylaxis treatment after birth to prevent haemorrhagic disease.
13. Alternative name for tongue tie.
14. Number of blood spots required on the specimen sample for completion of newborn screening.

Find out more

Below is a list of things you can find out about to enhance your knowledge of the issues and topics covered in this chapter. Make notes using the chapter content, the references and further reading identified, local policies and guidelines and discussions with colleagues.

1. What are the normal ranges for pulse, blood pressure and respiratory rate in the mother during the postnatal period?

2. Find out what other postnatal services are available in the area to support the transition to parenthood.

3. Find out what advice is given to mothers regarding care of their caesarean section and perineal wounds.

4. Read the Hospital Trust Policy and Guidelines relating to the provision of postnatal care.

Glossary of terms

Afterpains   Pain caused by uterine contractions after childbirth, especially during breastfeeding, due to release of oxytocin. More common in multiparous women.

Autolysis   Destruction of cells through the action of own enzymes.

Diuresis   Increased secretion of urine.

Endometritis   Inflammation or infection of the endometrium.

Endometrium   Inner mucous membrane lining the uterus.

Epithelium   Layer of cells lining organs and glands.

Fibroid   Benign tumours of smooth muscle tissue growing in or around the uterus.

Fundus   The part of an organ opposite or the furthest from its opening.

Haemostasis   Stopping of bleeding involving blood coagulation and contraction of damaged blood vessels.

Haematological   Disorders associated with the study of blood.

Hypercoaguable   Propensity for the body to develop thrombosis.

Hypervolaemia   Blood volume is increased.

Hypotension   Abnormally low arterial blood pressure.

Involution   Physiological process of the uterus returning to be a pelvic organ.

Ischemia   Inadequate blood supply to tissues caused by blockage of the blood vessels.

Lochia   The decidual lining of the uterus degenerates and is shed in the postpartum blood loss through the vagina.

Myometrium   Middle layer of the uterus.

Phagocytosis   Digestion of bacteria and removal of pathogens.

Proteolytic enzyme   Digestive enzyme causing breakdown of protein.

Puerperal infection   Infection of the genital tract arising in the postnatal period.

Puerperium   The six to eight week period following childbirth, during which the mother's body returns to its physiological pre-pregnant state.

Pyrexia   Rise in body temperature above the normal.

Symphysis pubis   Joint between the pubic bones of the pelvis.

Tachycardia   Abnormal increase in the heart rate.

(Adapted from Martin 2010.)

References

Acosta, C.D., Kurinczuk, J.J., Nuala Lucas, D., Tuffnell, D.J., Sellers, S., Knight, M. (2014) *Severe Maternal Sepsis in the UK, 2011–2012: A National Case-Control Study*. POLS Medicine. DOI: 10.1371/journal.pmed .1001672.

Azulay Chertok, I.R. (2013) The postpartum period and lactation physiology In: Tucker Blackburn, S. (2013) *Maternal, Fetal, & Neonatal Physiology: A Clinical Perspective*, 4th edn. Philadelphia: Elsevier Saunders.

Bastos, M.H., McCourt, C. (2010) Morbidity during the postnatal period: impact on women and society. In: (eds) Byrom, S., Edwards, G., Bick, D. *Essential Midwifery Practice: Postnatal Care*. Oxford: Wiley Blackwell.

Bick, D., MacArthur, C. (1995) The extent severity and effect of health problems after childbirth. *British Journal of Midwifery* 3(1), pp. 27–31.

Bick, D., MacArthur, C., Winter, H. (2009) *Postnatal care Evidence and Guidelines for Management*. Edinburgh: Churchill Livingstone Elsevier.

Bick, D. (2012) Reducing postnatal morbidity. *The Practising Midwife* 6 (5), pp. 29–31.

Bhavnani, V., Newburn, M. (2010) *Left to your own devices: the postnatal care experiences of 1260 first-time mothers*. London: The National Childbirth Trust.

Calder, A.B. (1912) Lectures on midwifery, 2nd edn, cited in Marchant, S. (2010) The history of postnatal care, national and international perspectives. In: (eds) Byrom, S., Edwards, G., Bick, D. *Essential Midwifery Practice: Postnatal Care*. Oxford: Wiley Blackwell.

Care Quality Commission (2014) *Safeguarding People* [online] Available: http://www.cqc.org.uk/public/ what-are-standards/safeguarding-people

Care Quality Commission (2013) *National findings from the 2013 survey of women's experiences of maternity care*. London: CQC.

Cattrell, R., Lavender, T., Wallymahmed, A., Kingdon, C., Riley, J. (2005) Postnatal care: what matters to midwives. *British Journal of Midwifery* 13 (4), pp. 206–213.

Confidential Enquiry into Maternal and Child Health (2007) *Saving Mothers Lives: reviewing maternal deaths to make motherhood safer (2003–2005)*. London: RCOG.

Centre for Maternal and Child Enquiries (2011) Saving mothers' lives: reviewing maternal deaths 2006–2008. *British Journal of Obstetrics and Gynaecology* 118 (Suppl. 1), pp. 1–203.

Coad, J., Dunstall, M. (2011) *Anatomy and Physiology for Midwives*. Edinburgh: Churchill Livingstone.

Day, M. (2003) Recognizing and managing deep vein thrombosis. *Nursing* 33 (5), pp. 36–41.

Department of Education (2011a) *Safeguarding Children Across Services: Message to Adult Services Professionals Working with Parents*. London: Department of Education [online]. Available: https://www.gov.uk/government/uploads/system/uploads/attachment_data/file/197705/DFE–RB164d_1_.pdf.

Department of Education (2011b) *Safeguarding Children Across Services: Message to Health Professionals Working with Children*. London: Department of Education. Available:https://www.gov.uk/government/uploads/system/uploads/attachment_data/file/197703/DFE–RB164b_1_.pdf

Department of Health (2004) *National Service Framework for Children, Young People and Maternity Services*. London: Department of Health.

Department of Health (2007) *Maternity Matters: Choice, Access and Continuity of Care in a Safe Service*. London: Department of Health.

Dixon, L. (2013) Observation of mother and baby in the immediate postnatal period: implications for midwifery practice. *Midwifery News* March, pp. 12–13.

Dykes, F. (2005) A critical ethnographic study of encounters between midwives and breast–feeding women in postnatal wards in England. *Midwifery* 21, pp. 241–252.

England, C. (2014) Recognizing the healthy baby at term through examination of the newborn screening. In: (eds) Marshall, J., Raynor, M. *Myles Textbook for Midwives*, 16th edn. Edinburgh: Elsevier.

Fatherhood Institute Pushing Fatherhood up the agenda: Annual Report 2012–2013 [online] Available: http://www.fatherhoodinstitute.org/wp-content/uploads/2013/11/FI-Annual-Report-12-13-Final-Web.pdf

Fisher, D. (2007) *Including New Fathers: A Guide for Maternity Professionals* [online] Available www.fatherhoodinstitute.org.uk

Glazener, C., Abdalla, M., Stroud, P., Naji, S., Templeton, A.., Russell, I.T. (1995) Postnatal maternal morbidity: extent, causes, prevention and treatment. *An International Journal of Obstetrics & Gynaecology* 102 (4), pp. 282–287.

Gutteridge, K. (2010) Transition into parenthood: ideology and reality. In: (eds) Byrom, S., Edwards, G., Bick, D. *Essential Midwifery Practice: Postnatal Care*. Oxford: Wiley Blackwell.

Hardacre, S. (2005) Routine enquiry into domestic abuse – The all Wales Clinical Pathway. *British Journal of Midwifery* 13 (11), pp. 697–701.

House of Commons Health Committee (2005) *The prevention of venous thromboembolism in hospitalized patients*. London: The Stationary Office.

Hunter, L. (2004) The views of women and their partners on the support provided by community midwives during postnatal visits. *Evidence Based Midwifery* 2 (1), pp. 20–27.

Jackson, P. (2011) Content and organisation of postnatal care. In: (eds) MacDonald S., Magill-Cuerden, J. *Mayes Midwifery*, 14th edn. Edinburgh: Bailliere Tindall.

Jomeen, J. (2010) *Choice, Control and contemporary childbirth: understanding through women's stories*. Oxford: Radcliffe Publishing.

Jones, C.C.G., Jomeen J., Hayter M. (2013) The impact of peer support in the context of perinatal mental illness: A meta-ethnography midwifery. [online] Available: http://dx.doi.org/10.1016/j.midw.2013.08.003i

Lewis, L. (2009) Postnatal clinics: women's and midwives' experiences. *British Journal of Midwifery* 17 (12), pp. 791–795.

MacArthur, C., Winter, H., Bick, D., Henderson, C., Knowles, H. (2002) Effects of re-designing community postnatal care on women's health 4 months after birth: a cluster randomised controlled trial. *Lancet* 359, pp. 378–85.

Martin, E.A. (2010) *Concise Oxford Colour Medical Dictionary*. Oxford: Oxford University Press.

Meetoo, D. (2010) In too deep: understanding, detecting and managing DVT. *British Journal of Nursing* 19 (16), pp. 1021–1027.

Mills, T., Lavender, T. (2011) Advanced maternal age. *Obstetrics, Gynaecology and Reproductive Medicine* 21 (4), pp. 107–111.

186

National Institute for Health and Clinical Excellence (2006) *Routine postnatal care of women and their babies*, Guideline 37. London: NICE.

National Institute for Health and Clinical Excellence (2009) *When to Suspect Child Maltreatment*. London: NICE.

National Institute for Health and Clinical Excellence (2011) *Caesarean Section Clinical, Guideline 132*. London: NICE.

National Institute for Health and Clinical Excellence (2010) *Venous thromboembolism – reducing the risk CG92*. London: NICE.

National Institute for Health and Care Excellence (2013) *Information for people who use NHS postnatal care services*. Manchester: NICE.

NICE (2014) *Domestic violence and abuse: how health services, social care and the organisations they work with can respond effectively Public Health Guidance 50*. London: NICE.

Nursing and Midwifery Council (2009) *Standards for Pre Registration Midwifery Education*. London: NMC.

Nursing and Midwifery Council (2012) *Midwives rules and standards*. London: NMC.

Office of National Statistics (2013) *Births in England and Wales 2012: Statistical bulletin*. Office of National Statistics [online] Available: http://www.ons.gov.uk/ons/dcp171778_317196.pdf

Raynor, M., England, C. (2010) *Psychology for Midwives, Pregnancy, Childbirth and Puerperium*. Maidenhead: Open University Press.

Royal College of Midwives (2013) Concern women not told about potentially life-threatening postnatal problems [online] Available http://www.rcm.org.uk/college/about/media-centre/press-releases/concern-women-not-told-about-potentially-life-threatening-postnatal-problems-10-11-13/

Royal College of Midwives (2014) Pressure Points: The case for better postnatal care [online] Available: http://www.rcm.org.uk/college/campaigns-events/pressurepoints/

Royal College of Midwives (2011a) *Reaching out: Involving fathers in Maternity Care*. London: RCM.

Royal College of Midwives (2011b) *Top Tips for Involving Fathers in Maternity Care*. London: RCM.

Rowe, J., Barnes, M., Suthers, S. (2013) Supporting Maternal Transition: Continuity, Coaching and Control. *The Journal of Perinatal Education* 22 (3), pp. 145–155.

Royal College of Obstetricians and Gynaecologists (2009) *Reducing the risk of thrombosis and embolism during pregnancy and the puerperium, Green-top Guideline number 37a*. London: RCOG.

Saunders, H. (2004) *Twenty Nine Child Homicides: Lessons still to be learned on domestic violence and Child Protection*. Bristol: Women's Aid Federation of England.

Sinha, P., Otify, M. (2012) Genital tract sepsis: early diagnosis, management and prevention. *The Obstetrician & Gynaecologist* 14, pp. 106–114.

Smythe, E.A., Payne, D., Wilson, S., Wynyard, S. (2013) The dwelling space of postnatal care. *Women and Birth* 26, pp. 110–113.

Schmied, V., Cooke, M., Gutwein, R., Steinlein, E., Homer, C. (2008) Time to listen: Strategies to improve hospital-based postnatal care. *Women and Birth* 21, pp. 99–105.

Steen, M., Downe, S., Bamford, N., Edozien, L. (2012) Not patient and not-visitor: A meta-synthesis of fathers encounters with pregnancy, birth and maternity care. *Midwifery* 28 (4), pp. 362–371.

UNICEF UK (2013) Baby Friendly Initiative statement on *Bed-sharing when parents do not smoke: is there a risk of SIDS? An individual level analysis of five major case–control studies* [online] Available: http://bmjopen.bmj.com/content/3/5/e002299.full

Walsh, D. (2011) A review of evidence around postnatal care and breastfeeding. *Obstetrics, Gynaecology and Reproductive Medicine* 21 (12), pp. 346–350.

Warren, P.L., McCarthy, G. (2011) maternal parental self-efficacy in the postpartum period. *Midwifery* 27, pp. 802–810.

White, G. (2007) You cope by breaking down in private: fathers and PTSD following childbirth. *British Journal of Midwifery* 15 (1), pp. 39–45.

Wilson, A. (1995) *The Making of Man – Midwifery: Childbirth in England 1660–1770*. Massachusetts: Harvard University Press.

Williams, H., Foster, D., Watts, P. (2013) Perinatal domestic abuse: Midwives making a difference through effective public health practice. *British Journal of Midwifery* 21 (12), pp. 852–858.

Wray, J., Bick, D. (2012) Is there a future for universal midwifery postnatal care in the UK. *MIDIRS Midwifery Digest* 22 (4), pp. 495–498.

187

Chapter 9

Care of the newborn

Liz Smith
University of Hull, Hull, UK

Brenda Waite
Diana Princess of Wales Hospital, Grimsby, UK

Learning outcomes

By the end of this chapter the reader will be able to:

- explain the links between physiological processes in the early days of life and the wellbeing of the newborn baby
- discuss the care of the newborn immediately after birth
- discuss the care of the newborn in the postnatal period
- monitor the wellbeing of the newborn and recognise deviations from the normal
- provide evidence-based information for parents.

Introduction

Although the majority of the care provided to newborn babies is given by their mothers, the midwife still plays an important role in ensuring that the health and wellbeing of the baby is monitored and that mothers and their families are provided with evidence-based information to support them in caring for their new baby. Some babies, although generally healthy, will need extra care and interventions from midwives such as basic resuscitation and screening tests. This chapter will provide an overview of the key aspects of care of the newborn infant. It does not address the care of the preterm or sick neonate, but aims to address the needs of the healthy, term baby whilst providing some insight into recognition of deviations from the normal in the early neonatal period.

Transition to extra-uterine life

Care of the baby following birth and in the postnatal period should be underpinned by knowledge of the process of change associated with a transition from uterine to extra-uterine life. The majority of neonates progress through this complex process without any problems, but those

Fundamentals of Midwifery: A Textbook for Students, First Edition. Edited by Louise Lewis.
© 2015 John Wiley & Sons, Ltd. Published 2015 by John Wiley & Sons, Ltd.
Companion website: www.wileyfundamentalseries.com/midwifery

who do experience difficulties will require appropriate and prompt intervention to minimise the effects on their development. In some cases delay or difficulties associated with transition can be as a result of congenital abnormality such as cardiac anomalies, prematurity or as a result of maternal ill health during pregnancy. These issues are generally known about prior to labour and delivery and therefore the care needs of the infant can be planned for. However it is important that the transition to extra-uterine life is not taken for granted in the absence of known risk factors. Midwives need to be prepared for and skilled in providing newborn resuscitation and recognising deviation from normal progress during the postnatal period. Resuscitation equipment should always be checked regularly to ensure that it is ready for use at all times.

Fetal circulation

Fetal circulation differs from adult circulation in order to facilitate oxygenation and nutrition via the placenta. This is achieved by means of three temporary structures which are:

* **The ductus venosus** which shunts oxygenated blood from the placenta away from the liver.
* **The foramen ovale** which allows oxygenated blood entering the right atria from the placenta via the inferior vena cava to shunt across to the left atria and therefore to enter the systemic circulation and bypass the pulmonary circulation.
* **The ductus arteriosus** which shunts blood from the pulmonary artery into the aorta; this also facilitates oxygenated blood exiting from the right side of the heart entering the systemic circulation and therefore mostly bypassing the lungs.

These fetal structures are essential for ensuring that oxygenated blood is circulated to where it is needed for growth and development. See Figure 9.1 for an illustration of the fetal circulation.

Transition

The transition from fetal circulation to extra-uterine circulation takes approximately a week to 10 days following birth. During labour the contractions and compression of the umbilical cord cause a rise in carbon dioxide and a fall in oxygen levels in the fetal blood; this situation is further exacerbated by clamping and cutting the cord at birth. As a result of this the respiratory centre is stimulated and this along with compression and release of the chest wall during birth stimulate the infant to take its first breath. The lungs expand with the first breaths and there is an associated fall in pulmonary vascular resistance. The decrease in pressure in the right atrium results in constriction and then closure of the ductus venosus. Cutting the umbilical cord causes a rise in systemic blood pressure. The increased flow of blood to the lungs and back to the left atria causes a change of pressure within the heart which causes the 'trapdoor' of the foramen ovale to close; this occurs within 24–48 hours after birth. In some infants this closure does not occur and this may cause problems with disrupted flow of blood in early childhood, or may remain undetected until adulthood. Changes in flow and pressure also cause minimal flow in the ductus arteriosus. The oxygen saturations rise to normal limits as the extra-uterine circulation takes over and this causes a fall in the production of prostaglandin E_2 which results in closure of the ductus during the first week or 10 days of life (see Figure 9.2, which illustrates this process). The ductus is usually obliterated by three weeks of age.

Apgar scoring

The Apgar score was devised by the anaesthetist Virginia Apgar in 1952 and was introduced as a grading system of the newborn to allow a comparison and discussion of the results of obstetric

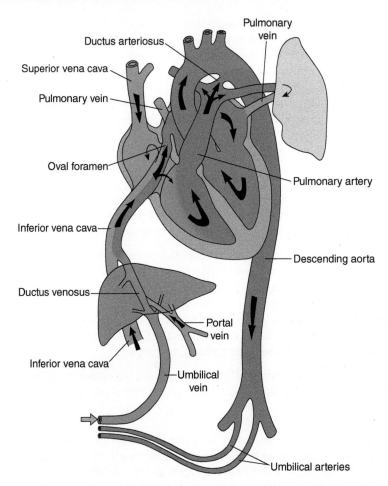

Figure 9.1   Fetal circulation. Source: Sinha et al. 2012, Figure 1.2, p. 3. Reproduced with permission of John Wiley & Sons.

practice, maternal analgesia and effects of resuscitation (Apgar 1953). It utilises a simple scoring system of five features of the infant at birth, which are assessed and recorded at one minute of age and then at five-minute intervals for the duration of any resuscitative measures. These features are heart rate, respiratory effort, response to stimulus, muscle tone and colour, each of which is scored out of two to give an overall score out of ten (Table 9.1).

The National Institute for Health and Care Excellence guideline for intrapartum care (NICE 2007) instructs that the Apgar score at one and five minutes should be recorded routinely, although its value has been questioned and debated (Marlow 1992) because the assessment is made by those involved in the resuscitation and is rarely used contemporaneously to direct how the resuscitation should proceed, but retrospectively using recollection of those present. Other reports suggest that the person conducting the birth should not be the one to evaluate the score as they are often performing other duties and may introduce bias (Montgomery 2000), but in some maternity units this may be the only professional present at the birth. It should not be considered a measure of outcome or prognosis; the score does provide a useful indicator of condition at birth and highlights those babies who need closer monitoring in the early neonatal period. A score of under seven is considered low and under four very low with the lower scores

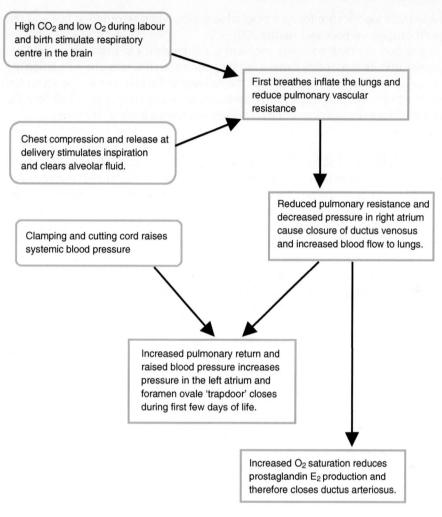

Figure 9.2   Transition to extra-uterine life.

Table 9.1   Agpar scoring

	0	1	2
Heart rate	Absent	<100 bpm	>100 bpm
Respiratory effort	Absent	Slow, irregular	Regular, crying
Tone	Flaccid	Some flexion	Active
Response to stimulus	None	Grimace	Cough, cry
Colour	Blue/pale	Body pink, limbs blue	Pink

having more significance for neurological sequalae when recorded at five and ten minutes of age (Thorngren-Jerneck and Herbst 2001).

In practice, the most common problem is the tendency to evaluate the initial score sooner than one minute as in reality this is a longer period than it seems. The evaluation at five minutes of age may coincide with the timing of the delivery of the placenta and again is often calculated retrospectively, but if no resuscitative measures have been required by this time then the infant has not given any cause for concern and will not have a low Apgar score.

Basic resuscitation of the newborn

It is estimated that only 10% of newborns will require some form of resuscitation (Fernandes 2012), but it is not always possible to predict which babies these will be prior to birth. Midwives Rules and Standards (Nursing and Midwifery Council (NMC) 2012) state that a practising midwife is responsible for care of both woman and child during childbirth therefore every midwife has a responsibility to keep up to date with the principles of basic resuscitation.

If a baby is born and does not spontaneously establish respiration within one minute, further assessment is required. During this first minute the actions of drying the baby and changing to fresh warm towels gives the opportunity to assess colour, tone, heart rate and respiratory effort. The heart rate is the most important of these signs and if this remains above 100 bpm in a baby with reasonable tone, some further time may be allowed for the baby to breathe spontaneously. Most will achieve this within 90 seconds.

If a baby at birth is pale, floppy and bradycardic, then it is likely to need resuscitation, so help should be called for if not already in attendance. Even though this would seem to call for more immediate action, it is important to remember that the initial action of drying and changing to dry warm towels is still vital as hypothermia has a significant effect on the success of resuscitative measures. The only caveat to this is in the event of prematurity where it may be the policy to wrap the infant in an occlusive material such as plastic rather than drying the skin, or if there has been meconium present in the liquor as this is the one situation where suction is indicated and stimulus is initially kept to a minimum.

For a baby with no obvious risk factors prior to birth, who does not commence spontaneous respiration, there are a few basic measures to undertake, the first of which is correct positioning. A newborn skull has a large occiput due to the moulding of the birth process and this has the effect of pushing the head forward when laid flat, thus causing the chin to drop and the airway to become occluded. Placing the head in the neutral position, with the nose pointing directly at the ceiling will correct this, open the airway and may allow spontaneous respiration to occur. If this measure is not enough, the airway may still be partially occluded by the back of the tongue. Poor muscle tone that can be seen in the limbs is likely to be affecting internal structures equally so it is necessary to perform a chin lift by placing a finger under the bony tip of chin (making sure not to press on the soft tissues) or a jaw thrust manoeuvre to pull the bottom jaw forward and move the tongue. This is achieved by applying gentle pressure each side behind the angle of the lower mandible, just below the ears, in a forward motion. This action can be performed with the fingers whilst the thumbs are placed on the cheek bones.

A baby that is still not breathing despite an open airway will need to have their lungs inflated for them. This is performed using a face mask and positive pressure, in the hospital setting provided by a resuscitaire; in the community setting this may be by bag and face mask or portable ventilation equipment. The recommendations are that this is initially performed using air, with the addition of oxygen only if required (World Health Organization (WHO) 2012; Resuscitation Council (UK) 2010).

As it is not possible to predict which babies are going to need assistance to establish respiration, it is important that the equipment has been checked prior to birth and the pressures set
appropriately. The pressure required for initial inflation of the newborn lungs of a term baby is
30 cm/H_2O and to enable the fluid to be pushed back into the circulating volume this needs to
be maintained for two to three seconds. This should be repeated for five inflations and then
reassessment can take place. It is important to watch for chest movement during this procedure
to confirm air entry, but the more certain indicator of successful lung inflation is an increase in
the heart rate. Once lung inflation has been achieved many babies will begin regular respirations, but if not further assistance will be required with ventilation or they will once again
become hypoxic and bradycardic. The same technique is used but these ventilation breaths are
at a rate of 30 per minute so are a shorter duration of only one second with one second gaps.

If regular respiration still does not occur, then further intervention may be required and personnel with further training may need to take over the resuscitation, but efficient use of these
basic methods will maintain the airway until appropriate staff is available. It is important to
inform any personnel involved if the mother has received opiates during her labour as this may
have a respiratory depressant effect on the baby. Other information that may indicate an
increased risk of infection or respiratory problems such as prolonged rupture of membranes or
meconium stained liquor must also be passed on to any incoming personnel (see Figure 9.3,
which illustrates the basic care and resuscitation algorithm for the newborn).

Immediate care of the newborn

For the majority of babies who do not require resuscitation, the immediate transition into extra-
uterine life can be accomplished in a more natural way. The NICE Guideline for Intrapartum Care
(Hutton and Hassan 2007) suggests that if the Apgar score at one minute is five or less then the
cord should be double clamped to enable the collection of paired cord samples to analyse cord
gases; however in other cases early cord clamping is not recommended. Very early cord clamping has been suggested to contribute to hypovolaemia and anaemia and a delay in cord clamping of at least two minutes has been shown in a review of controlled trials to improve the
haematological and iron status of the term infant in both the short and long term, up to six
months of age (Hutton and Hassan 2007). The concerns of a higher haematocrit and increased
jaundice due to the placental transfusion resulting from delayed clamping were not found to
have any clinical significance even when active management of the third stage is undertaken.
The Resuscitation Council UK (2010) recommend for uncompromised babies, a delay in cord
clamping of at least one minute from the complete delivery of the infant.

A further important contributor towards this transition is the use of skin-to-skin contact with
the mother. which involves placing the naked infant prone on the mother's chest. Studies have
found numerous benefits of skin-to-skin contact immediately after birth for mother and baby
including stabilisation of the cardiovascular system, better thermoregulation, higher blood
glucose levels, earlier initiation of breastfeeding, and a reduction in crying and improved breastfeeding rates up to four months of age (Moore et al. 2012). It is important to note that this same
review highlighted some factors that may impact on the effectiveness of skin-to-skin care such
as room temperature, modesty and lack of privacy. Therefore the midwife should endeavour to
create an environment conducive to this practice whilst respecting the fact that the decision to
do so is ultimately the mother's choice. If undertaken, it is important to ensure a few simple
measures are utilised. The infant will need to be dried and a cover placed over mother and baby
as heat loss will occur via wet skin due to evaporation and from cooler air draughts through
convection. To prevent heat loss via conduction and radiation, the contact with the mother

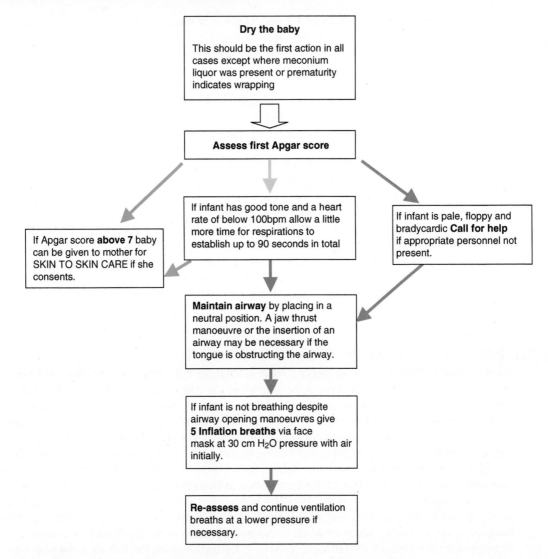

Figure 9.3 Basic care and resuscitation of the newborn.

should be directly on the skin and not through clothing or bed covers. The head will need to be covered with either a cover or hat as this area loses the most heat. (See Table 9.3 for more information regarding heat loss mechanisms.) Necessary procedures such as weighing the baby (see Figure 9.5) should ideally occur prior to commencement of skin-to-skin or very soon afterwards with the infant being returned to mother directly, to enable the early initiation of breast-feeding where appropriate; other procedures such as measurements and initial examination may be performed whilst allowing skin-to-skin contact to continue.

An initial examination of the newborn infant for any obvious abnormalities should be carried out by the midwife following birth. This should include a head to toe check done with the parents' consent and ideally in their presence (NICE 2006). A more comprehensive examination will be carried out prior to discharge, but this initial examination remains vital in the early

Table 9.2   Examining the newborn infant

Head	Moulding (overriding of the bones of the skull) and caput succedaneum (oedema of the scalp) are common but generally resolve within 48 hours. Parents will often need reassurance that their baby's misshapen head is not a sign of abnormality. However excessive moulding or cephalhaematoma (bleeding between the periosteum and the bone) should be noted and the baby observed for any signs of cerebral birth trauma.
Face	Abnormal facial appearance may indicate conditions such as palsy or syndromes (e.g. Edward's) but it is sensible to see both parents before placing too much weight on appearance alone. Any marks from instrumental delivery should be explained to parents.
Eyes	Always check that both eyes are present as this cannot be ascertained when the eyelids are closed.
Ears	The position of the ears should be noted as low set ears are associated with some syndromes.
Mouth	Checking that the palate is properly formed without a cleft is important. Inserting a clean to feel the palate is a common method of choice or inspect with a light which may reveal a sub-mucus cleft. Visualisation is essential to ensure smaller clefts are not missed. Inspection of the mouth also gives the midwife some idea of the sucking reflex (see Figure 9.4).
Genitalia	Check for any obvious abnormality.
Anus	Check for position and apparent patency.
Back	Run a finger down the spine to check for any indentations or swellings. Some babies may have an area of blue discolouration around the sacrum and buttock area; this is particularly common in some racial groups and is normal.
Limbs	Check fingers and toes for missing or extra digits and for any webbing.

recognition of gross abnormality and also in beginning the process of parent education in the care of their new infant.

In addition to examining the baby as detailed in Table 9.2, the baby should be weighed and measurements of head circumference (occipito-frontal circumference) and length should be taken. These measurements should be considered against 'norms' for gestational age, but it should be remembered that moulding may affect head circumference. It is generally accepted practice to gain consent for administration of vitamin K at this time (NICE 2006). Vitamin K is essential for effective blood clotting and is given to prevent rare but life-threatening haemorrhagic disease of the newborn. It is ideally given as an intramuscular injection (1 mg) but if parents are unwilling to consent to this method of administration NICE guidance (NICE 2006) suggests offering oral treatment as an option (see Chapter 15: 'Pharmacology and medicines management' and refer to the monographs where vitamin K is discussed in more depth). If parents decline vitamin K, they should be provided with advice about symptoms that would indicate possible vitamin K deficiency bleeding. These symptoms include: bleeding, bruising or petichiae unrelated to any known trauma and symptoms associated with intracranial bleeding (irritability, high pitched crying, pallor, loss of appetite, vomiting).

Maintaining health in the first few days of life

It is essential in the first few days of life that the infant is kept warm and that feeding is established. Any deviations from the normal should be recognised quickly and appropriate action taken. The care provided should be aimed at keeping the baby PINK, WARM AND SWEET. This is because

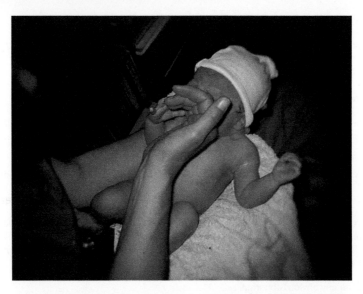

Figure 9.4   Illustrates finger insertion to examine for cleft palate. Source: Chapman and Charles 2013, Figure 5.3, p. 94. Reproduced with permission of John Wiley & Sons.

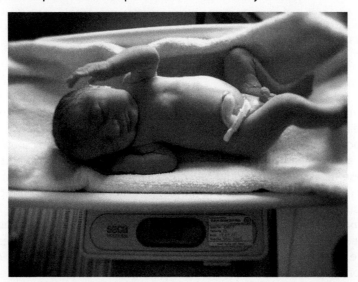

Figure 9.5   Newborn being weighed. Source: Chapman and Charles 2013, Figure 5.2, p. 90. Reproduced with permission of John Wiley & Sons.

these factors will are closely linked to the overall health of the baby. A cold baby will use up energy trying to keep warm; this will burn up the limited energy stores causing low blood sugars (hypoglycaemia) and will also increase oxygen demand which therefore increases respiratory rate. The increased respiratory rate will also increase energy demand and lower blood sugars even further and the lack of available energy to burn will reduce temperature further making the baby significantly hypothermic, hypoglycaemic and demonstrating signs of respiratory distress including cyanosis. As shown in Figure 9.6, the cycle can start at any point as the interactions between temperature, blood sugar and respiratory effort work in both directions.

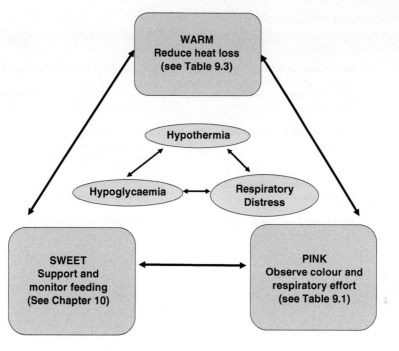

Figure 9.6 The relationship between temperature, blood sugar and respiratory function.

Infant feeding is addressed in Chapter 10; therefore the focus here is in keeping the baby at an appropriate temperature and the recognition of respiratory symptoms.

WHO (1997) recommend that the normal temperature of an infant in the first few days of life should be between 36.5 and 37.5°C; however since good practice requires neonatal tempera-tures to be taken under the axilla, slightly lower temperatures are acceptable. NICE (2006) rec-ommend the normal temperature for a baby should be around 37°C. A baby with cool skin, pallor and any increase in respiratory rate and/or grunting should have his/her temperature checked. Newborn babies are at risk of heat loss because they have a relatively high surface area in comparison with their weight; however the risk of chilling can be reduced by under-standing how heat is lost (see Table 9.3).

At rest the newborn respiratory rate is around 30–40 breaths per minute (England 2010a) Normal respiration should be easy and relatively quiet.

It is important that midwives should be able to recognise abnormal breathing behaviour in order that early intervention minimises further deterioration (see Box 9.1).

Postnatal care of the baby should therefore be to ensure that feeding is established and the baby is in a suitably warm, draught free environment. Regular checks of wellbeing should be made to monitor colour and breathing. Parents should be provided with advice and guidance with regard to the right environment for the baby at home (too hot is also detrimental to well-being) and about reporting any concerns regarding breathing and feeding to their midwife and/or General Practitioner.

Skin care and hygiene of the newborn

There has been much debate over the years regarding bathing and general skin care in relation to neonates. Bathing the baby as soon as possible after delivery was thought to reduce the risk

Table 9.3   Mechanisms of heat loss in newborn infants

Mechanism	Description	Prevention
Evaporation	Occurs when the baby is wet and the water on the skin is converted to vapour on contact with the air with associated loss of heat	Drying the baby at delivery and wrapping in warm towels. Similarly if the baby is bathed prompt drying and dressing will reduce heat loss.
Conduction	Heat is lost by contact with a cooler surface.	Weighing scales, resuscitaires and hands should be warmed before coming into contact with the baby.
Convection	Heat is lost due to movement of air over the surface of the skin.	Doors and windows should be closed and draughts avoided.
Radiation	Heat is lost from the exposed skin of the baby to surrounding cooler surfaces.	Ensure the baby is not placed near cooler surfaces such as windows.

Box 9.1   Symptoms of respiratory distress

- Tachypnoea – respiratory rate higher than 40 breaths per minute usually 60 or above.
- Nasal flaring – as the baby tries to draw more air in to meet its increasing needs there is flaring of the nostrils.
- Recession – the extra effort made to increase respiratory rate and air entry causes recession of the intercostals muscles.
- Grunting – this is an expiratory sound made by breathing against a closed glottis.
- Poor colour – this may be demonstrated by mottling, central cyanosis or pallor.

of infection, particularly that due to blood-borne pathogens such as HIV, and the use of products such as baby powder was commonplace. A better understanding of neonatal skin and infection has changed practice, particularly in respect of immediately after birth, but there is still debate about the use of bathing and skin care products (Hale 2007).

Newborn skin is thinner than adult skin and is more prone to irritation or allergic reactions. As skin is a significant part of the infant's limited immune system it is vital that it is protected as much as possible. However, there is only limited evidence in relation to whether the use of bathing and skin care products disrupt the function and/or integrity of the skin, and parental choice has to be a factor in decision-making (Hale 2007; Hughes 2011). WHO (2006) recommend that the newborn baby is not bathed for at least six hours following birth and that any vernix is not removed as it has antiseptic as well as moisturising properties. NICE (2006) recommends that infants are bathed in plain water only, but some authors (Walters et al. 2008; Blume-Peytavi et al. 2009) suggest that plain water is inadequate for ensuring cleansing of the nappy area and that the high mineral content of some tap water may cause irritation. Steen and Macdonald (2008) suggest that parents may want to use skin cleansers because they believe they are more effective and due to the influence of gifts and free samples. It is important therefore that parents are provided with as much advice as possible with regard to their choice of skin products for their baby. Box 9.2 summarises some of the guidance around newborn skin care.

Box 9.2   Skin care product guidance

- Soap should be avoided as it disrupts the skin's natural lipid barrier.
- When skin cleansers and products are gradually introduced, they should be free from sulphates, colours and perfumes.
- Avoid the use of cloths or sponges as these may rub and damage the skin.
- Hand washing the baby or using cotton wool or a natural sponge is gentler.
- Baby wipes should be avoided in the first month. Once gradually introduced, they should be alcohol and fragrance free.
- It is safer to bath the newborn in plain water for at least the first month of life.
- Oils containing perfume or dye should not be used and nut and petroleum-based oils should be avoided.

(Trotter 2010)

Nappy care

Gentle cleansing of the nappy area at each nappy change with plain, warm water and cotton wool is key to preventing or at least minimising the risk of nappy rash. Trotter (2010) recommends washing the nappy area with warm water and the application of a thin layer of a barrier cream. Trotter (2008) suggests any barrier cream should be fragrance and antiseptic free. As noted in Box 9.3, the use of baby wipes are not recommended for at least the first month of life (Trotter 2008; 2010).

Cord care

The evidence available currently clearly suggests that the best method of cord care is to keep it as clean and dry as possible without the use of sprays, creams and powders as these may well inhibit rather than assist natural separation (Trotter 2010; Hughes 2011; Zupan et al. 2012). Hand washing before handling the cord is essential to minimise the risk of colonisation by pathogens and keeping the cord free of the nappy area to prevent contamination by urine or faeces. A small amount of moisture at the base of the cord is normal, and should not be mistaken for infection (Trotter 2010).

Parents are often nervous of the umbilical cord stump and should be reassured about drying it carefully when bathing the baby. They should also be provided with information regarding the normal process of separation, both to prevent unnecessary worrying and to allow them to recognise potential infection.

Jaundice

Physiological jaundice

Physiological jaundice is a common newborn problem that rarely needs active intervention, although it can sometimes require investigation and active management (Gordan and Lomax (2011). The presence of certain risk factors can increase the severity and frequency of physiological jaundice, for example; low birth weight and prematurity (Gordan and Lomax 2011). It arises due to the immaturity of the liver at a time when there is increased production of bilirubin due to the breakdown of excess red blood cells. In utero the fetus needs extra red blood cells to accommodate the relatively low oxygenation provided by the placenta, but once delivered and breathing spontaneously a reduction of approximately 20% is made to bring the cell count to normal limits. The liver is responsible for bilirubin metabolism and its immaturity in the neonatal period means that the process is inefficient leading to circulating bilirubin being deposited in the subcutaneous fat – it is this deposition under the skin that causes the yellow discolouration of jaundice. Bilirubin processed by the liver changes from being fat soluble (unconjugated) to water soluble (conjugated) and is passed into the gastrointestinal system via the gall bladder. Some conjugated bilirubin will be absorbed via the gut wall and will be excreted via the kidneys giving the urine its characteristic straw colour. The rest is excreted in the faeces. In the newborn, however, the intestinal process is impeded by the lack of gut bacteria and relatively slow peristalsis and this results in conjugated bilirubin being converted back to unconjugated and reabsorbed to be returned to the liver. This process is illustrated in Figure 9.7. Physiological jaundice generally occurs around the third after birth and peaks around the fourth and fifth day resolving by the seventh to tenth day (England 2010b). Visible early jaundice in the first 24 hours of life is strongly associated with haematological disease such as rhesus incompatibility or red cell abnormality.

Physiological jaundice is not usually dangerous in itself, as it is self-limiting in that once the reduction in red blood cells has been achieved, the production of bilirubin will return to levels the liver can manage effectively. However, there is always a risk that it masks a more pathological process associated with liver or haematological disorder or congenital abnormality. It is vital therefore that any jaundice in the newborn is taken seriously and that babies who may be at greater risk from complications are identified. NICE (2010) recommend a pathway approach to the care of babies with visible jaundice and that all such babies have the serum bilirubin measured. The measurement of serum bilirubin in jaundiced babies is important as high levels can result in a condition known as kernicterus or bilirubin encephalopathy, which will have neurodevelopment consequences for the affected baby. Levels of bilirubin which do not cause encephalopathy can nevertheless cause auditory impairment.

Levels of serum bilirubin can be measured by means of a capillary blood sample (obtained by a heel prick) or by transcutaneous bilirubinometer. Although the latter is non-invasive, it is an expensive piece of equipment and midwives need training in its use; therefore this method may not be available in all units. A reading deemed high on a bilirubinometer would necessitate a blood test to provide a more accurate clinical picture. NICE (2010) guidance provides a graph with regard to levels of bilirubin that require treatment in the term baby to better standardise initiation of treatment and thereby improve outcomes for significantly affected babies. Treatment, should it be required, is to use blue-green light to break down bilirubin in the skin. The blue-green light can either be delivered by an overhead phototherapy unit placed over the cot or incubator in which the baby is nursed, naked except for a nappy and eye protection, or a slightly less effective biliblanket which can be wrapped around the baby who does not need eye protection from this method.

Breastfeeding jaundice

Some babies who are breastfed may demonstrate higher bilirubin levels than formula-fed infants, and their jaundice may be more prolonged. This is thought to be due to the lower fluid and calorific intake associated with breastfeeding in the first few days of life which increases entero-hepatic shunting. The slower colonisation of the gut with bacteria in breastfed babies also contributes to higher bilirubin levels. It is thought that this may occur to utilise the antioxidant properties of unconjugated bilirubin and provided that the baby is feeding well and gaining sufficient calories and the jaundice is monitored carefully, there will be no adverse

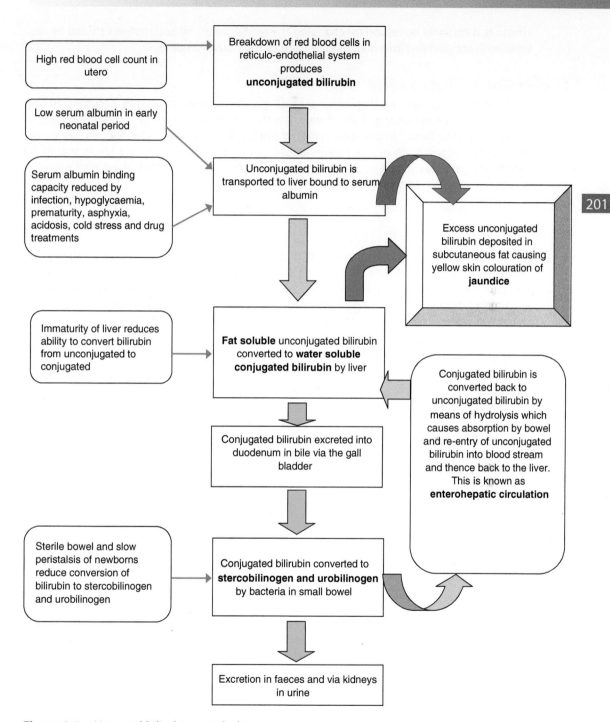

Figure 9.7   Neonatal bilirubin metabolism.

effects. It is certainly no reason for changing the feeding method and mothers should be provided with support and information in relation to their breastfeeding.

Breastmilk jaundice syndrome

This jaundice is later in onset than either physiological or breastfeeding types, occurring around 4 days postnatal and peaking at 10–15 days. It is thought that this type of jaundice is related to be due to specific factors in the breastmilk and can last for between 3–12 weeks. Babies should be medically assessed to rule out pathological causes of the jaundice and levels should be monitored, but the syndrome is rarely associated with complications. Again there is no evidence to support cessation of breastfeeding.

Neonatal screening

It is the role of the midwife to ensure that women are provided with accurate information regarding newborn screening tests so that they can make informed choices for their babies. This information giving should commence antenatally but should also be provided postnatally in a timely fashion to allow screening tests to be carried out at the optimum time.

The blood spot test

This test is offered to all mothers and should ideally be taken on day 5 (taking the day of delivery as day 0) (UK Newborn Screening Centre, 2012) but should be within 5–8 days of birth in term infants who have been feeding normally (there are specific guidelines for preterm or sick infants who have not been enterally feeding). Recommendations from the UK Newborn Screening Centre (UK NSC) suggest that it provides screening for:

* phenylketonuria (PKU)
* congenital hypothyroidism (CHT)
* sickle cell disease (SCD)
* cystic fibrosis (CF)
* medium-chain acyl-CoA dehydrogenase deficiency (MCADD).

Throughout the UK the blood spot test is used to screen for PKU, cystic fibrosis and hypothyroidism with some areas adding tests for MCADD, unusual haemoglobins (e.g. sickle cell) and galactosaemia (Wylie 2010). The purpose of the universal screening by this means is to detect disease as early as possible and therefore gain early referral and treatment which improves the outcome for the affected baby. Informed parental consent is essential and the blood sample must be taken safely and according to the protocol or there will be a requirement to repeat the sample causing both baby and parents unnecessary distress. The UK Newborn Screening Centre (2012) has published clear and detailed guidelines for professionals and information for parents and families (Activity 9.1).

Further reading activity

Read the Newborn Bloodspot Guidelines [Available online] http://newbornbloodspot.screening .nhs.uk/bloodspotsampling

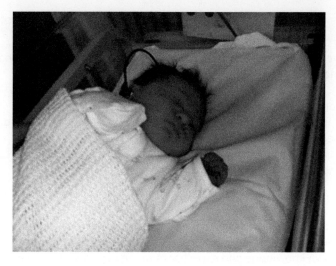

Figure 9.8   Baby receiving a hearing screen in the hospital, note the ear piece.

Newborn hearing screening

It is estimated that 1–3 of every 1000 newborn babies will be affected by congenital hearing loss which can be caused by neurological or conductive disorder. The hearing loss is mostly genetic in origin, but can also be caused by intrauterine infection (particularly cytomegalovirus) or prematurity. The universal screening programme has been in place in the UK since 2005, as early detection of deafness reduces its impact on language development. The test is generally carried out before the baby leaves hospital by trained personnel but can also be carried out in the home by health visitors and involves a small earpiece being inserted into the baby's ear (see Figure 9.8). Two painless screening tests are carried out – the otoacoustic emissions test and the automated auditory brainstem response test – These will diagnose moderate to profound hearing loss.

✐ Further reading activity

Read about the NHS Newborn Hearing Screening Programme [Available online] http://hearing.screening.nhs.uk/

Advice for parents

Parents rely on healthcare professionals, particularly midwives, to provide them with relevant information to enable them to keep their babies as safe as possible. As with all midwifery care this has to be tailored to individual needs. It should always include the information listed in Box 9.3, but questioning parents about issues that may concern them is also good practice. It is important to make sure that they feel they can discuss their worries without feeling silly as many parents feel that they should know how to care for their baby but in reality they have little knowledge and experience of small babies.

Box 9.3   Advice for parents

- Cot death prevention information particularly in relation to positioning and co-sleeping (see Chapter 8 for more details)
- Car safety
- Appropriate room temperature and clothing guidance
- Sterilising equipment (even if breastfeeding as breast pumps and bottles for expressed breast milk may be used)
- How to contact appropriate health care professionals in the event of any concerns about the health of the baby

All the advice provided to parents must be based on current evidence and where necessary midwives should utilise other members of the multidisciplinary team to provide information outside their own knowledge and expertise. A range of printed material is available and should be used to support the information given where appropriate; it is essential this is provided in appropriate format e.g. large print and other languages if necessary.

Detailed neonatal examination by the midwife

The more comprehensive examination advised by the National Screening Committee (NSC) (2008; Public Health England 2013) has traditionally been undertaken by a paediatrician, but has now been incorporated as an extended role of the midwife who has undertaken further training to qualify for this. Some of the reasons reported why a midwife was preferred were: they impart more information whilst performing the examination; they spend more time at it; and they are often someone the mother knows. Part of the preparation for the examination should be gaining a good history, including a review of the maternal medical notes to highlight any risk factors that may need to be discussed with the parents (Tappero and Honeyfield 2003). It is here that a midwife undertaking the examination may also have an advantage over a paediatrician as they are likely to be already aware of the history from antenatal and intrapartum care.

The recommendation is for this full examination to be performed within 24 hours of birth, but some consideration should be given to the timing of the procedure. NICE 2006 guidelines recommend the full examination is done within 72 hours of birth and is repeated at the end of the postnatal period. As this examination has a greater chance of detecting a problem, it is of benefit to have both parents present or some alternative support for the mother. The midwife who is ward-based is more likely to be able to alter her schedule to enable this rather than a paediatrician with other time constraints and neonatal unit commitments.

On introduction to the parents, an explanation of and consent for the examination must be undertaken. Informed consent is a requirement for any procedure undertaken by a midwife (NMC, 2008) and for this consent to be valid, a number of facts must be made clear to the parents. It is important that parents are made aware that it is a midwife with further training who is undertaking the examination. Baston and Durward (2010) highlight that if parents are expecting a procedure to be performed by a doctor and are not made aware that it is not, this will render the consent invalid. Where it is an option, they should be offered the opportunity to have a paediatrician perform the examination if preferred. It should be explained that this is a screening test and as such may detect a problem. It has been suggested that similar to the ultrasound scans that are undertaken in early pregnancy, the parents are often not prepared for the fact an abnormality may be detected (Baston and Durward 2010). This information should be given along with an explanation that if any concerns are highlighted they will be given further opportunity to discuss the problems and ask questions with a paediatrician. It is important to inform the parents that this examination may not detect some conditions which do not become apparent until later and they will be offered a further examination at 6 to 8 weeks (Davis and Elliman 2008). It should also be explained that if the examination is being performed after only six hours, there may be some anomalies detected that will not be found on a subsequent examination, such as a lax hip joint or soft heart murmur. It is useful to detail the four areas which will be examined in more detail than the initial examination: eyes, heart, hips and testes in boys with a brief explanation of the conditions being screened for. This intro-duction period also presents a useful time for more history gathering as the parents can be asked about any family history or observation of their new baby that has given them any cause for concern. Another good reason for waiting until both parents are present is that during this time observation of the parents' facial features may explain what could otherwise have been considered anomalies in the infant (Baston and Durward 2010).

Communication appeared to be the key area where the midwives performing this examina-tion were appreciated more than the doctors (Murray et al. 2006). Having to break bad news to new parents is a very difficult thing to do and Robb (1999) suggests that parents do not always remember the exact words used to inform them of their baby's disability, but they do remember the general approach and the staff's attitude so this is a vital time and there is only one chance at it.

Although it would seem midwives are ideally placed to undertake this role, many midwives once qualified to perform this examination do not continue to practise this extended role (Steele 2007). Midwives have expressed a great deal of satisfaction in being able to deliver a complete package of care to their women (Mitchell 2003a) but a number of reasons why they did not perform this task were highlighted in a study by Steele (2007) and included a lack of support from peers and managers, work pressures and staffing levels. Interestingly, the pre-sumed fear of litigation if an abnormality is not detected (Baston and Durward 2010) was not put forward as a reason, but is a point worth clarifying as all professionals undertaking this role must be aware of their responsibility. The EMREN study (Townsend et al. 2004) which evaluated this extension to the midwives' role concluded that there was no statistical difference between SHO paediatricians and midwives, either in appropriate or inappropriate referrals, or in prob-lems identified or not identified. So if mothers are expressing more satisfaction with the mid-wives, this is a valuable role for midwives to undertake, and they should endeavour to liaise with medical colleagues and midwifery management to provide opportunities to keep up their skills (Mitchell 2003b).

Key points

- Care of the newborn baby requires knowledge of normal physiology during the neonatal period in order to recognise any deviation from the normal.
- Midwives should provide parents with appropriate, evidence-based information in order for the them to make informed choices and provide safe care for their baby.
- Care needs to be individualised and take into account maternal history, needs and understanding.

Conclusion

Care of the newborn baby is an essential element of the midwives' role and includes both monitoring the health and wellbeing of the baby and educating and supporting parents in caring for their new baby. Understanding normal physiology, particularly in relation to the transition from intrauterine to extrauterine life, is vital in recognising deviations from the normal. A good knowledge of the evidence supporting care of the newborn is also essential to effective midwifery care. Care needs to take into account antenatal and intrapartum issues that may affect the neonate and the individual needs of the parents and family. Good communication and record keeping are as ever central to good midwifery practice.

206

End of chapter activities
Crossword

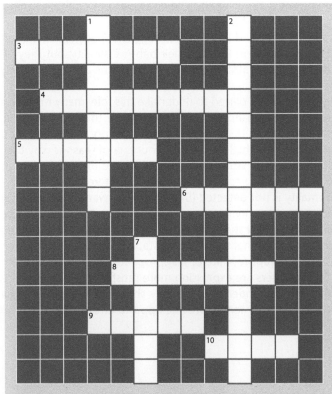

Across

3. The ductus which shunts blood away. from the liver in utero.
4. Jaundice is caused by this substance.
5. This action should be the first element of immediate care of the newborn baby.
6. A cold baby will use this to try and keep warm.
8. Screening test offered to all newborns since 2005.
9. Scoring method used for infant's condition at birth.
10. Ideal colour for a newborn.

Down

1. Overriding of the skull bones is known as this.
2. One of the diseases the blood spot screening test detects.

7. One of the measurements taken following delivery.

Find out more

Below is a list of things you can find out about to enhance your knowledge of the issues and topics covered in this chapter. Make notes using the chapter content, the references and further reading identified, local policies and guidelines, and discussions with colleagues.

1. Familiarise yourself with the neonatal resuscitation equipment in your placement delivery suite.

2. Reflect on the determination of Apgar scores for births you have attended particularly in relation to timing and accuracy.

3. Find out what advice is given to mothers regarding skin care products for babies in your placement area.

4. Find out about your local guideline for the management of neonatal jaundice.

5. Find out more about local practices for screening of the newborn.

Glossary of terms

Apgar score   An internationally recognised scoring system for the condition of the baby at birth which scores heart rate, respirations, muscular tone, colour and response to stimulus.

Caput succedaneum   Oedematous swelling of the scalp due to pressure during delivery.

Cephalhaematoma   Bleeding under the periosteum (outer layer) of a skull bone.

Conduction   Heat loss to cold surfaces.

Convection   Heat loss due to cold draughts.

Evaporation   Heat loss due to wet skin.

Grunting   The sound of expiration when the glottis is partially closed which is associated with respiratory distress.

Hypoglycaemia   blood sugar below normal limits

Hypothermia   A body temperature below normal limits.

Hypothyroidism   Low levels of thyroid hormone which can cause intellectual impairment if untreated.

Jaundice   Yellow discolouration of the skin and mucous membranes due to subcutaneous bilirubin deposits.

Moulding   Slight overlapping of the skull bones to facilitate passage through the birth canal.

Phenylketonuria (PKU)   A metabolic disease that untreated will cause brain damage.

Physiological jaundice   Jaundice due to immaturity of the neonatal liver and the breakdown of fetal haemoglobin which should not reach levels sufficient to cause harm in an otherwise well baby.

Radiation   Heat loss to surrounding cooler surfaces.

Transition   The physiological changes necessary for the baby to progress from intrauterine to extrauterine life.

References

Apgar, V. (1953) A proposal for a new method of evaluation of the newborn infant. *Current Researches in Anesthesia and Analgesia* July–August, pp. 260–267.

Baston, H., Durward, H. (2010) *Examination of the Newborn. A Practical Guide*. London: Routledge.

Blume-Peytavi, U., Cork, M.J., et al (2009) Bathing and cleansing in newborns from day 1 to first year of life: recommendations from a European round table meeting. *Journal of the European Academy Dermatology and Venereology* 23 (7), pp. 751–759.

Chapman, V., Charles, C. (2013). The *Midwife's Labour and Birth Handbook*, 3rd edn. Oxford: John Wiley & Sons Ltd.

Davis, A., Elliman, D. (2008) Newborn Examination: Setting Standards for Consistency. *Infant* 4 (4) pp. 116–120.

England, C. (2010a) Neonatal respiratory problems. In: Lumsden, H., Holmes, D. (eds) (2010) *Care of the Newborn by Ten Teachers*. London: Hodder Arnold.

England, C. (2010b) Care of the jaundiced baby In: Lumsden, H. Holmes, D. (eds) (2010) *Care of the Newborn by Ten Teachers*. London: Hodder Arnold.

Fernandes, C.J. (2012) Neonatal resuscitation in the delivery room [online] Available: http://www.uptodate.com/contents/neonatal-resuscitation-in-the-delivery-room

Gordan, M., Lomax, A. (2011) The Neonatal Skin: examination of the Jaundiced Newborn and Gestational Age Assessment In (Lomax, A. (2010) (ed.) *Examination of the newborn: an evidenced-based guide*. Chichester: Wiley-Blackwell.

Hale, R. (2007) Protecting neonates' delicate skin. *British Journal of Midwifery* 15 (4), pp. 231–235.

Hughes, K. (2011) Neonatal skin care: Advocating good practice in skin protection. *British Journal of Midwifery* 19 (12), pp. 773–775.

Hutton, E.K., Hassan, E.S. (2007) Late vs. early clamping of the umbilical cord in full-term neonate: systematic review and meta-analysis of controlled trials. *Journal of the American Medical Association (JAMA)* March 297 (11), pp. 1241–1252.

Marlow, N. (1992) Do we need an Apgar score? *Fetal and Neonatal Edition Archives of Disease in Childhood* 67, pp. 765–769.

Mitchell, M. (2003a) Midwives conducting the neonatal examination: part 1. *British Journal of Midwifery* 11 (1), pp. 16–21.

Mitchell, M. (2003b) Midwives conducting the neonatal examination: part 2. *British Journal of Midwifery* 11 (2), pp. 80–84.

Montgomery, K.S. (2000) Apgar scores: examining the long-term significance. *Journal of Perinatal Education* 9 (3), pp. 5–9.

Moore, E.R., Anderson, G.C., Bergman, N., Dowswell, T. (2012) Early skin-to-skin contact for mothers and their healthy newborn infants Cochrane Library [online] available: http://onlinelibrary.wiley.com/doi/10.1002/14651858.CD003519.pub3/full 18th March 2013.

Murray, K., Hamilton, S., Martin, D. (2006) Delivering Effective Communication. *The Practising Midwife* 9 (4), pp. 24–26.

National Institute for Health and Clinical Excellence (NICE) (2006) Postnatal Care: Routine postnatal care of women and their babies (CG37). London: NICE.

National Institute for Health and Clinical Excellence (NICE) (2008) Intrapartum care: care of healthy women and their babies during childbirth. London: NICE:

National Institute for Health and Clinical Excellence (NICE) (2010) Quick Reference Guide: Neonatal Jaundice CG98. London: NICE.

National Screening Committee (2008) Newborn and Infant Physical Examination Standards and Competencies. London: NSC.

Nursing and Midwifery Council (NMC) (2008) The Code: Standards of Conduct, Performance and Ethics for Nurses and Midwives. London: NMC.

Nursing and Midwifery Council (NMC) (2012) Midwives Rules and Standards. London: NMC.

Public Health England (2013) NHS Newborn and Infant Physical Screening Programme [online] Available: http://newbornphysical.screening.nhs.uk

Resuscitation Council (UK) (2010) Resuscitation at Birth: Newborn Life Support. London: Resuscitation Council UK.

Robb, F. (1999) Congenital malformations: breaking the bad news. *British Journal of Midwifery* 7 (1), pp. 26–31.

Sinha, S., Miall, L., Jardine, L. (2012). *Essential Neonatal Medicine*, 5th edn. Oxford: John Wiley & Sons.

Steele, D. (2007) Examining the Newborn: Why don't Midwives use their skills? *British Journal of Midwifery* 15, pp. 748–752.

Steen, M., Macdonald, S. (2008) A review of baby skin care. Midwives [online] Available: http://www.rcm.org.uk/midwives/in-depth-papers/a-review-of-baby-skin-care/

Tappero, E.P., Honeyfield, M.E. (2003) *Physical Assessment of the Newborn. A Comprehensive Approach to the Art of Physical Examination*, 3rd edn. California: Nicu.Ink.

Thorngren-Jerneck, K., Herbst, A. (2001) Low 5-minute Apgar Score: A Population-Based Register Study of 1 Million Term Births. *The American College of Obstetrics and Gynaecologists* 98 (1), pp. 65–70.

Townsend, J., Wolke, D., Hayes, J., et al. (2004) *Health Technology Assessment* 8 (14), Health Technology Assessment NHS R&D HTA Programme.

Trotter, S. (2010) Neonatal skin care. In: Lumsden, H., Holmes, D. (eds) (2010) *Care of the Newborn by Ten Teachers*. London: Hodder Arnold.

Trotter, S. (2008) *Baby Care – Back to Basics*. Troon: TIPS Ltd.

UK Newborn Screening Centre (2012) Guidelines for Blood Spot Sampling. London: UK NSC.

Walters, R.M., Fevola, M.J., LiBrizzi, J.J., Martin, K. (2008) Designing cleansers for the unique needs of baby skin. *Cosmet Toilet* 123 (12), pp. 53–60.

World Health Organization (WHO) (2012) Guidelines on Basic Newborn Resuscitation. Geneva: WHO.

WHO (2006) *Pregnancy, Child Birth, Postpartum and Newborn Care*, 2nd edn. Geneva: WHO.

WHO (1997) Thermal Protection of the Newborn: A Practical Guide. Geneva: WHO:

Wylie, L. (2010) Newborn screening and immunization. In: Lumsden, H., Holmes, D. (eds) (2010) *Care of the Newborn by Ten Teachers*. London: Hodder Arnold.

Zupan, J., Garner, P., Omari, A.A.A. (2012) Topical umbilical cord care at birth. *The Cochrane Collaboration*. Chichester: John Wiley & Sons.

209

Chapter 10

Infant feeding

Louise Lewis
University of Hull, Hull, UK

Liz Mason
Women and Children's Hospital, Hull, UK

Learning outcomes

By the end of this chapter the reader will be able to:

- apply the Baby Friendly Initiative best practice standards to clinical practice
- recognise why breastfeeding is important for mother and baby
- understand the basic anatomy of the breast and physiology of lactation
- recognise the bio-psycho-social needs of mothers in their infant feeding choices
- identify how midwives and other healthcare workers can support mothers to initiate and sustain effective breastfeeding
- identify and manage common breastfeeding problems
- explain the principles of safe formula feeding.

Introduction

Infant feeding choices are entrenched within an array of social, cultural and political factors and are influenced by knowledge, expectations and the support received. Consequently infant feeding seems to elicit emotive responses in mothers, healthcare professionals and society. It is central to the role and responsibilities of a midwife to ensure that babies are receiving adequate nutrition and hydration, and that mothers are receiving information and educational intervention which supports effective infant feeding. This chapter provides evidence-based knowledge and practical skills to apply in maternity care, supporting the principles of safe infant feeding with the use of professional standards and relevant evidence.

Fundamentals of Midwifery: A Textbook for Students, First Edition. Edited by Louise Lewis.
© 2015 John Wiley & Sons, Ltd. Published 2015 by John Wiley & Sons, Ltd.
Companion website: www.wileyfundamentalseries.com/midwifery

Why breastfeeding is important

Breastfeeding is an interdependent relationship between the mother and baby, often described as a dyad. It is viewed as the gold standard for infant nutrition during the first 6 months of life (Godfrey and Lawrence 2010). The benefits to both mother and baby of breast over formula milk are universally acknowledged, with well-developed evidence quantifying the risks of not breastfeeding for both the baby and the mother. Breastfeeding the baby is associated with a reduction in acute otitis media, gastrointestinal disease, respiratory disease, dermatitis, asthma, obesity in later life, type 1 and 2 diabetes mellitus, childhood leukaemia, sudden infant death syndrome and necrotising enterocolitis in the pre-term baby (Fewtrew 2004; Ip et al. 2007; Riordan 2010; Lawrence and Lawrence 2011). More recent studies have demonstrated breast-feeding is related to improved neurological development (Herba et al. 2012; Quigley 2013) and an increased chance of upward social mobility (Sacker et al. 2013), with increased risk of poorer cognitive development and behavioural problems in children who are not breastfed (Heikkilä et al. 2011).

211

The World Health Organization (WHO) recommends exclusive breastfeeding from birth to six months of age, with breastfeeding continuing to be part of the infant's diet until at least two years of age (WHO 2002). However, some mothers may make an informed choice to express their breastmilk and feed it to their baby by a bottle and teat; practitioners also need to be knowledgeable in supporting mothers who choose this method. Although the benefits to mothers are not as well-researched, there is enough evidence to confirm that women who breastfeed up to and beyond one year can have reduced risk of breast cancer, type 2 diabetes, cardiovascular disease, some reproductive cancers, rheumatoid arthritis (Godfrey and Lawrence 2010; Lawrence and Lawrence 2011) and postnatal depression (Donaldson-Myles 2011). Other studies have demonstrated that infant suckling at the breast reduces the short-term response against stress in the mother (Heinrichs et al. 2001), and encourages more oxytocin pulses in the early postpartum period leading to increased uterine contraction (Matthiesen et al. 2001). Breastmilk is also easily accessible, a low cost option and environmentally friendly.

Economic implications and potential health risks associated with not breastfeeding has prompted service planners and government policy makers to improve breastfeeding rates, with the aim of reducing health inequalities. It has been estimated in a report commissioned by UNICEF (2012b) that if there were a moderate increase in breastfeeding rates, over £17 million could be gained per annum by treating fewer cases of acute conditions in infants and breast cancer in mothers. All pregnant women should be given the opportunity to discuss the impor-tance of breastfeeding and recognising and responding to their baby's needs (UNICEF 2012a).

Factors influencing the initiation and duration of breastfeeding

Despite the benefits of breastfeeding being well-documented, the most recent Infant Feeding Survey identified the United Kingdom as having one of the lowest breastfeeding rates in Europe (McAndrew et al. 2012). Although the initiation rates of breastfeeding have risen, there are still ongoing issues with high rates of early cessation and low rates of exclusive breastfeeding up to 6–8 weeks (McAndrew et al. 2012). Breastfeeding rates are typically low amongst disadvantaged white women, particularly teenage women, first time mothers or lone parents (Dyson et al. 2006; McAndrew et al. 2012).

It is reported that breastfeeding mothers still continue to experience conflicting advice, intrusive assistance, and under resourced postnatal wards affecting their experiences of breast-feeding (McInnes and Chambers 2008; Care Quality Commission 2013). Lack of knowledge and understanding about the mechanisms of breastfeeding; perceived insufficient breastmilk supply; infant feeding too frequently; inadequate family support; painful breasts or nipples; social norms and the sexualisation of breasts portrayed in the media; all shape a woman's decision whether to initiate and continue breastfeeding (Burns et al. 2010; Brown et al. 2011; Andrew and Harvey 2011; Dodds 2013). This suggests infant feeding decisions are deep rooted in socio-cultural-economic influences, shaped by opportunities, experience, personal confidence, levels of self-efficacy and the support available.

Understanding the social–cultural context of infant feeding

The literature indicates the decision to initiate and continue breastfeeding is much more complex than simply the practicalities of providing nutrition to the baby; rather it is influenced by a social and cultural construct. Many women appear to have the understanding that 'breast is best', but many other factors impinge on the decision to breastfeed (Burns et al. 2010). Some mothers, particularly in Western societies, view formula feeding as the more practical and convenient option (Lee 2007; Brown et al. 2011). However, the experiences of some mothers who have chosen to formula feed have been reported as being negative, with emotions of anger, guilt and a sense of failure as a mother (Lakshman et al. 2009; Guyer et al. 2012). Mothers may experience conflict through a perceived moral duty to breastfeed viewed as good mothering, and the cultural norms of formula feeding, requiring less intensive mothering and a quicker independence of the baby. It is questionable how useful the 'breast is best' slogan really is in supporting mothers in their choice of infant feeding.

Health professionals and care givers need to understand the complexities, and meanings attributed to the mothers' infant feeding intentions at different times during childbearing. It is argued by Sheehan et al. (2010) that care needs to be individualised to suit women's needs rather than being embedded in the dominant 'breast is best' message, with the needs of the infant superseding that of the mother. It has been suggested that the focus on the productivity of breastfeeding; the mother supplying a product based on a baby's demand, implies a disembodied experience likely to cause doubt in the mother's ability to produce enough milk (Dykes 2005; Dykes and Flacking 2010). Similarly, the language used by health professionals could inadvertently undermine a woman's confidence and natural mothering ability, with the focus on frequency, duration and timings of breastfeeds. Teaching and observing techniques guided by hospital policies may give the impression that breastfeeding is difficult, prone to problems and supports the 'I'll give it a go' culture reinforced by the formula companies advertising their products (Marsden and Abayomi 2012). Culturally, shared knowledge of breastfeeding has been lost within communities. It has become a health behaviour that needs to be promoted, taught, observed, learned and guided by healthcare professionals, rather than it being an accepted cultural norm as a result of shared learning and development of tacit knowledge.

Activity 10.1

Go to these newspaper articles and think about what they say about society's views of breastfeeding.

[Available online] http://www.theguardian.com/media/2008/dec/30/facebook-breastfeeding-ban and http://www.dailymail.co.uk/femail/article-2356952/Breastfeeding-mother-humiliated-train-conductor-told-to-toilet-feed-daughter.html?ITO=1490&ns_mchannel=rss&ns_campaign=1490

Activity 10.2

Find magazines aimed at pregnant women and mothers and think about what the images say about infant feeding. How do you think they might influence women and families in their decisions?

Supporting mothers to initiate breastfeeding and continue exclusive breastfeeding for longer

Focusing simply on the biological benefits of breastfeeding can cause many dilemmas for women, increasing their susceptibility to psychological ill health affecting the maternal-infant bond (Guyer et al. 2012). It is important for health professionals and supporters involved in the care of the woman and families, to apply a bio-psycho-social approach in assessing individual needs, being sensitive to individual values and beliefs whilst promoting and supporting breast-feeding. Health professionals could improve a mothers' experience by paying more attention to emotional issues and setting realistic achievable goals, rather than focusing on the technicalities of breastfeeding. A family-centred approach should be achieved by listening, respecting values and encouraging breastfeeding for as long as the mother feels she can, celebrating her individual success and achievable goals.

The way breastfeeding works

For midwives and other health professionals to feel confident in supporting mothers to breast-feed, an understanding of the physiology of the breast and lactation is important. Figure 10.1 illustrates the physiology and anatomy of the breast.

Physiology of lactation

Lactogenesis I

Lactogenesis I begins during the second trimester of pregnancy and is characterised by the proliferation of the ductal and alveoli tissue within the breast in preparation for milk production at term. These developments are directed by the circulating hormones of pregnancy, namely oestrogen, progesterone and human placental lactogen (HPL). Lactocytes (milk producing cells), begin to synthesise small amounts of early milk (colostrum) from components: glucose, amino acids, fatty acids, vitamins and minerals, diffusing from the surrounding blood capillary network across the alveolar cell membrane (Kent 2007). The high levels of progesterone, oestrogen and HPL also serve to inhibit the release of prolactin from the anterior pituitary gland during pregnancy, thus preventing the onset of copious milk production at this stage (Lawrence and Lawrence 2011).

Lactogenesis II

Lactogenesis II is hormone driven under endocrine control and is triggered by the rapid fall in circulating oestrogen, progesterone and HPL, following the expulsion of the placenta and membranes (Lawrence and Lawrence 2011). This allows prolactin secretions to be released in response to milk removal by frequent and effective breastfeeding or breast expression in the first few postnatal days. Close skin-to-skin contact, and stimulation of the nipple tissue by the baby's tongue just prior to attachment to the breast, results in a neuro-hormonal reflex called the milk ejection reflex (MER), commonly known as the 'let-down reflex' which some mothers

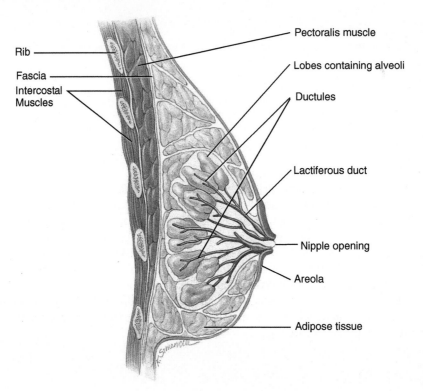

Sagittal section of lactating breast

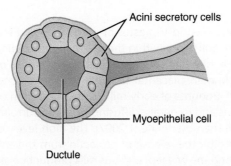

Figure 10.1   Anatomy of the breast. Source: Adapted from Tortora and Derrickson 2009, Figure 28.6, p. 1088, with permission of John Wiley and Sons, Inc.

feel as a tingling sensation. Oxytocin is released into the circulation from the posterior pituitary gland in pulsatile waves, causing the myoepithelial cells surrounding the alveoli to contract, pushing the milk out into the ductal system towards the nipple pore openings (Lawrence and Lawrence 2011). Lactogenesis II is also dependant on a delicate balance of insulin, thyroxin and adrenal cortisol and blood supply (Kent 2007). The combination of frequent milk removal and subsequent prolactin releases ensures that the prolactin receptor cells within the alveoli of the breast are triggered, i.e. 'switched on' and copious milk production ensues. The mother

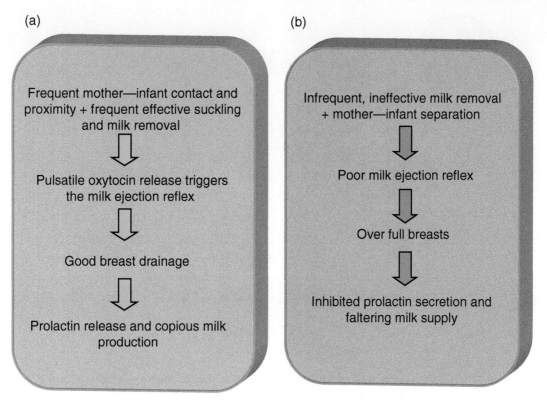

(a)

Frequent mother—infant contact and proximity + frequent effective suckling and milk removal

⇩

Pulsatile oxytocin release triggers the milk ejection reflex

⇩

Good breast drainage

⇩

Prolactin release and copious milk production

(b)

Infrequent, ineffective milk removal + mother—infant separation

⇩

Poor milk ejection reflex

⇩

Over full breasts

⇩

Inhibited prolactin secretion and faltering milk supply

Figure 10.2   Recognising (a) optimal and (b) suboptimal hormonal responses and effect on milk production during breastfeeding.

experiences these changes by feeling the breasts increase in size, weight and warmth 48–72 hours after the birth of the baby. This process is often referred to as the 'milk coming in'.

Lactogenesis III

Lactogenesis III refers to the maintenance of the milk supply which takes place gradually from about 10 days to 6 weeks postnatally. It involves a change from endocrine control to autocrine control within the breast, and is a reflection of the baby's appetite and its ability to attach well and feed frequently and effectively (Riordan 2010). The effective attachment by the baby ensures the breasts are drained well, thus maintaining a continual supply of milk, which changes according to the baby's changing appetite over time. Figure 10.2 illustrates the maternal hormonal responses in response to effective and ineffective milk removal and the effects on milk production.

Prolactin Releasing Factor (PRF)

Prolactin from the anterior pituitary gland (APG) is the hormone responsible for establishing and maintaining effective milk supply. The removal of breastmilk by the suckling baby or expressing increases levels of circulating prolactin; this binds to the walls of the acini cells (lactocytes) triggering milk production. Figure 10.3 illustrates the positive feedback mechanism between the mother and the baby. When the breasts are overfull with milk and the alveolar

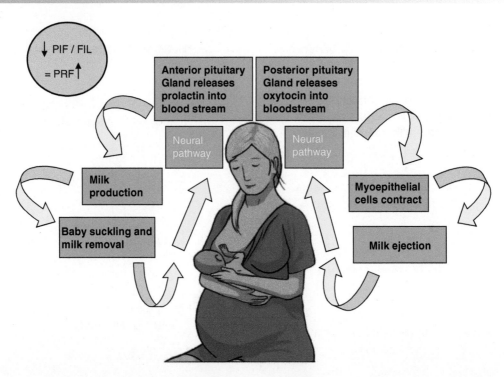

Figure 10.3 Summary of the neuroendocrine reflexes involved in effective lactation. Source: Reproduced with permission from J. Green.

walls are stretched, prolactin is unable to attach to the receptor sites and cannot enter the lactocytes, resulting in decreased milk production (Pollard 2012). Skin-to-skin contact and effective frequent breastfeeds in the early postnatal days increases the production of prolactin to prime the prolactin receptor sites. This mechanism is referred to as *'opening up the factory'* to put in the order for milk supply throughout the lactation period, maximising the long-term success of lactation (UNICEF 2008).

Feedback Inhibitor of Lactation

Feedback Inhibitor of Lactation (FIL) locally controls milk synthesis; the specific mechanism is not clear, but it appears to be a compound within the milk. When the milk is not removed, because of reduced breastfeeding, or reduced breast expression, FIL builds up in the milk-filled breasts and slows prolactin secretion from the APG (Riordan 2010). Figure 10.3 illustrates the hormonal control and mechanism of lactation.

Prolactin Inhibitory Factor

Prolactin Inhibitory Factor (PIF) is a hypothalamic trigger which may be related to dopamine or a related substance that builds up and suppresses prolactin secretion from the anterior pituitary gland when breasts are not emptied, decreasing milk production and vice versa (Lawrence and Lawrence 2011).

Prolactin increases milk synthesis and emptying of the breast by the baby suckling or by the use of hand or breast pump expression, enhances plentiful milk production.

Oxytocin is responsible for milk release, enhanced by stimulation of the breast by touch; by sight, smell or cry of the baby and by effective suckling of the baby.

Skin-to-skin

Skin-to-skin contact soon after birth is a natural transition for the mother and baby, facilitating the adaptation from intrauterine to extrauterine life and should be recommended for all mothers, irrespective of their infant feeding choice. Skin-to-skin contact helps by regulating the baby's heart rate, breathing and establishment of thermoregulation (Anderson et al. 2006; Jonas et al. 2007), whilst also triggering the immune system as the skin bacteria from mother colonises the skin of the baby. Babies are extremely alert and responsive to the mother's touch and smell soon after birth. Breast odour is a strong stimulus driving the baby towards the nipple, encouraging neurodevelopment and the baby's pre-feeding behaviours (Porter and Winberg 1999). The nipple secretions are a similar smell to a substance in amniotic fluid and the baby begins to salivate once he realises food is available.

Skin-to-skin contact promotes bonding between mother and baby and stimulates pulsatile oxytocin secretion in the mother, initiating milk ejection from the cells of acini, facilitating effective milk transfer to the baby when the baby is attached well and suckling effectively. Research has shown that newborns use their hands as well as their mouths to stimulate maternal oxytocin release after birth (Matthiesen et al. 2001). Skin-to-skin contact continues to be beneficial in the postnatal period for mothers and fathers. Figure 10.4 illustrates a mother feeding her baby skin-to-skin in the postnatal period.

217

Supporting effective infant feeding

The new UNICEF UK Baby Friendly Initiative (BFI) standards for maternity, neonatal, health visiting, children centres and other community services, reflect the latest evidence to support practitioners in providing the best outcomes for mother and babies in the UK (UNICEF 2012a).

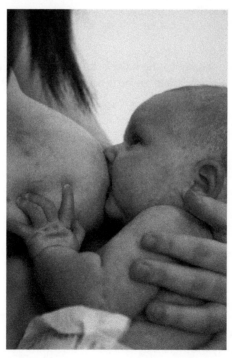

Figure 10.4 Skin-to-skin contact in the postnatal period. Source: Reproduced with permission from Philip Batty, www.ibreastfeed.co.uk.

Activity 10.3

Read the New UNICEF UK BFI standards and observe how these are implemented in organisations working towards or maintaining BFI accreditation [Available online] http://www .unicef.org.uk/Documents/Baby_Friendly/Guidance/Baby_Friendly_guidance_2012. pdf?epslanguage=en

Practical skills to support mothers to breastfeed

Learning and developing practical skills to support effective breastfeeding are considered to be a fundamental part of the midwives role in supporting infant feeding. Boxes 10.1 and 10.2 outline the key principles to teach mothers using a hands off approach as recommended by UNICEF Baby friendly Initiative.

Box 10.1 Key principles for positioning and attachment

Positioning – see Figure 10.5

1. The baby is held close to the mother's body.
2. The baby's head and body are in alignment making sure the baby has freedom to tilt the head back.
3. The baby's shoulders are supported, not the back of the head.
4. The baby's nose starts opposite the nipple.
5. The position is sustainable.

Attachment – see Figure 10.6

1. When the baby's mouth opens wide the baby is brought towards the breast quickly.
2. Chin and tongue leading, nipple goes towards the junction of soft and hard palate.

(UNICEF 2008)

Box 10.2 Recommendations for recognising effective attachment to enable sufficient milk transfer

- The baby's mouth is wide open with the bottom lip curled back.
- The baby has a large mouth full of breast.
- Cheeks look full and rounded.
- The baby's chin touching the breast.
- More of the darker skin of the areola is visible above the baby's top lip than below the baby's bottom lip – lower portion of areola is not visible.
- Feeding is pain free. Initially mothers may feel some discomfort at the start of the feed.

(UNICEF 2008)

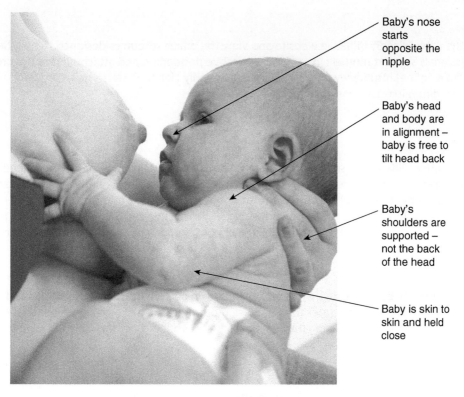

Baby's nose starts opposite the nipple

Baby's head and body are in alignment – baby is free to tilt head back

Baby's shoulders are supported – not the back of the head

Baby is skin to skin and held close

Figure 10.5 Demonstrates key principles of effective positioning as outlined in Box 10.1. Source: Reproduced with permission from Philip Batty, www.ibreastfeed.co.uk.

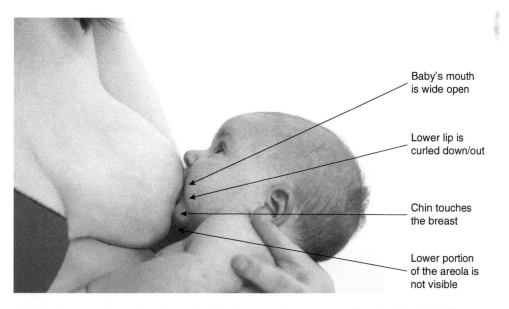

Baby's mouth is wide open

Lower lip is curled down/out

Chin touches the breast

Lower portion of the areola is not visible

Figure 10.6 Demonstrates key signs of effective attachment as outlined in Box 10.2. Source: Reproduced with permission from Philip Batty, www.ibreastfeed.co.uk.

Activity 10.4

Visit the Baby Friendly Initiative website and view the online resources designed to help health professionals support mothers in achieving effective positioning and attachment at the breast. [Available online] http://www.unicef.org.uk/BabyFriendly/Health-Professionals/Care-Pathways/ Breastfeeding/First-days/Positioning-and-Attachment/

Different positions for breastfeeding

Adopting different positions for breastfeeding allows sustainability of the breastfeed and can be used as part of a feeding plan to manage different breastfeeding challenges, e.g. breast engorgement. Some of the different positions used by mothers may include the underarm hold shown in Figure 10.7 or the cross cradle hold shown in Figure 10.8 using the same key principles (outlined in Boxes 10.1 and 10.2) for initially positioning the baby at the breast for effective attachment.

Breastfeeding pattern

When the baby is attached effectively there is a characteristic pattern of sucking and swallowing. When the baby first goes to the breast, rapid short sucks can be observed to stimulate the MER and get the milk moving through the lactiferous ducts. Once the milk is flowing the feeding

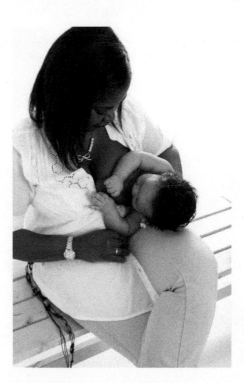

Figure 10.7   Underarm hold. Source: Reproduced with permission from Philip Batty, www. ibreastfeed.co.uk.

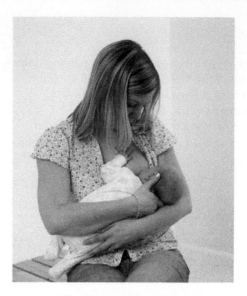

Figure 10.8   Cross cradle hold. Source: Reproduced with permission from Philip Batty, www. ibreastfeed.co.uk.

pattern changes to longer, more rhythmical sucks with audible swallowing of the milk and pauses. The sucking/swallowing ratio should be approximately 1:1 or 2:1 indicative of sufficient milk transfer (UNICEF 2008). Four or more sucks per swallow can be an indication the baby is not attached effectively to the breast or there is insufficient milk transfer.

At the end of the feed, the sucking pattern can be less vigorous and flutter sucking can be observed whereby swallowing may be less frequent. This is indicative of the baby receiving higher fat content in the breastmilk (UNICEF 2008).

Biological nurturing – a different breastfeeding approach

Babies are born with an innate ability to smell, locate and latch onto a food source (Porter and Winberg 1999). With the rise of formula feeding in developed countries, it is argued by Colson (2010) that we have lost faith in a baby's natural ability to find the breast itself. UNICEF (2008) recommends using conventional practical skills to teach mothers positions to support the transition to effective breastfeeding as outlined in Boxes 10.1 and 10.2. It is challenged by Colson (2010) that upright positions of the mother apply pressure to the baby's back, which counteracts gravity, decreasing primitive neonatal reflexes that assist in helping the baby to establish successful breastfeeding. Colson's research argues that babies are 'abdominal feeders' and that mothers may benefit from neither sitting upright or laying on their sides, but by adopting a semi-recumbent position leaning back and encouraging the baby to lie prone in close frontal apposition with maternal body contours. It is argued that these positions encourage primitive neonatal reflexes pivotal to the establishment of breastfeeding (Colson et al. 2008).

Box 10.3   Assessing sufficient milk transfer

- Within the first 24 hours after birth, baby should be passing urine and stools.
- At least 1–2 voids of urine in the first 24 hours.
- At least 2–3 voids of urine in the first 48 hours.
- Increasing to 6 voids of urine per day by day 4–5.
- 1 or 2 stools of meconium in the first 24 hours.
- Increasing to at least two stools per day by day 4 changing through black/green/brown and then to yellow by day 5.

(UNICEF 2010, Breastfeeding Assessment Tool)

222

Further reading activity

Access and read the following articles by Suzanne Colson, where you can see images of laid-back breastfeeding.

Colson, S. (2008) optimal positions for the release of primitive neonatal reflexes stimulating breastfeeding *Early Human Development* 84, pp. 441–445.

Colson S (2010) what happens to breastfeeding when mothers lie back *Clinical Lactation* 1, pp. 9–12.

Visit biological nurturing [available online] www.biologicalnurturing.com

Getting enough milk

A mother needs to be able to recognise sufficient milk transfer to feel confident in being able to provide adequate nutrition for her baby. Health professionals need to be aware of the key factors indicative of sufficient milk transfer, outlined in Box 10.3. Early skin-to-skin contact, initiation of breastfeeding and frequency of breastfeeds with effective attachment is the foundation for sustained effective feeding.

Further reading activity

Access and read the breastfeeding Assessment Tools on the Baby Friendly Initiative website to assist you in being able to recognise insufficient milk transfer in the baby [available online] http://www.unicef.org.uk/BabyFriendly/Resources/Guidance-for-Health-Professionals/Forms-and -checklists/Breastfeeding-assessment-form/

Physiological delayed lactogenesis

There are physiological factors in the mother that can affect the mother's ability to lactate sufficiently to meet the requirements of the baby. Possible factors affecting this include: anaemia, postpartum haemorrhage, polycystic ovarian syndrome, caesarean section, retained products, acute maternal illness, certain medications, diabetes, breast surgery, or anxiety in the mother (Powers 2010). However, the majority of mothers do have the physiological ability to lactate adequately. Ineffective removal of milk from the breast affecting the normal physiology of

Box 10.4 Reasons for poor milk supply

- Interruption of skin to skin contact
- Delay in the first breastfeed
- Ineffective attachment and positioning of the baby
- Inappropriate use of supplement feeds
- Separation of the mother and baby
- Infrequent feeding
- Absence of baby-led feeding
- Use of pacifiers, plastic teats, and nipple shields

Box 10.5 Recognising insufficient milk transfer in the baby

- Poor urine output
- Abnormal stool pattern
- Weight loss is not within normal parameters
- Poor weight gain
- Jaundice
- Lethargy, not waking to feed regularly
- Baby quickly falls asleep at the breast
- Baby consistently feeds for less than 5 minutes or longer than 40 minutes
- Unsettled baby after feeds
- Baby on and off the breast frequently during the feed
- Difficulty in attaching the baby to the breast
- No change in sucking pattern observed
- Noisy feeding (clicking sounds heard)
- Mother's nipples sore or damaged
- Mother's breasts engorged or mastitis

lactation, separation of mother and baby and supplementary feeds are some of main reasons for delayed or impaired lactogenesis. Box 10.4 outlines some of the reasons for poor milk supply and Box 10.5 highlights key factors for recognising insufficient milk transfer in the baby.

The aim is to maintain the health of the baby, ensuring adequate nutrition and preventing dehydration. Supporting the mother to stimulate milk production, ensuring the breasts are drained adequately, maintains optimal neurohormonal balance to support successful feeding. Box 10.6 outlines some key ways to stimulate milk production.

Ankyloglossia (tongue tie)

Approximately 1 in 10 babies is born with a short, thick or tight lingual frenulum (ankyloglossia) which may restrict the forward protrusion, upward lift and or lateral mobility of the tongue (Riordan 2010). Babies initiating breastfeeding can experience difficulty gaining a deep enough attachment to the nipple/areola complex of the breast to transfer milk effectively (Dollberg

Box 10.6   Stimulating milk production and managing insufficient milk transfer

- Obtain breastfeeding history (Pollard 2012).
- Obtain medical and obstetric history.
- Ascertain the baby's feeding behaviours.
- Ascertain the frequency of urine and colour of stools of the baby.
- Observe a complete breastfeed.
- Assess the baby's general clinical condition – refer to paediatrician if concerned.
- Ascertain the use of supplementary feeds, dummies, teats, nipple shields.
- Consider maternal physiology factors that may delay lactogenesis.
- Encourage skin-to-skin contact.
- Ensure effective positioning and attachment of the baby.
- Encourage more frequent, effective feeds, throughout day and night, to increase prolactin release.
- Offer both breasts at each feeding.
- Express by hand or pump after feeds to increase milk removal and increase prolactin release.
- If supplementary feed required, give baby expressed breastmilk (EBM) ideally, via a cup or syringe. Or formula milk if mother unable to express milk.
- Support the mother by instilling confidence in her abilities.

et al. 2008). This can be attributed to the reduced mobility of the tongue preventing the baby from being able to protrude the tongue over the lower lip and gum ridge (Algar 2009).

Breastfeeding mothers with a tongue-tied baby frequently experience breast pain and nipple damage due to difficulty latching the baby effectively onto the breast, which, subsequently, can result in reduced milk supply in the mother and poor weight gain in the baby (Messner et al. 2000; Ballard et al. 2002; Griffiths 2004; Mettias et al. 2013). The suboptimal drainage of the breast also increases the risk of mastitis in the mother. Bottle feeding babies with a significant tongue tie can also find it difficult to create a good seal around the bottle teat, resulting in excessive dribbling, prolonged feeds, spillage of milk and reflux (Hogan et al. 2005; Finigan 2014).

It is important to note that the observation of a lingual frenulum underneath the tongue does not necessarily mean that the baby is 'tongue tied'. It is the assessment of the tongue function which determines whether the baby is tongue tied. If a tongue tie is suspected and all other strategies for achieving comfortable and effective breastfeeding or efficient milk transfer from a bottle have been unsuccessful, then urgent referral to a health professional who is a qualified Frenotomy Practitioner should be sought. Frenotomy (division of tongue tie) offers a safe, simple procedure to release the tongue tie to enable the baby to feed effectively with the normal range of tongue movement restored (Hogan et al. 2005; NICE 2005; Sethi et al. 2013).

Reasons for expressing breastmilk

Every breastfeeding mother should be taught how to express by hand, as part of her initiation of breastfeeding, in the first few days after giving birth.

- To stimulate the baby to attach for a breastfeed by expressing a few drops onto the baby's lips.

- To collect colostrum, to syringe or cup feed, to a newborn baby which has not yet established effective baby-led breastfeeding.
- To collect colostrum for a premature or sick baby on the neonatal unit and to stimulate the onset of copious lactation when the baby is unable to breastfeed directly.
- To relieve an overfull or engorged breast.
- To improve breast drainage post-feed, if engorgement is still an issue/if the mother has mastitis or a blocked duct/or if the baby is unable to achieve adequate breast drainage due to prematurity, sickness or other clinical condition which may affect the baby's ability to suckle effectively and transfer milk, e.g. Down syndrome; cleft lip and palate.
- To encourage an increase in milk production by expressing post-feed, when lactation is faltering as part of a detailed feeding plan.
- To support a mother's choice of feeding, which may be to give her baby expressed breastmilk by bottle and teat. This may be undertaken occasionally, to enable others (including the father) to feed the baby (reflecting cultural changes to a more family-centred approach to newborn feeding), or regularly, at every feed time if the mother chooses not to put her baby to the breast but wishes to use her breastmilk as the ideal infant milk.
- To provide breastmilk for the baby's feeds, if the mother is going to be away from the baby for period of time.
- To maintain the breastmilk supply, when separated from the baby, by expressing at the times the baby would usually feed.

Hand expression

A clear explanation should be given to the mother, as to why this skill is important to enable her to learn how to manage breastfeeding and the variety of situations and challenges she may encounter. Gaining the ability to hand express, will help the mother to develop confidence and autonomy in relation to breastfeeding and will provide her with one of the 'self-help' strategies if a breastfeeding challenge arises.

For mothers whose baby is being cared for on the neonatal unit, learning how to hand express effectively and frequently, gives both parents something very positive to do every few hours and helps them to feel as though they are contributing to their baby's wellbeing. For premature babies, every drop of colostrum is regarded as an essential medicine to provide the safest milk to line the gut and reduce the risk of necrotising enterocolitis (McGuire and Anthony 2003; Heiman and Schanler 2006). It also provides vital immune factors produced by the mother to protect the baby from infections; hormones, which help maintain physiological stability; and enzymes, which aid digestion and absorption of nutrients. For this group of mothers, commencing hand expression as soon as possible after the birth (within 6 hours wherever possible), is vital to facilitate the onset of copious lactation over the next few days. It is crucial to remove all available colostrum frequently, in order to trigger surges of prolactin from the anterior pituitary gland, which targets and 'switches on' the prolactin receptor cells for milk production. Delay in stimulation of these cells can lead to suboptimal lactation. This group of mothers should be encouraged to express at least 8 times in 24 hours, including once in the night to capitalise on the higher nocturnal prolactin levels.

The same is true for mothers who have their newborn baby by their side, where the baby is not waking and breastfeeding well enough to remove colostrum frequently and trigger the release of prolactin. A baby will often pummel or pad the breast with its hands and bang its head on the breast, brushing past the nipple before latching on. These actions provide tactile skin stimulation to the nerve supply of the breast and nipple, increasing levels of oxytocin.

However, the secretion of oxytocin is inhibited by circulating adrenaline, which is released in response to fear, anxiety or stress. It is important, therefore, to use strategies to calm and relax the mother prior to commencing expressing and ensure she has privacy and comfort, otherwise it is unlikely that her milk will flow for collection, as a result of a lack of the MER reflex. Difficulty in producing milk at an expression can increase concern and anxiety in the mother who may become tearful and despondent.

Key points for teaching hand expression

1. It is vital to teach this technique in a quiet and unhurried manner, using a 'hands off' approach in order to achieve the optimal responses.
2. Show the mother how to stroke/massage her breast to trigger the tactile stimulation. [A knitted breast is useful to demonstrate with. A pattern to make one is available on Lactation Consultants of Great Britain website.
3. Ask her to gently stimulate the nipple tissue between the pad of her thumb and first finger. This encourages the muscle cells in the nipple tissue to contract, making it protrude more.
4. The mother should 'cup' the breast and form a 'C' shape with her thumb above the nipple, on the areola and her first finger below. Larger breasted mothers may benefit from supporting the weight of the breast with her other hand.
5. To locate the correct area on the breast to elicit a productive flow of milk, the mother needs to gently feel where the lower milk cells are, by compressing the tissue with her thumb and first finger, beginning just behind the firm nipple tissue which usually feels quite soft and working backwards, away from the nipple until she can feel a change in texture – a firmness or knobbly texture.
6. She should be guided to press backwards into the breast tissue, towards her rib cage, and then maintaining this backwards pressure, gently compress the breast tissue for a few seconds between her thumb and first finger, and then release the pressure whilst retaining contact in the same place on the skin. Repeat the compress/release technique until the MER has been triggered and milk begins to flow, slowly at first and then more quickly. Continue in this area until the flow slows then rotate the thumb and finger and locate the correct area in the next segments of the breast and repeat the technique until sufficient milk has been expressed to meet the clinical need.
7. Depending on the reason for hand expressing, the mother may be encouraged to express both breasts to drain and collect all available colostrum/milk.
8. Small amounts of colostrum are best collected in a 1 mL or 2 mL syringe, by whoever is helping the mother. If the milk is not being used immediately and requires storing in the designated fridge at 4°C or taking to the neonatal unit, a sterile 'stopper' needs to be placed on the end of the syringe and the body of the syringe needs to have a label attached which identifies the mother/hospital case note number/ward/bed/date and time of collection.

Equipment for breast pump expressing
Using a hand pump

The choice of hand pumps is extensive but all work in a similar way. They require the user to follow the manufacturer's instructions for safe cleaning, sterilisation of parts and correct assembly. Hand pumps are significantly cheaper than electric pumps and for intermittent or occasional expressing, they are ideal. The mother may benefit from triggering a 'milk ejection reflex' using the technique described above in Key Points for Teaching Hand Expression, points 2–6, prior to placing the funnel of the breast pump against her breast.

Once the milk is beginning to flow, the mother places the funnel of the breast pump against her breast ensuring that the nipple is placed in the centre of the aperture, to avoid any rubbing or chafing. Some manufacturers provide a choice of funnels and apertures to accommodate different sized nipples. The funnel should be held close enough to provide a good seal, but the mother should be guided to avoid excessive pressure because this could restrict the flow of milk along the ducts.

She will need to hold the funnel and support the breast with one hand and depress the lever of the pump with the other. Initially, repeated depressions will need to be made, to create a vacuum and then the milk will begin to drip and then spurt. Once this is underway, the mother can manage the milk removal, by only depressing the lever far enough to create the vacuum pull. Milk can be observed spurting out like jets of milk.

It is very important that the mother does not create too much vacuum pressure because that can cause nipple pain and nipple tissue trauma. Mothers should be warned against the temptation to try and pump too fast and too vigorously as this can be counterproductive, leading to poor milk drainage as a result of increased levels of anxiety. Much better milk expression is achieved if the mother expresses slowly and gently, in a private and calm environment, which enhances oxytocin secretion. When the milk flow slows right down and or the breast feels well drained, she can repeat the whole process on the other breast, depending on the reason for her expressing milk.

When the expression is completed, the breastmilk should be stored safely or fed to the baby, according to the clinical situation. The pump parts must be separated, cleaned and sterilised according to the manufacturer's instructions.

Further reading activity

For more information about hand expressing and safe storage of expressed breastmilk look at the following resources [Available online] www.mothersguide.co.uk and http:// www.unicef.org.uk/BabyFriendly/Resources/Resources-for-parents/ Off to the best start: Information about feeding your baby

Using an electric pump

As with hand pumps, there are many manufacturers of electric breast pumps and the choice of pump should be based on clinical effectiveness, ease of assembly, guidance from knowledgeable lactation consultants and the price. For regular or long-term expressing, an electric pump is probably more suitable.

The mother should ensure the pump parts have been appropriately cleaned and sterilised following any previous expression and then assemble them. A minute or two of pre-expressing breast massage can begin to stimulate oxytocin secretions. Having some calming music playing, or watching a favourite TV programme can help the mother remain relaxed during the expression and if she is separated from her baby, for example the baby is on the neonatal unit, then looking at a photograph of her baby can enhance oxytocin secretions.

After placing the assembled breast pump gently against her breast, she should switch on the stimulation phase button, if the pump has one, and wait for the MER and then proceed to the expression phase. If the mother is expressing to relieve a blocked duct, engorgement or mastitis, it is helpful to use her spare hand to gently massage the breast tissue beneath the skin in the area which feels congested, as this can aid the flow of the milk down through the lactiferous ducts and out through the nipple pore openings. Sometimes, milk which has been blocked in

227

the breast over many hours can look thick and congealed as it begins to be released, but will gradually return to normal consistency as it flows more freely. It is all safe to be fed to the baby.

It is important to ensure the mother understands that to turn the vacuum button up to maximum, is unlikely to achieve optimum milk flow or good breast drainage because if the vacuum is too high it will create too much suction, drawing the walls of the lactiferous ducts closer to each other and restricting the flow of milk. In addition, excessive vacuum may also cause nipple tissue damage and pain. Some mothers who are expressing frequently and over a lengthy period can be drawn into thinking that to turn the pump up to maximum vacuum will result in reducing the time taken to complete the expression, but this will more likely result in reduced milk flow, poor breast drainage, pain and disappointment. Each mother should determine the most effective settings, for each of her breasts. The breasts are two separate organs, which are likely to have different speeds of MER and need slightly different levels of vacuum to achieve optimal expression.

It is milk removal from the breast, either by the baby feeding effectively or by using a breast pump, which triggers the secretion of prolactin from the anterior pituitary gland, which in turn stimulates the prolactin receptor cells in the cells of acini in the breast tissue. This results in milk production to replace what has been removed.

Identifying and managing common breastfeeding problems

Many of the pathological conditions can be traced back to either:

- poor positioning and attachment of the baby
- infrequent feeding and ineffective milk removal
- poor breastfeeding management
- nipple tissue damage, or
- a combination of all the above.

It is important mothers receive support from midwives, lactation consultants, peer support-ers, health visitors, and GPs, ensuring early recognition and appropriate management if com-plications occur. As part of assessment, the midwife should take a lactation history and observe a breastfeed before planning the care (Pollard 2012). Some of the common conditions include; breast engorgement, mastitis (non-effective or infective), sore nipples, and thrush (*Candida albicans*).

Breast engorgement

This is an accumulation of milk, congestion and increased vascularity in the breast (Lawrence and Lawrence 2011). It usually presents with both breasts feeling hot and painful, hard and full of milk, with difficulty in attachment. The aim is for the mother to achieve effective attachment and avoid increase in FIL by encouraging drainage of the breasts regularly. The feeding may be mother-led rather than baby-led to ensure the milk is removed from the breast; the mother may need to express for comfort (UNICEF 2008). Hand expression prior to the feed is helpful to soften the breast, prior to the baby attaching. The mother will need to be advised on appropriate analgesia if required.

Mastitis

Mastitis can develop if engorgement remains untreated. It is an inflammatory condition of the breast in response to breastmilk leaking into the tissue (Noonan 2010); it is usually unilateral affecting one or more lobes or segments, but can be seen in both breasts (Pollard 2012). The mastitis may be either non-infected or infected. Mastitis presents as a blocked lactiferous duct/s, with evidence of localised inflammation and breast pain experienced by the mother. Flu-like symptoms present in the mother with body aches and pyrexia due to the inflammatory response. The aim is to achieve effective attachment of the baby using different positions to ensure drainage of the breast, ensuring baby's lower jaw is on the same side as the area of mastitis. Avoid increase in FIL by encouraging drainage of the breasts regularly, expressing after feeds if necessary, particularly from the affected breast for the mother to feel comfortable. Kent (2007) indicates that not all milk available is consumed at every breastfeed. The breast should feel softer and lighter after a feed, including the areas affected (UNICEF 2008). Expressing after feeds to ensure optimal breast drainage may encourage higher milk yield, but by gradually reducing the expressing once the inflammation has subsided, the supply will return to normal (UNICEF 2008).

UNICEF (2008) highlight it is difficult to determine whether infection is present, but recommend that if measures to drain the milk do not quickly relieve the mother's symptoms within 24 hours, infection should be suspected. The mother will require urgent referral to the GP for antibiotic, anti-inflammatory and analgesic medications and should be encouraged to rest, increase fluid intake, and be supported to ensure there is effective removal of the milk from the breasts. Warm compresses prior to feeding and cold compresses after the feed may help to relieve the discomfort (Pollard 2012). Untreated mastitis can lead to breast abscesses and puerperal sepsis (CMACE 2011).

Candida albicans

Candida albicans is a commensal organism that causes oral thrush (Lawrence and Lawrence 2011). Infection may be precipitated by the mother or baby taking antibiotics, and/or the use of dummies, teats and nipple shields. In the mother, the condition usually presents in both breasts, as a sudden onset of shooting pain in the breast during and after feeds, which may develop following days or weeks of pain-free breastfeeding. The nipple/areola complex may suddenly become more sensitive and itchy with a delay in healing of sore nipples (Breastfeeding Network 2009). There is usually no inflammation of the breast and no maternal pyrexia. The mother will need to be referred to the GP for antifungal treatment and appropriate analgesia. Regular handwashing and appropriate sterilisation of any feeding equipment should be reiterated to the mother. The baby may present with white patches on the tongue or inside the cheeks, with nappy rash and may be unsettled. The baby will also need to be referred to the GP to be simultaneously treated with the mother. It is important that both mother and baby are treated, even if only one of them has signs and symptoms, otherwise the infection is likely to pass from one to the other.

Further reading activity

Access the Breastfeeding Network website for further information on managing common breastfeeding problems [Available online] http://www.breastfeedingnetwork.org.uk/

When breastfeeding is not recommended

Certain blood-borne viruses, such as human immunodeficiency virus (HIV) are passed through the breastmilk and may infect the child. In such cases, breastfeeding is not recommended (WHO 2010), where replacement feeding is acceptable, feasible, affordable, sustainable and safe. Certain medications the mother is taking may be contraindicated due to their effects on the baby (Hale 2012) (see Chapter 15: 'Pharmacology and medicines management', for further information).

229

Babies with the metabolic disorder phenylketonuria (PKU) can be prescribed supplementary phenylalanine (PHE)-free formula and have breastfeeds. The lactation consultant and paediatrician would work closely together to manage the feeding plan for the baby with PKU. It is recommended that the PHE-free formula is given prior to the breastfeeds (Page-Goertz and Riordan 2010).

Supporting mothers to formula feed

Although breastfeeding is promoted as the best form of nutrition for infants, most babies receive some formula milk in the first year of life. The most recent UK infant feeding survey in 2010 showed 76% of mothers who initially breastfed had used formula milks, either in combination with breastmilk or alone, by the time their infant was aged 4–6 months (McAndrew et al. 2012). Research has shown that many mothers receive little information on formula feeding and mistakes in preparation of feeds are common (Lakshman et al. 2009). Mothers choosing to formula feed their babies need support to ensure they are confident with sterilising equipment, preparing and storing feeds, and feeding the baby. Inadequate information, support for mothers and partners with formula feeding can lead to health complications for the baby. Prior to preparing formula feeds, handwashing should be undertaken. The Department of Health (2013) and the Food Standards Agency have reiterated the advice on safe preparation of formula feeding. Some of the key elements being restated include the following:

- Make up powdered infant formula using water at a temperature of 70°C or above to ensure any pathogens in the milk powder are destroyed.
- The advice is to boil at least 1 litre (1.7 pints) of fresh tap water and then allow it to cool in the kettle for no more than 30 minutes, so that it will have reached a temperature of at least 70°C.
- Follow the manufacturer's instructions to make up the feed correctly; the water is always added to the bottle first, before adding the powdered infant formula (UNICEF 2012c).
- Once the feed is prepared, it is important to cool the formula appropriately so that it is not too hot for the baby to drink. The bottle can be cooled by holding the bottom half of the bottle under cold running water or placing the bottle in a cold water bath (UNICEF 2012c). Readers are encouraged to read the DH and UNICEF guidelines on safe preparation of infant formula, outlined in the Further Reading Activity below.
- Feeding the baby away from home, or using ready-to-feed liquid formula which is sterile, can help to reduce the risk of infections (UNICEF 2012c). Information can also be accessed from reading the UNICEF guidelines.
- Parents may need to be reminded that formula feeds should never be heated up in a microwave, due to risk of creating hot spots and scalding the baby's mouth.

Further reading activity

Access and read the guidelines from Department of Health (2011, 2013) and UNICEF (2010a; 2010b; 2012c) on safe preparation of formula milk [Available online] http://www.unicef.org.uk/babyfriendly/ and https://www.gov.uk/government/publications/start4life-updated-guide-to-bottle-feeding

Activity 10.5

Find out what resources are available on postnatal wards, to teach mothers about sterilising feeding equipment and safe preparation of formula feeds.

Key points

- Infant feeding choices are influenced by social, cultural and emotional factors.
- Providing evidence-based information and support to a mother and partner to ensure their baby receives adequate nutrition is a fundamental role of the midwife.
- Understanding the physiology of the breast and lactation is necessary to be able to support mothers effectively to initiate and maintain breastfeeding.
- Early recognition and appropriate management of breastfeeding complications is a fundamental skill of the midwife.
- Understanding the principles of safe formula preparation and feeding is necessary to be able to give parents evidence based information.

Conclusion

Evidence suggests that improving the initiation and duration of breastfeeding will help towards reducing health inequalities. Midwives and health professionals need to be aware of the factors influencing a woman's decisions in infant feeding and ensure that the best available evidence is applied to clinical practice. The care provided should be culturally sensitive, family-centred and responsive to individual needs, respecting values and beliefs. All women need to be supported in their choice of infant feeding and receive consistent information and guidance in order to maintain the infant's nutritional requirements and to foster confidence in the mother and her partner.

End of chapter activities
Crossword

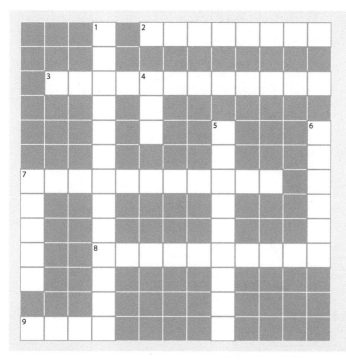

Across

2. Hormone released by the posterior pituitary gland causing myoepithelial cells to contract.
3. Lactogenesis II is stimulated by a sudden drop in this hormone.
7. Ducts that are found 5–8 millimeters from the nipple opening.
8. The alveoli consist of a single layer of milk-producing secretory cells called
9. Decreased milk production is due to the lactocytes being too

Down

1. Cells surrounding the alveoli.
4. The fat content of a breastfeed is higher at the
5. Hormone responsible for milk synthesis.
6. Has a negative effect on milk production.
7. Glandular tissue within the breast are arranged in these.

Label the diagram

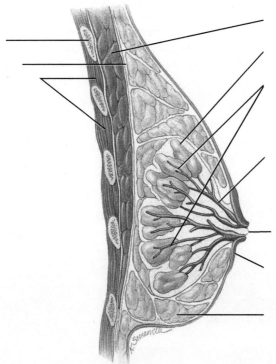

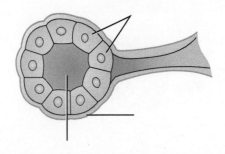

Find out more

Below is a list of things you can find out about to enhance your knowledge of the issues and topics covered in this chapter. Make notes using the chapter content, the references and further reading identified, local policies and guidelines and discussions with colleagues.

1. Read the infant feeding policy in the local hospital.

2. Seek the opportunity to spend time with a breastfeeding peer supporter and infant-feeding co-ordinator or lactational consultant.

3. Read the International Code of Marketing of Breastmilk Substitutes and consider how this applies to clinical practice. [Available online] http://www.unicef.org/nutrition/files/nutrition_code_english.pdf

4. For more information visit:
   http://www.unicef.org.uk/babyfriendly/
   www.tongue-tie.org.uk/
   http://www.ibreastfeed.co.uk/
   http://www.breastfeedingnetwork.org.uk/
   http://www.lcgb.org/

Glossary of terms

Acute otitis media   Inflammation, usually due to infection of the middle ear. Symptoms include pain and high fever.

APG   Anterior pituitary gland.

Asthma   Condition which involves narrowing of the bronchial airways which changes in severity over short periods of time, leads to cough, wheezing and difficulty breathing

Dermatitis   Inflammatory condition of the skin.

Diabetes mellitus   Disorder of carbohydrate metabolism in which sugars in the body are not metabolised to produce energy.

FIL   Feedback inhibitor of lactation.

HPL   Human placental lactogen.

Lactiferous ducts   Ducts responsible for transporting milk from the alveoli lumen to the nipple opening.

Lactogenesis   Production of milk by the mammary glands.

Leukaemia   Group of malignant disease; the bone marrow and other blood forming organs produce increased numbers of white blood cells.

MER   Milk ejection reflex.

Myoepithelial cells   Encourage the secretion of milk into the ductal system.

Necrotising enterocolitis (NEC)   Life-threatening disease affecting the bowel of the newborn during the first few weeks of life, more common in pre-term babies.

Neuroendocrine   Control of certain activities of the body by the nervous system and circulating hormones.

Obesity   Condition in which excess fat has accumulated in the body, mostly in the subcutaneous tissues.

Oxytocin   Hormone produced by the posterior pituitary gland causing contraction of the myoepithelial cells around the alveoli lumen which stimulates milk flow from the breasts after the birth, in response to the baby suckling at the breast.

PIF   Prolactin Inhibiting Factor.

Postnatal depression   Depression that starts after childbirth.

PPG   Posterior pituitary gland.

PRF   Prolactin Releasing Factor.

Prolactin   Hormone that stimulates milk production after childbirth.

(Martin 2010.)

References

Algar, V. (2009) Should an infant who is breastfeeding poorly and has a tongue tie undergo a tongue tie division? *Archives of Disease in Childhood* 94, pp. 911–912.

Anderson, G.C., Moore, E., Hepworth, J., Bergman, N. (2006) Early skin-to-skin contact for mothers and their healthy newborn infants. *The Cochrane Database of systematic reviews Issue 3.*

Andrew, N., Harvey, K. (2011) Infant feeding choices: experiences, self-identity and lifestyle. *Maternal & Child Nutrition* 7, pp. 48–60.

Ballard, J.L., Auer, C.E., Khoury, J.C. (2002) Ankyloglossia: assessment, incidence, and effect of frenuloplasty on the breastfeeding dyad. *Pediatrics* 110 (5), pp. 63–67.

Brown, A., Raynor, P., Lee, M. (2011) Healthcare professionals' and mothers' perceptions of factors that influence decisions to breastfeed or formula feed infants: a comparative study. *Journal of Advanced Nursing* 67 (9), pp. 1993–2003.

Breastfeeding Network (2009) [available online] www.breastfeedingnetwork.org.uk

Burns, E., Schmied, V., Sheehan, A., Fenwick, J. (2010) A meta-ethnographic synthesis of women's experience of breastfeeding. *Maternal & Child Nutrition* 6, pp. 201–219.

Care Quality Commission (2013) *National findings from the 2013 survey of women's experiences of maternity care.* London: CQC.

Centre for Maternal and Child Enquiries (2011) Saving mothers' lives: reviewing maternal deaths 2006–08. *British Journal of Obstetrics and Gynaecology* 118 (Suppl. 1), pp. 1–203.

Colson, S.D. (2010) What happens to breastfeeding when mothers lie back? *Clinical Lactation* 1, pp. 9–12.

Colson, S.D,. Meek, J.H., Hawdon, J.M. (2008) Optimal positions for the release of primitive neonatal reflexes stimulating breastfeeding. *Early Human Development* 84, pp. 441–449.

Department of Health (2013) *Equality Analysis: Chief Medical Officer and Director of Public Health Nursing – Communication about 'Best Practice preparation of formula milk'.* Department of Health: London.

Department of Health (2011) *A guide to bottle feeding.* London: Department of Health.

Dodds, R. (2013) UK Infant Feeding Survey: Good news for breastfeeding. *British Journal of Midwifery* 21 (3), pp. 179–186.

Dollberg, S., Botzer, E., Grunis, E., Mimouni, F. (2008) Immediate nipple pain relief after frenotomy in breast-fed infants with ankyloglossia: a randomised, prospective study. *Journal of Pediatric Surgery* 41, pp. 1598–1600.

Donaldson-Myles, F. (2011) Postnatal depression and infant feeding: A review of the evidence. *British Journal of Midwifery* 19 (10), pp. 619–624.

Dykes, F. (2005) Supply and demand: breastfeeding as labour. *Social Science & Medicine* 60, pp. 2283–2293.

Dykes, F., Flacking, R. (2010) Encouraging breastfeeding: A relational perspective. *Early Human Development* 86, pp. 733–736.

Dyson, L., Renfrew, M., McFadden A., McCormick, F., Herbert, G., Thomas, J. (2006) *Promotion of breastfeeding initiation and duration.* London: National Institute for Health and Clinical Excellence:

Fewtrew, M.S. (2004) Long-term benefits of being breastfed. *Current Paediatrics* 14, pp. 97–103.

Finigan, V. (2014) Overcoming tongue-tie. *Midwives* Issue 3. London: Royal College of Midwives.

Godfrey, J.R., Lawrence, R.A. (2010) Towards optimal health: the maternal benefits of breastfeeding. *Journal of Women's Health* 19 (9), pp. 1597–1602.

Griffiths, D.M. (2004) Do tongue-ties affect breastfeeding? *Journal of Human Lactation* 20 (4), pp. 409–413.

Guyer, J., Millward, L.J., Berger, I. (2012) Mothers breastfeeding experiences and implications for professionals. *British Journal of Midwifery* 20(10), pp. 724–733.

Hale, T. (2012) *Medications and Mothers Milk: A Manual of Lactational Pharmacology*, 15th edn. Amarillo: Hale Publishing.

Heikkilä, K., Sacker, A., Kelly, Y., Renfrew, M.J., Quigley, M.A. (2011) Breastfeeding and child behaviour in the millennium cohort study. *Archives of Disease in Childhood* 96, pp. 635–642.

Heiman, H., Schanler, J. (2006) Benefits of maternal and donor human milk for premature infants. *Early Human Development* 82, pp. 781–787.

Heinrichs, M., Meinlschmidt, G., Neumann Wagner, I., Kirschbaum, C., Ehlert, U., Hellhammer, D. (2001) Effects of suckling on hypothalamic–pituitary–adrenalaxis responses to psychosocial stress in postpartum lactating women. *Journal of Clinical Endocrinology & Metabolism* 86 (10), pp. 4798–4804.

Herba, C.M., Roza, S., Govaert, P., Hofman, A., Jaddoe, V., Verhulst, F.C., Tiemeier, H. (2012) Breastfeeding and early brain development: the Generation R study. *Maternal & Child Nutrition* 9 (3), pp. 332–349.

Hogan, M., Westcott, C., Griffiths, M. (2005) Randomized, controlled trial of division of tongue–tie in infants with feeding problems. *Journal of Paediatrics and Child Health* 41, (5/6), pp. 246–250.

Ip, S., Chung, M., Raman, G., Chew, P., Magula, N., Devine, D., Trikalinos, T., Lau, J. (2007) *Evidence Report/ Technology Assessment No: 153*. Rockville MD: Agency for Healthcare Research and Quality.

Jonas, W., Wiklund, I., Nissen, E., Ransjo-Arvidson, A.B., Uvnas-Moberg, K. (2007) Newborn skin temperature two days postpartum during breastfeeding related to different labour ward practices. *Early Human Development* 88, pp. 55–62.

Kent, J.C. (2007) How breastfeeding works. *Journal of Midwifery & Women's Health* 52 (6), pp. 564–570.

Lakshman, R., Ogilvie, D., Ong, K. (2009) Mothers experiences of bottle-feeing: a systematic review of qualitative and quantitative studies. *Archives of Disease in Childhood* 94, pp. 596–601.

Lawrence, R.A., Lawrence, R.M. (2011) Breastfeeding: A Guide for the Medical Profession. Maryland Heights, MO: Elsevier Mosby.

Lee, E. (2007) Infant feeding in risk society. *Health Risk & Society* 9 (3), pp. 295–309.

Matthiesen, A.S., Ransjo-Arvidson, A.B., Nissen, E., Uvnas-Moberg, K. (2001) Postpartum maternal oxytocin release by newborns: effects of infant hand massage and sucking. *Birth* 28 (1), pp. 13–19.

Martin, E.A. (2010) *Concise Oxford Colour Medical Dictionary*. Oxford: Oxford University Press.

Marsden, A., Abayomi, J. (2012) Attitudes of employees working in public places toward breastfeeding. *British Journal of Midwifery* 20 (4), pp. 271–277.

McAndrew, F., Thompson, J., Fellows, L., Large, A., Speed, M. (2012) *Infant Feeding Survey 2010: Summary*. London: The Information Centre for Health and Social Care.

McGuire, W., Anthony, M.Y. (2003) Donor human milk versus formula for preventing necrotising enterocolitis in preterm infants: systematic review. *Archives of Disease in Childhood Fetal and Neonatal Edition* 88, pp. F11–F14.

McInnes, R.J., Chambers, JA. (2008) Supporting breastfeeding mothers: qualitative synthesis. *Journal of Advanced Nursing* 62 (4), pp. 407–427.

Messner, A.H., Lalakea, M.L., Aby, J., Macmahon, J., Bair, E. (2000) Ankyloglossia incidence and associated feeding difficulties. *Archives Otolaryngology Head Neck Surgery* 126, pp. 36–39.

Mettias, B., O'Brien, R., Mohamed, M., Khatwa, A., Nasrallah, L., Doddi, M. (2013) Division of tongue tie as an outpatient procedure. Technique, efficacy and safety. *International Journal of Pediatric Otorhinolaryngology* 77, pp. 550–552.

National Institute for Health and Clinical Excellence (NICE) (2005) *Division of Ankyloglossia (Tongue-Tie) for Breastfeeding*. London: NICE.

Noonan, M. (2010) lactational mastitis: recognition and breastfeeding support. *British Journal of Midwifery* 18 (8), pp. 503–508.

Page-Goertz, S., Riordan, J. (2010) The ill child: breastfeeding implications. In: (eds) Riordan, J., Wambach, K. *Breastfeeding and Human Lactation*, 4th edn. Boston: Jones and Bartlett.

Powers, N.G. (2010) Low intake in the breastfeeding infant: maternal and infant considerations. In: (eds) Riordan J., Wambach, K. *Breastfeeding and Human Lactation*, 4th edn. Boston: Jones and Bartlett.

Porter, R.H., Winberg, J. (1999) Unique salience of maternal breast odours for newborn infants. *Neuroscience and Biobehavioral Reviews* 23, pp. 439–449.

Pollard, M. (2012) *Evidence based care for breastfeeding mothers: A resource for midwives and allied healthcare professionals*. London: Routledge.

Quigley, M.A. (2013) Breastfeeding, casual effects and inequalities. *Archives of Disease in Childhood* [online] Available: Archives of Disease in Childhoodadc.bmj.com doi: 10.1136/archdischild-2013-304188

Riordan, J. (2010) The Biological Specificity of Breastmilk. In: (eds) Riordan J., Wambach, K. *Breastfeeding and Human Lactation*, 4th edn. Boston: Jones and Bartlett.

Sacker, A., Kelly, Y., Lacovou, M., Cable, N., Bartley, M. (2013) Breastfeeding and intergenerational social mobility: what are the mechanisms? *Archives of Disease in Childhood* [online] Available: doi: 10.1136/archdischild-2012-303199.

Sethi, N., Smith, D., Kortequee, S., Ward, V.M.M., Clarke, S. (2013) Benefits of frenulotomy in infants with ankyloglossia. *International Journal of Pediatric Otorhinolaryngology* 77, pp. 762–765.

Sheehan, A Schmied, V., Barclay, L. (2010) Complex decisions: theorizing women's infant feeding decisions in the first 6 weeks after birth. *Journal of Advanced Nursing* 66 (2), pp. 371–380.

Tortora, G.J., Derrickson, B.H. (2009) *Principles of Anatomy and Physiology*, 12th edn. Hoboken: John Wiley & Sons, Inc.

UNICEF UK Baby Friendly Initiative (2010a) *A guide to infant formula for parents who are bottle feeding*. London: UNICEF.

UNICEF UK Baby Friendly Initiative (2010b) *The health professional's guide to: A guide to infant formula for parents who are bottle feeding*. London: UNICEF.

UNICEF UK (2008) *Three-day course in breastfeeding management*. London: UNICEF.

UNICEF (2012a) Guide to Baby Friendly Initiative Standards. London: UNICEF.

UNICEF (2012b) *Preventing disease and saving resources: the potential contribution of increasing breastfeeding rates in the* UK. London: UNICEF.

UNICEF (2012c) *A guide to bottle feeding start 4 life*. London: UNICEF.

UNICEF Baby Friendly Initiative [online] Available: http://www.unicef.org.uk/babyfriendly/

World Health Organization (2002) *Nutrient adequacy of exclusive breastfeeding for the term infant during the first six months of life*. Geneva: WHO.

World Health Organization (2010) *Principles and recommendations for infant feeding in the context of HIV: A summary of evidence*. Geneva: WHO.

236

Chapter 11

Public health and health promotion

Olanma Ogbuehi

University of Hull, Hull, UK

Fiona Robinson

Women and Children's Hospital, Hull, UK

Catriona Jones

University of Hull, Hull, UK

Acknowledgement: *Lizzy de Angelis, Specialist Obesity Dietician, Angel Nutrition, Visiting Lecturer at the University of Hull (Maternal Nutrition, Midwifery) and Sheffield Hallam University (MSc Sports Science), London, UK*

Learning outcomes

By the end of this chapter the reader will be able to:

* explain different concepts of health
* define public health, health promotion, epidemiology and demography
* describe major contributing factors public health among the population of childbearing women and their babies
* explain the importance of good maternal health to the future health of populations
* recognise the midwife's unique contribution to public health of childbearing women and infants.

Introduction

In this chapter, the concept of public health will be defined, first exploring the meaning of health and then the origin, development, notion and practice of public health, in the United Kingdom (UK). In doing this, the disciplines of epidemiology and demography will be introduced. The domains of public health will be outlined, along with a discussion of the determinants of health and illness in populations. Health inequalities in the UK will be explored with this in mind. The

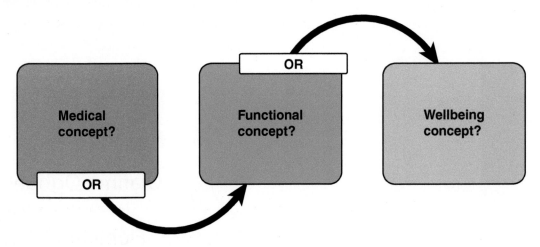

Figure 11.1 Differing Concepts of Health adapted from Bowden (2006).

midwife's role in public health and health promotion will be investigated. This chapter will also show that public health is a longstanding sphere of midwifery practice, rather than a 21st century innovation. Contemporary public health issues for mothers and infants, which come under the remit of midwifery care, will then be explored.

The concept and definition of health

Before the 18th century, health was seen as a function of metaphysical and spiritual theories (Tripp 1997). Societal attitudes and beliefs evolved, so that the body was viewed more mechanistically. Mordacci and Sobel (1998, p. 34) stated that defining 'health' is as 'slipper-as-mercury'. Any group of individuals has a variety of shared and diverse life experiences, which may result in their adopting very different views of health, or wellness. Bowden (2006) explains a tripartite, construction of health (see Figure 11.1). These are:

- a medical concept
- a functional concept
- a wellbeing concept.

The medical concept of health refers to the absence of illness and is characterised by the avoidance and destruction of pathogens and the slowing or prevention of disease progression. This is the predominant understanding of UK health service personnel (Bowden 2006). This is a mechanistic or biomedical approach to health, in which the body is a machine that needs repair and maintenance. Diseases are defined as disruptions in bodily systems or organ structure with characteristic signs and symptoms, aetiological agents and anatomical changes (Porth 2009). Poor health, in this system, is purely physical, measurable and treatable. Clarke (2011) creates two categories in the medical concept of health:

1. The *absence of clinically verifiable disease*: diagnosis dwells on biophysical abnormalities (Martin 2010; Clarke 2011).
2. The *absence of illness*: focusing on subjective perceptions – symptoms (Martin 2010; Clarke 2011).

However, as early as the mid-20th century, the model was shown to be incomplete. The World Health Organization (1948) adopted a broader definition of health calling it:

>...a state of complete physical, mental and social wellbeing and not merely the absence of disease or infirmity.

This is idealistic (Porth 2009), encompassing bodily, psychological and social contexts of life and has been criticised for lacking any real meaning and being 'hopelessly utopian' (Mordacci and Sobel 1998, p. 34); simultaneously, totally comprehensive and meaningless (Lewis 1953). It may be more desirable to use definitions of health which extend beyond biophysical parameters but which relate realistically with people's lived experiences and aspirations.

'Functional health' is the ability to practically function within society (Bowden 2006), viewed from the perspective of either the individual or society (Clarke 2011). This is found in the 'social model of disability' discourses, which emphasise the cooperative actions of society in removing disabling factors from within it, above individual impairment (Oliver 1983). A functional concept of health might be defined by a person's ability to engage in the activities of daily living (Chamberlain and Gallop 1988), which may be achieved by people with chronic ill-health, such as bronchial asthma or type-I diabetes mellitus, with appropriate management.

Western medicine has recently experienced a shift towards more holistic thinking, relating bodily function to the mind and soul (Tiran 2008; Martin 2010). Health is conceptualised as wellbeing, or 'feeling good about yourself' (Bowden 2006). Illness is possible in the absence of a biophysical disease: clinical dysfunction is possible in the absence of subjectively experienced illness (Mordacci and Sobel 1998). Wellbeing encompasses individuals' experiences of central wholeness and harmony, regardless of biophysical diagnoses and harnesses physiological, psychological and spiritual aspects (Guttmacher 1979).

Health could be viewed as any one of these three concepts (see Figure 11.1). Beldon and Crozier (2005) argue that midwives tend to prefer holistic concepts of health, which could be represented as the sum of all three aspects (see Figure 11.2), or possibly the intersection between the three (see Figure 11.3).

239

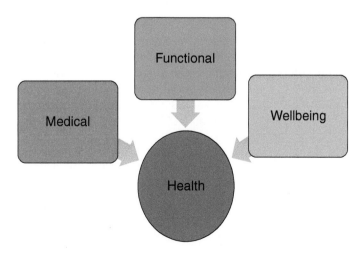

Figure 11.2   Diagram representing how different Concepts of Health contribute to the overall concept (adapted from Bowden, 2006).

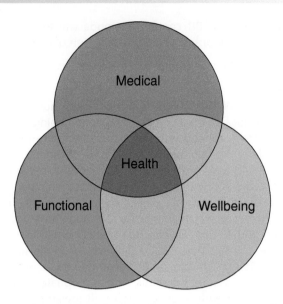

Figure 11.3 Venn diagram showing health as the intersection between the three concepts (adapted from Bowden, 2006).

Public health

Public health has been defined as:

> ...*The science and art of promoting and protecting health and well-being, preventing ill-health and prolonging life through the organised efforts of society*...
>
> (UK's Faculty of Public Health 2010)

This is:

> ...*inclusive of all interventions designed to improve the health of the public*...
>
> (Wanless 2003, p. 49)

Public health requires whole societal involvement, harnessing individual choices, capabilities and actions, in partnership with health services. Prolonging life implies progressive improvements in a society's health. Historically, scientific research, innovation and dissemination, public sanitation, healthcare developments, social welfare, social reform and legislation, have all contributed to public health improvements (Sydenstricker 1935; McCormick 1993). General Secretary of the Royal College of Midwives (RCM), Audrey Wood (1957) identified British midwives' public health role through antenatal care as having had a major role in preventing prematurity, stillbirths and neonatal deaths. The RCM (2001) position paper on the Midwife's Role in Public Health responded to the prevailing policy direction of the National Health Service (NHS) (DH, 2000). Public health incorporates social and political factors, not just individualistic medical perspectives, exploring the roots and causes of health and ill health in populations (RCM 2001; Martin 2010).

Epidemiology

Epidemiology, literally, *'studies upon people'* is foundational to public health (Farmer et al. 2004; Omran 2005). Epidemiology traces how disease and ill-health is distributed through populations, discovering influencing factors, measuring, reporting and interpreting the causes of disease (morbidity) and death (mortality) (Farmer and Lawrenson 2004; Gordis 2009). Epidemiology informs the prevention of the spread of disease and the control of societal health problems (Carr et al. 2007). Puerperal sepsis (childbed fever) was a major cause of maternal mortality in the early 19th century (Gordis 2009). Ignaz Semmelweis (in Austria) and Florence Nightingale (in England) were instrumental in demonstrating the links between place of birth, hygiene, caregivers' practices and rates of maternal mortality from puerperal sepsis, contributing to its significant decline (Nightingale 1871; Dunn 1996; Gordis 2009).

Demography

Demography measures populations, providing records of size, location and characteristics, such as age, gender, social class, migration and ethnicity (Bowling 2009; Martin 2010), which is essential for effective planning of health services and guiding public health interventions. Maternity statistics include conception rates, fertility rates, birth rates, maternal and infant mortality rates. The National Health Service Act (1977) requires births to be notified within 36 hours to the relevant area Director of Public Health by a midwife or doctor in attendance. Birth registration must be conducted within 42 days of birth by the parents or midwives (and others classified as owning the premises) if the child's parents have not done so (Sidebotham and Walsh 2011).

Conception rates

Conception statistics include pregnancies that result in one or more live births, stillbirths or a legal abortion under the Abortion Act 1967. They do not include miscarriages or illegal abortions. These relate to women of childbearing (age 15–44 years old), who could give birth in any year (Office for National Statistics (ONS) 2012a).

Fertility rates

The *General Fertility Rate* (GFR) equates to '… the number of children per 1000 women born to a population or sub-population' (ONS 2012a, p. 7). For example, a GFR of 56 in 2007 for the UK means that for every 1000 women of childbearing age in the UK, 56 babies were born. The *Total Fertility Rate* measures the average number of children that a group of women would each have if they experienced the age-specific fertility rates for a particular year throughout their childbearing lives. For example, a TFR of 1.90 in 2007 means that a group of women would have an average of 1.90 children each during their lifetimes based solely on 2007's Age-specific Fertility Rates (ONS 2012a). *Age-specific Fertility Rates (ASFR)* are measures of fertility specific to the age of the mother obtained by dividing the number of live births in a year, to mothers in each age group, by the number of females in the mid-year population of that age, these are expressed per 1000 women in the age group (ONS 2012a).

Birth and death statistics

Live birth refers to a baby born, showing spontaneous signs of life after birth regardless of gestational period (ONS 2012b; WHO 2013). Figure 11.4 shows the number of Livebirths in the England and Wales over a 50 year period (between 1961 and 2011). Other statistics quantify maternal and infant deaths, which are important for discovering risks and identifying preventative strategies (Table 11.1).

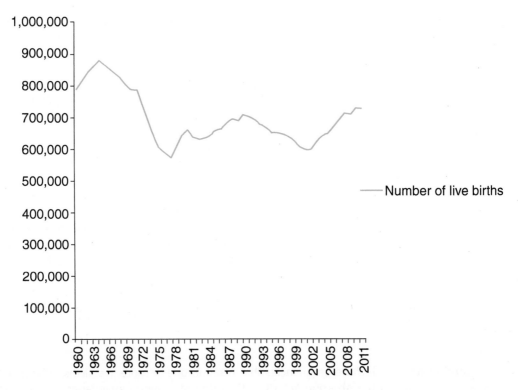

242

Figure 11.4 Graph showing number of live births in the England and Wales over a 50-year period (between 1961 and 2011) (ONS, 2012c).

Table 11.1 Maternal and infant deaths

Measure	Definition
Stillbirth	Since 1992: a child born from the 24th completed week of gestation, who never showed any signs of life.
Stillbirth rate	Number of stillbirths per 1000 total births (live births plus stillbirths).
Early neonatal deaths	Deaths under seven days.
Perinatal deaths	Stillbirths and early neonatal deaths.
Maternal mortality	The death of a woman within 42 days of the end of pregnancy from any cause related to or aggravated by the pregnancy or its management, but not from accidental or incidental causes.
Maternal mortality rate	Number of maternal deaths of mothers, from direct and indirect causes, within the first 42 days after the end of pregnancy per 100,000 maternities (pregnancies).
Maternal mortality ratio	Number of maternal deaths of mothers, from direct and indirect causes, within the first 42 days after the end of per 100,000 live births.
Neonatal deaths	Deaths under 28 days.
Post-neonatal deaths	Deaths between 28 days and 1 year.
Infant deaths	Deaths under 1 year.

Domains of public health

The UK Faculty of Public Health (2010) has identified three interrelated domains of public health (see Figure 11.5) (Griffiths et al. 2005). These are:

- health improvement
- health protection
- health services (quality improvement).

Health improvement concerns socioeconomic aspects, health promotion, and determinants of health (Thorpe et al. 2008). This encompasses reducing health inequalities in partnership with multiple sectors (Griffiths et al. 2005). *Health protection* includes the control of infectious and communicable diseases and environmental hazards; strategies include immunisation pro- grammes (Thain and Hickman 2004). *Health service (quality improvement)* relates to the role of healthcare systems, service planning and quality, clinical effectiveness, clinical governance and health economics. These include prioritisation and equity of services, clinical audit, evaluation and research (Thorpe et al. 2008; UK's Faculty of Public Health 2010).

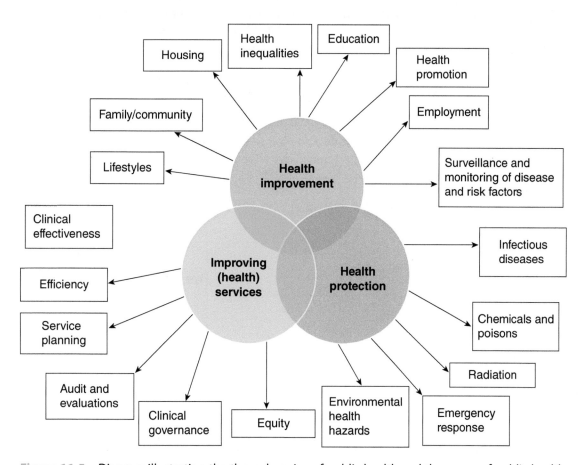

Figure 11.5   Diagram illustrating the three domains of public health and the scope of public health practice.

Health improvement: the midwife and health promotion

Health promotion is defined as activities designed to maintain optimum health and quality of life for groups of people; these involve engaging the community in their personal health whether individually or collectively (Martin 2010). Childbirth, as a normal life event, fits within a health promotion framework (Beldon and Crozier 2005). Health education uses persuasive methods to inform groups or individuals about adopting healthier lifestyles and rejecting unhealthy habits; the educator determines what changes will be beneficial for the population (Martin 2010). Piper (2005) proposes four categories of health promotion strategies used by midwives; these are the *behaviour change agent*, the *collective empowerment facilitator*, *strategic practitioner* and *collective empowerment* facilitator (see Figure 11.6).

The *behaviour change agent*, or *health persuasion* approach uses health education where an expert clinician (e.g. midwife) identifies areas within the medical model of health requiring change in the recipients of care (Piper 2005). Disease prevention is emphasised, using orthodox medical approaches (Furber 2000; Whitehead 2003). Pregnancy is seen as the pre-eminent *'teachable moment'* (Herzig et al. 2006, p. 230): women are highly motivated and responsive, within a context of relatively intensive and continuous care from health professionals. Preventative measures may be *primary, secondary* or *tertiary*, these relate respectively to avoidance of disease (or wider public health problems), control of an identified condition, or preventing worsening of an identified issue.

An *empowerment facilitator* uses non-coercive, democratic, women-centred methods to achieve health promotion through constructive partnership with women (e.g. in the use of the

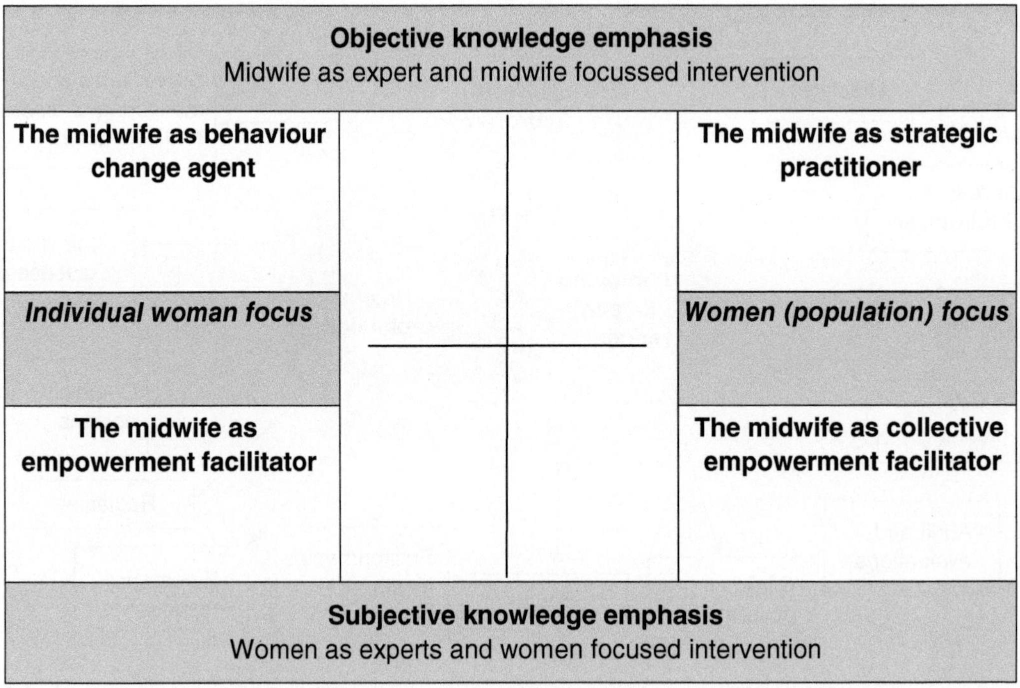

Objective knowledge emphasis Midwife as expert and midwife focussed intervention		
The midwife as behaviour change agent		**The midwife as strategic practitioner**
Individual woman focus		*Women (population) focus*
The midwife as empowerment facilitator		**The midwife as collective empowerment facilitator**
Subjective knowledge emphasis Women as experts and women focused intervention		

Figure 11.6   Diagram displaying the difference between models of health promotion (Piper 2005).

expert patient, patient advice, liaison services and engagement of service users (Piper 2005). A *strategic practitioner* uses the legislative action to evaluate wider socio-political issues which affect the health of individuals, but are beyond their direct control. These include, health inequalities and unequal distribution of wealth and capital (Furber 2000; Piper 2005). This is a top-down approach to health promotion. The *collective empowerment facilitator* employs the 'community development method' of health promotion (Furber 2000; Piper 2005), focusing on societal factors as the main determinant of health. However, these operate a bottom-up approach, responding to the collectively expressed, subjective health needs of women and their families. Examples include the facilitation of peer support schemes for mothers, such as breast-feeding drop-in peer support groups (Piper 2005).

Health surveillance

Health surveillance aims to, '*provide the right information, at the right time, in the right place to inform decision-making and action-taking*' (DH 2013a, p. 5). Screening is part of health surveillance which is part of routine antenatal midwifery care. Screening is where apparently healthy members of a population are assessed for their susceptibility to diseases and conditions (Tiran 2008; Martin 2010). Antenatal screening may include determining a mother's carrier status for recessive genetic disorders, which the baby could inherit or the mother's susceptibility to certain infectious diseases. UK childbearing women are offered a programme of routine antenatal screening and diagnostic testing in pregnancy for certain infectious diseases in the mother, which may be at a pre-clinical stage, but still infectious (Tiran 2008; Porth 2009; Martin 2010). Additional screening and diagnostic testing are made available when there is a clear history of exposure or susceptibility. This programme aims to improve health outcomes in the population of childbearing women and their babies (see Chapter 6: 'Antenatal midwifery care', where antenatal screening is discussed in greater depth).

Improving health services through clinical audit: confidential enquiries into maternal and child health

A major way in which clinical audit has been used to inform maternal public health is the Confidential Enquiries into maternal deaths instituted in the UK in 1952 and subsequently infant mortality (Weindling 2003; Kee 2005). These gather statistical data on maternal and infant mortality over a three year period (e.g. Centre for Maternal and Child Enquiries (CMACE) 2011). These enquiries revealed key areas of risk, compelling midwives to act to reduce maternal mortality in relation to key issues including:

- sepsis (see Chapter 8)
- serious illness (see Chapter 16)
- smoking
- mental health (see Chapters 4 and 13)
- obesity
- age (younger and older mothers) (see Chapter 5)
- ethnicity
- asylum status
- literacy

Table 11.2   Social class definitions used in the Black Report (1980)

Class definition	Descriptions	Percentage of the population in 1980
I. (Professional)	Professional (e.g. accountant, doctor, lawyer)	5%
Ii. (Intermediate)	Intermediate (e.g. manager, schoolteacher, nurse)	18%
Iiin. (Skilled, Non-Manual)	Skilled non-manual (e.g. clerical worker, secretary, shop assistant)	12%
Iilm. (Skilled, Manual)	Skilled manual (e.g. bus driver, butcher, coal face worker, carpenter)	38%
IV. (Partly Skilled)	Partly skilled (e.g. agricultural worker, bus conductor, postman)	18%
V. (Unskilled)	Unskilled (e.g. labourer, cleaner, dock worker)	9%

- substance misuse
- domestic abuse. (Jewell 2005; Lewis 2007; Centre for Maternal and Child Enquiries (CMACE) 2011)

Health inequalities

DH (2007, p. 16) stated:

> …Health inequalities stem from inequalities in people's early life experience, their education and occupational status, exposure to lifestyle and the environmental risks and diseases to which their life courses predispose them. People in disadvantaged groups and areas tend to experience the poorest health…

The Black Report (1980) identified the persistence of inequalities in health between people of different social classes in the UK, despite major health service reforms and advancements. These included higher mortality rates, lower life expectancy, and lower birth weight of infants, for people in social classes IV and V (Table 11.2). Some of this could be attributed to different habits and lifestyle choices of people in different social classes. Cancer Research UK (2011) reported the persistently higher prevalence of smoking among manual workers, compared with non-manual workers (see Figure 11.7). The European Foundation for the Improvement of Living and Working Conditions (2003) reported links between poverty and ill health (see Figure 11.8) and showed that lower income areas had demonstrably poorer health outcomes. Complex relationships exist between wealth, employment and ill-health which contribute to the polarisation of health outcomes in different social classes (see Figure 11.9). Similarly, Osmond et al. (1989) showed that place of birth predicted likelihood of future ill-health, independent of current place of residence. This featured in the seminal work 'Fetal and Infant Origins of Adult Disease' (Barker 1989) showing correlations between events in early life, and the development of chronic ill health in later life (e.g. type-2 diabetes mellitus and coronary heart disease, resulting in lower life expectancy). Maternal health status and infant nutrition were implicated in shaping outcomes for offspring (Barker 1997; Barker 2001; Morley 2006). Social class is also correlated with relative breastfeeding initiation and continuation rates (see Chapter 10: 'Infant feeding', where socio-economic influences on infant feeding choices are discussed in greater depth).

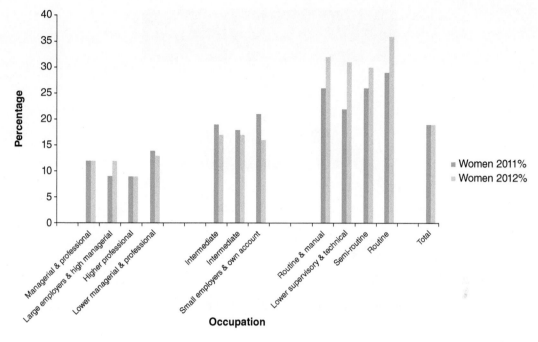

Figure 11.7   The relationship between occupation and prevalence of smoking, in women 2011 and 2012 (ONS, 2013).

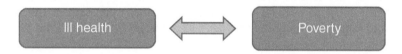

Figure 11.8   Diagram illustrating the relationship between poverty and ill health.

The Acheson Report (1998) made recommendations for supporting healthy maternal and child nutrition and reducing risks to children through unhealthy maternal lifestyles, such as smoking in pregnancy and maternal obesity, geared towards positively influencing the long term health of children and adults. These recommendations were reflected in the NHS Plan (Department of Health (DH) (2000), identifying midwives as an integral part of its public health strategy. A strong public health focus, involving midwives within maternal and child health services, was preserved throughout the New Labour administration. The National Service Frameworks (NSF) for Children, Young People and Maternity Services (DH 2004) placed a strong emphasis on health promotion, from pre-conceptual stages, pregnancy, childhood, through to adulthood. Strategies included high quality care throughout pregnancy and the initiation of 'Sure Start' programmes in order to deliver public health targets. Community midwives' relocation to Children's Centres enhanced their visibility and accessibility to local communities, with the intention of reducing health inequalities (DH 2004).

Determinants of health

Health inequalities are related to wider societal factors defined by Dahlgren and Whitehead (1992) as 'Determinants of Health'. A person's individual characteristics, such as genetic make

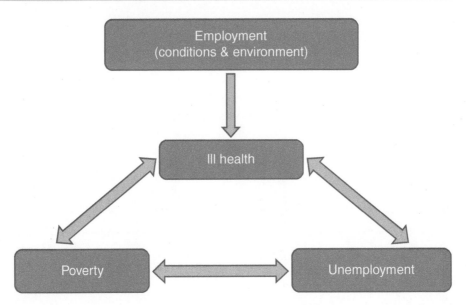

Figure 11.9   Diagram illustrating the possible relationships between poverty, ill-health and employment.

up, sex and age are central. These are then influenced by multiple factors, including lifestyle choices and living and working conditions. When discussing each of the issues below it is important to remember that many of these do not occur in isolation from one another, in any childbearing woman. For example, socioeconomic status and ethnicity is related to both smoking and obesity. Some of these are interrelated complex social needs in one woman, such as: domestic abuse, young motherhood, substance misuse and mental illnesses. Women who do not speak English have been identified as having complex social needs; they and their children have poor perinatal health outcomes (CMACE 2010; NICE 2010a). It should also become apparent that there is much overlap between the different domains of public health.

Guidance for public health

The National Institute for Clinical Excellence (NICE) was established in 1999, as a special health authority ensuring better consistency in availability and quality of NHS treatments and care. Following a merger with the Health Development Agency in 2005, NICE became the National Institute for *Health* and Clinical Excellence incorporating public health guidance, for preventing ill health and promoting healthier lifestyles. Numerous NICE guidelines focus on the care of childbearing women and babies (Table 11.3). In April (2013) NICE became the National Institute for Health and Care Excellence. Public Health England was established in 2013 to '*protect and improve the nation's health and to address inequalities*' as an executive agency of the DH (DH 2011). The Health and Social Care Act (2012) instituted health and wellbeing boards through which key stakeholders from the Health and Social Care sectors could collaborate to improve the health and wellbeing of local populations and reduce health inequalities, using community knowledge to prioritise needs and work more cooperatively (Local Government Association 2014).

Table 11.3   NICE guidelines for the care of childbearing women and babies

Name of guideline	Identifier (CG – Clinical Guideline; PH – Public Health Guideline)	Year of publication
Antenatal Care Guideline	(CG62)	2008
Postnatal Care Guideline	(CG47)	2006
Antenatal and Postnatal Mental Health Guideline	(CG45)	2007
Diabetes in pregnancy: management of diabetes and its complications from pre-conception to the postnatal period	(CG63)	2010
Quitting smoking in pregnancy and following childbirth	(PH26)	2010
Weight management before, during and after pregnancy	(PH27)	2010
Pregnancy and complex social factors	(CG110)	2010
Ectopic pregnancy and miscarriage: Diagnosis and initial management in early pregnancy of ectopic pregnancy and miscarriage	(CG154)	2012
Social and emotional wellbeing – early years	(PH40)	2012

Revisiting the midwife's role in public health

The independent Post-2010 Strategic Review of Health Inequalities 2009 'Fair Society, Healthy Lives' identified a 'social gradient' in health (p. 15), which causes people of lower social position, to experience poorer health (Marmot et al. 2010). Recommendations to reduce this social gradient were to ensure that children received the 'best start' in life (p. 94), through strategies such as promoting:

> …High quality maternity services, parenting programmes childcare and early years' education to meet need across the social gradient…

> (p. 94)

Using, a strong midwifery workforce:

> …to provide the infrastructure to support women and their partners during pregnancy, birth and early parenthood, for delivery of services that avoid unnecessary intervention, and for ensuring that those women who do, or may, require intervention are signposted at an early stage to specialist care…

> (p. 94)

The Public Health Work stream for Midwifery 2020 (Department of Health, Department of Health Safety and Social Services, Welsh Assembly Government Scottish Government 2010) made recommendations for midwives to strengthen their role in the public health agenda, as the first professional point of contact for childbearing women; they advocated a community-based practice. Midwives should be knowledgeable about the healthcare needs of the local population and work alongside social care services to identify and support women at risk and the wider family, engaging other services when necessary. The Coalition Government, White

Paper, 'Healthy Lives, and Healthy People' (DH 2010a) reiterated the priority of improving maternal health in order to:

> ...*give our children a better start in life, reduce infant mortality and the numbers of low birth-weight babies...*

(p. 5)

This was criticised for failing to explain midwives' important contribution to health promotion and early intervention, as the lead health professionals caring for pregnant women and young babies (RCM 2011). According to the International Confederation of Midwives (ICM) (2011) legally licensed midwives' scope of professional practice includes:

- making appropriate referrals to other agencies and practitioners
- taking preventative measures
- health education
- health counselling.

The Compassion in Practice report (Commissioning Board Chief Nursing Officer and DH Chief Nursing Adviser 2012), subsequently, recognised the importance of strengthening the public health role of the midwife. DH and Public Health England (2013a,b) explicitly describe midwifery public health actions aimed at an individual, community and population level aimed at improving health and wellbeing. The Maternity Matters report (DH 2007) promised women individualised and flexible care, led by a midwife, or the maternity team. The needs of women with complex social factors would be addressed through partnership with relevant agencies. Some contemporary maternal public health issues encountered by midwives are discussed below.

Maternal obesity

Tackling obesity has become a major focus of public health initiatives in the UK. The obese state, (body mass index [BMI] of $\geq 30\,\text{kg/m}^2$) is linked to many negative health outcomes in childbearing women, when compared with women who are not obese (Lewis 2007; see Figure 11.10). Obese women are more prone to experiencing prolonged pregnancies and fetal macrosomia. These issues require greater obstetric and neonatal interventions. Infants of obese mothers are significantly more likely to experience stillbirth or neonatal death, have congenital anomalies and premature birth. Children born to mothers who gained excessive weight in pregnancy were significantly more likely to be overweight at aged three years (Oken et al. 2007), possibly pre-programming childhood obesity. Maternal malnutrition has been linked to childhood disease in later life (Hales and Barker 2001; CMACE 2010). Lifestyle change is indicated to protect and improve present and future maternal and child health.

Nurses perceive weight as a sensitive issue to discuss and midwives have expressed concerns about how to communicate effectively with obese women without altering their relationship (Greener et al. 2010; Hansson et al. 2011; Mold and Forbes 2011; Schmied et al. 2011). This leads to potential avoidance of discussion of weight at antenatal booking and subsequent appointments. Specialist weight management services have been developed to support pregnant women who are overweight or obese which are being widely replicated. Since 2010, in Hull and East Yorkshire, for example, women are referred to a specialist 'Healthy Lifestyle Midwife' from community midwifery care (NICE 2011; Hull Clinical Commissioning Group 2013). However, NICE (2010) places the responsibility on all maternity care practitioners to educate, inform and support women with weight management during the childbearing period. The 'Healthy Start' scheme offers financial support to pregnant women and mothers with children under four, who

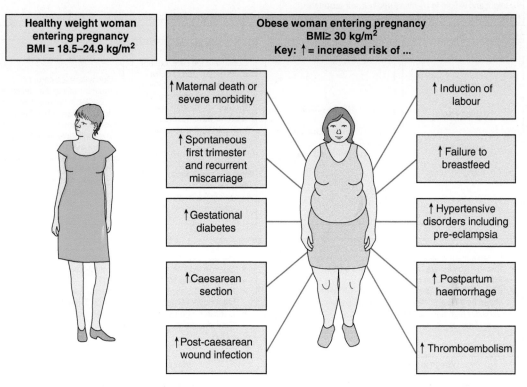

Healthy weight woman entering pregnancy BMI = 18.5–24.9 kg/m²

Obese woman entering pregnancy BMI≥ 30 kg/m²
Key: ↑ = increased risk of ...

↑ Maternal death or severe morbidity

↑ Spontaneous first trimester and recurrent miscarriage

↑ Gestational diabetes

↑ Caesarean section

↑ Post-caesarean wound infection

↑ Induction of labour

↑ Failure to breastfeed

↑ Hypertensive disorders including pre-eclampsia

↑ Postpartum haemorrhage

↑ Thromboembolism

Figure 11.10   Additional burden of illness and complications associated with maternal obesity in pregnancy (Lewis 2007).

251

are on low incomes, or aged under 18, to help provide them and their children a nutritious diet (Healthy Start no date). Figure 11.11 is an example of a local clinical guideline for all antenatal women, recommended by CMACE/Royal College of Obstetricians & Gynaecologists (RCOG) (2010).

Control of infectious diseases

Communicable or infectious diseases are diseases which can be transmitted from one person to another (i.e. contagious diseases) which may become endemic, epidemic or pandemic in nature (Martin 2010). Notifiable diseases must be reported to an officer of the local authority (e.g. a Consultant in Communicable Disease Control) (McCormick 1993). The virtual eradication of formerly devastating communicable diseases in the UK in the 20th century, relied upon almost universal uptake of vaccination programmes, improvements in housing and living conditions and a systematic and targeted public health prevention strategy, involving significant input from primary care professionals, including midwives, General Practitioners and health visitors. Indeed, the DH (2010a, p. 5) has stated that:

> ...clean air and water; enhanced nutrition and mass immunisation have consigned many killer diseases to the history books.

(DH 2010a, p. 5)

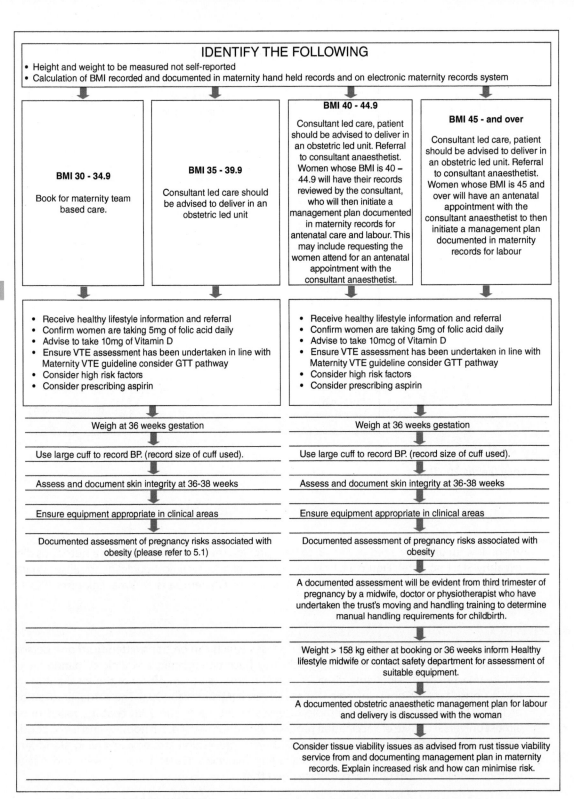

IDENTIFY THE FOLLOWING
- Height and weight to be measured not self-reported
- Calculation of BMI recorded and documented in maternity hand held records and on electronic maternity records system

BMI 30 - 34.9

Book for maternity team based care.

BMI 35 - 39.9

Consultant led care should be advised to deliver in an obstetric led unit

BMI 40 - 44.9

Consultant led care, patient should be advised to deliver in an obstetric led unit. Referral to consultant anaesthetist. Women whose BMI is 40 – 44.9 will have their records reviewed by the consultant, who will then initiate a management plan documented in maternity records for antenatal care and labour. This may include requesting the women attend for an antenatal appointment with the consultant anaesthetist.

BMI 45 - and over

Consultant led care, patient should be advised to deliver in an obstetric led unit. Referral to consultant anaesthetist. Women whose BMI is 45 and over will have an antenatal appointment with the consultant anaesthetist to then initiate a management plan documented in maternity records for labour

- Receive healthy lifestyle information and referral
- Confirm women are taking 5mg of folic acid daily
- Advise to take 10mg of Vitamin D
- Ensure VTE assessment has been undertaken in line with Maternity VTE guideline consider GTT pathway
- Consider high risk factors
- Consider prescribing aspirin

- Receive healthy lifestyle information and referral
- Confirm women are taking 5mg of folic acid daily
- Advise to take 10mcg of Vitamin D
- Ensure VTE assessment has been undertaken in line with Maternity VTE guideline consider GTT pathway
- Consider high risk factors
- Consider prescribing aspirin

Weigh at 36 weeks gestation

Weigh at 36 weeks gestation

Use large cuff to record BP. (record size of cuff used).

Use large cuff to record BP. (record size of cuff used).

Assess and document skin integrity at 36-38 weeks

Assess and document skin integrity at 36-38 weeks

Ensure equipment appropriate in clinical areas

Ensure equipment appropriate in clinical areas

Documented assessment of pregnancy risks associated with obesity (please refer to 5.1)

Documented assessment of pregnancy risks associated with obesity

A documented assessment will be evident from third trimester of pregnancy by a midwife, doctor or physiotherapist who have undertaken the trust's moving and handling training to determine manual handling requirements for childbirth.

Weight > 158 kg either at booking or 36 weeks inform Healthy lifestyle midwife or contact safety department for assessment of suitable equipment.

A documented obstetric anaesthetic management plan for labour and delivery is discussed with the woman

Consider tissue viability issues as advised from rust tissue viability service from and documenting management plan in maternity records. Explain increased risk and how can minimise risk.

Figure 11.11 Sample clinical pathway for weight management in pregnancy (courtesy of de Angelis and Robinson 2010 with permission).

The Health Protection Agency (HPA) (2010) issues a list of communicable diseases; this varies between regions and at different times. Some childhood infectious diseases have re-emerged as serious public health threats. HPA (2013) reported an eight-fold increase in confirmed cases of whooping cough (caused by the *Bordatella pertussis* bacterium), when comparing the fourth quarter of 2011 with the same period in 2012 in England and Wales. This is transmitted by droplet spread, causing serious illness and mortality among very young children (Martin 2010). Because 429 confirmed diagnoses were among infants aged less than three months old the Chief Medical Officer announced that pregnant women would be offered vaccinations to protect their newborn babies (DH 2012). Vaccination ensures the development of maternal antibodies to the infectious agent, conferring passive immunity in young infants, until their vaccination between six and eight weeks after birth. Similar strategies occurred with such infectious disease as influenza virus H1N1 (swine flu) (RCM 2012). Midwives are therefore, directly involved in both protecting and promoting health in the area of infectious diseases.

Noxious substances (teratogens and toxins)

Noxious substances are those which are harmful or have extremely unpleasant effects (Soanes et al. 2005). In childbearing woman these substances may present harmful effects to both mother and baby. Teratogens are substances which induce the formation of developmental abnormalities in the fetus (teratogenesis): these may be medically prescribed or recreational drugs, legal or illicit substances. Some pathogens (disease causing agents) (e.g. rubella) and exposure to some therapeutic treatments (e.g. ionizing radiation) may also be teratogenic (Martin 2010). Teratogens may be environmental (e.g. contamination or pollution of air, food or water supplies). These substances cross the placenta and enter the fetal circulation (see Figure 11.12).

Medications

Medications women consume in pregnancy, for pre-existing chronic health conditions and pregnancy induced health conditions (physical or psychological) may be teratogenic. Thalidomide and diethylstibestrol were prescribed to pregnant women, but were subsequently found to have caused fetal malformations (limb deformities) and the development of reproductive system malformations and cancers in women exposed in utero respectively (Lucchese et al. 2004).

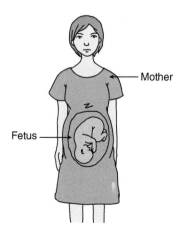

Mother

Fetus

Figure 11.12   Noxious substances, consumed by the mother, such as alcohol, may cross from the maternal to fetal circulation causing conditions like fetal alcohol syndrome.

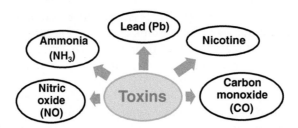

Figure 11.13   Toxins found in cigarette smoke.

Anti-epileptic treatments such as (sodium valproate and carbamazepime) are associated with a higher risk of fetal anomalies such as neural tube defects and cardiac malformations. However, close consultation, cooperation and monitoring within the interdisciplinary team is required to manage these conditions in pregnancy, to ensure that women receive accurate, evidence-based care, including advice regarding lactation. NICE produce care pathways for the management of care of people with certain conditions. It is important to avoid the potential harms to both the mother and the baby of abrupt withdrawal from therapeutic medications due to fear of harm to the fetus.

Cigarette and tobacco smoking in pregnancy

One quarter (26%) of mothers in the (UK) smoked at some point during pregnancy or in the previous 12 months (National Statistics and National Health Service Information Centre 2010); the highest prevalence was in Wales (33%), the lowest in England (26%): 54% gave up before birth. One eighth of all mothers (12%) smoked throughout their pregnancies. The overall prevalence has continually decreased, between 2005 and 2010. Pregnant smokers inhale numerous toxins (see Figure 11.13) exposing the fetus, via the maternal-feto-placental circulation, to fetal serum nicotine concentrations 15% higher than those in the maternal serum (Huizink and Mulder 2005).

Cigarette smoke impedes placental function, reducing uterine blood flow, causing fetal oxygen deprivation (fetal hypoxia-ischaemia) and malnutrition, resulting in intrauterine growth restriction (IUGR). Nicotine, carbon monoxide (CO) and tobacco tar can directly affect the fetal brain (Huizink and Mulder 2005; García-Algar 2008). Nicotine withdrawal has been noted in the early neonatal period (e.g. irritability, tremor and hypertonicity) and in childhood attention deficit hyperactivity disorder (ADHD) (Huizink and Mulder 2005; García-Algar 2008; Stroud et al. 2009). Furthermore, smoking increases risks of placental abruption, premature birth and sudden infant death syndrome (SIDS) (Hussein Rassool and Villar-Luís 2006).

Research using biochemical markers of smoking in postnatal women has demonstrated significant underreporting of smoking in mothers who gave birth to growth restricted babies (Delpisheh et al. 2007); this suggests fear of disclosure among mothers who smoke. Midwives are often willing to engage with smoking cessation strategies with childbearing women; however they sometimes feel ill-informed and ill-equipped to broach the issue, without stigmatising women and creating distrustful relationships (McLeod et al. 2003; Bull 2007). NICE (2010) and DH (2013b) recommend carbon monoxide breath tests to monitor women's levels of inhaled cigarette smoke as a cost-effective, non-invasive biochemical marker which helps the clinician identify and explore exposure to cigarette smoke with all women, which may reduce the risk of stigmatising some. These tests may also indicate exposure to second-hand smoke and other environmental pollutants (Bailey 2013). NICE (2010) produced guidance aimed at supporting childbearing women to stop smoking in pregnancy or following birth.

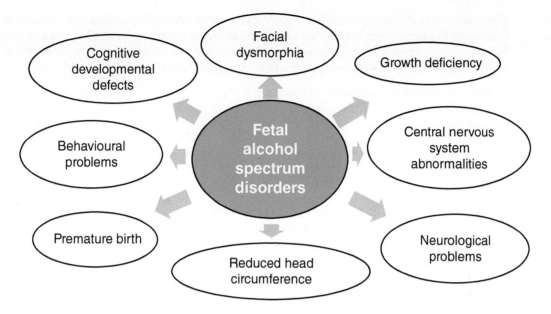

Figure 11.14   Diagram listing the characteristics associated with fetal alcohol spectrum disorders.

Alcohol consumption

Discussions about alcohol consumption in pregnancy are complex. As with smoking, drinking alcohol is legal and may be perceived as more culturally acceptable (pre and post-conception). Regular, moderate to heavy alcohol consumption in pregnancy is associated with neural, cranial and facial abnormalities seen in fetal alcohol spectrum disorders (Hutson et al. 2012; see Figure 11.14). Alcohol mimics the endocrine effects of maternal stress on the maternal hypothalamic–pituitary–adrenal (HPA) axis, leading to fetal growth restriction, underdevelopment and immunosuppression (Goldsmith 2004). The impact of these is chronic and irreversible. Since fetal alcohol spectrum disorders are entirely preventable, by abstinence, it is ethically problematic to conduct prospective studies to determine safe limits of alcohol consumption (Goldsmith 2004; Green 2007). Pregnant women and women planning to become pregnant should be advised to avoid drinking alcohol in the first three months of pregnancy, because there may be an increased risk of miscarriage (RCOG 2006).

- Non-abstinent pregnant women should drink no more than one–two UK units once or twice a week, since there is no evidence of harm to their unborn baby, at these levels (NICE 2008).
- Women should be advised not to get drunk or binge drink (drinking more than 7.5 UK units of alcohol on a single occasion) while they are pregnant because this can harm their unborn babies (NICE 2008).

However, the RCOG (2006) recommends total alcohol abstinence to avoid any risks to the pregnancy.

Illicit substances

Childbearing women may use opiates such as heroin which is snorted, smoked or injected. Its effects are to stimulate opiate receptors causing drowsiness and euphoria, but also nausea and respiratory depression (Hussein Rassool and Villar-Luís 2006). Heroin is physically addictive;

users experience increasing tolerance. People using heroin eventually require higher doses to experience the same effect. Withdrawal symptoms are experienced. Heroin crosses the placenta like many other psychoactive substances and in common with other opiates causes neurobehavioural teratogenicity. Maternal heroin use is associated with the following:

- Neonatal abstinence syndrome, including:
  - irritability
  - tremors
  - hypertonicity
  - tachypnoea
  - vomiting
  - diarrhoea. (Hussein Rassool & Villar-Luís 2006)

Injecting drug use also increases women's risk of contracting blood-borne viruses such as hepatitis B and C and human immunodeficiency virus (HIV) (Ornoy and Tenenbaum 2006; Thorne and Newell 2008; Sargent and Clayton 2010). Stimulants like cocaine provide increased energy and confidence, but have well-known physical effects such as tachycardia, hypertension and tachypnoea. Side effects include myocardial infarction (MI), cerebrovascular accident (CVA), seizures, depression, paranoia and venous injury. Due to its expense and illegality, cocaine has links to criminal behaviour. Its effects on the fetus and neonate are not well-established because the harmful effects cannot easily be isolated from those caused by concurrent aspects of health inequality like poverty, teenage pregnancy, single parenthood and common co-morbid factors such as: alcohol, tobacco, amphetamine and opiate abuse (Hussein Rassool and Villar-Luís 2006). Cannabis, or marijuana has also been reported to have negative consequences on the fetus, but no robust study has been conducted. There are numerous newer recreational or street drugs becoming available. Women seldom experience substance misuse in isolation from other complex social needs (NICE 2010). NICE (2010) recommends that all pregnant women be given lifestyle advice pertaining to smoking cessation, recreational drug use (implications) and alcohol consumption at the first contact with a health professional.

Domestic abuse

An area of increasing prominence in the maternal public health agenda is domestic abuse. Domestic abuse is:

> …any incident of threatening behaviour, violence or abuse (psychological, physical, sexual, financial or emotional) between adults who are or have been intimate partners, or family members; regardless of gender, sexuality, disability, race or religion…
>
> (British Medical Association (BMA) (2007, p. 1)

The scale of the issue is significant, in that it is increasingly recognised as a major contributor to poorer maternal, fetal and neonatal health outcomes (Lewis 2007; CMACE 2011; Table 11.4).

Women experiencing domestic abuse may demonstrate recognised patterns of behaviour (Department of Health [DH] 2005; Green and Ward 2010); these include late antenatal booking and poor attendance at antenatal appointments. They may present with repeated attendance in a minor injuries setting or have recurrent admissions with indefinable complaints, or unexplained. These women may demonstrate non-compliance (with treatment and management of various conditions). They may present to clinicians with mental health issues such as depression, anxiety or self-harm. They may exhibit injuries that are untended and of different ages, which they try to conceal or minimise. Women may also present with sexually transmitted infections

Table 11.4   The scale of domestic abuse

28% of women aged 15–59 have experienced domestic abuse.
About 10,000 women per week per week are sexually assaulted.
About 2000 women per week are raped.
34% of all reported rapes are on children under 16.
16% of children experienced sexual abuse in childhood.
More than five million women during childhood experienced sexual abuse.
People with a limiting illness or disability are more likely to experience abuse.

(STIs), urinary tract infections (UTIs) and vaginal infections; they may also have signs of poor obstetric history (Department of Health (DH) 2005; Green and Ward 2010). Women may find it difficult to escape the scrutiny of an abusive partner or relation. Between 2006 and 2008, CMACE (2011) identified 39 maternal deaths (12%) as displaying features of domestic abuse, a fifth by an intimate partner. The Task Force on Violence against Women and Children (2010) called for a national public health campaign on violence against women and children. Routine enquiry about domestic violence is now established midwifery practice, increasing frequency of disclosure (DH 2005; Price et al. 2007). Opportunity is sought for the pregnant women to consult with the midwife alone, at least once, which has been found highly acceptable to childbearing women. Midwives however, need training and education to help them better support women (Baird et al. 2011).

Midwives must promote the best interests of women and babies with complex social factors, through competent referrals (see Figure 11.15), providing appropriate advice, support and monitoring within the interprofessional team, and adopting a non-judgemental approach, making it possible for women to disclose their problems and complex social factors (NMC 2008; NICE 2010).

Activity 11.1

Think about how might you adapt the flow diagram in Figure 11.15 to help tackle the following issues:

- Smoking
- Mental health problems (see Chapters 4 and 13)
- Obesity
- Teenage mothers (see Chapter 5)
- Asylum seekers
- Non-English speaking women
- Domestic abuse

Conclusion

At some point, every baby had a mother; at some point every person was a baby. Therefore, midwives have a great responsibility and opportunity to support, and improve the health of the

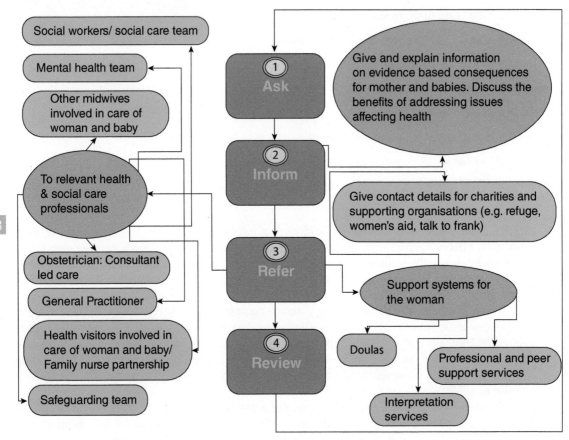

Figure 11.15   Referral pathway for women with complex social needs.

childbearing population and their babies. Any intervention aimed at reducing maternal and infant morbidity and mortality should be considered to be a major public health strategy. Midwifery care, as a whole could, therefore, be regarded as a public health intervention. It is recognised that there is a growing level of complexity in maternal and neonatal public healthcare. However midwives are strongly involved in delivering public healthcare.

Key points

- Public Health encompasses different dimensions of health and is a major facet of maternal and infant healthcare.
- Midwifery is a key public health profession because it is concerned with the health of childbearing women and infants, which may hold significant importance to the future health of the population.
- Health promotion is an important aspect of the public health role of the midwife and can be conducted individualistically, or strategically, top-down or bottom-up.
- A number of current public health issues affecting mothers and infants are set in the context of increasingly complex social factors: midwives must be aware of these and address them sensitively and with appropriate referrals within the interprofessional team.

End of chapter activities
Crossword

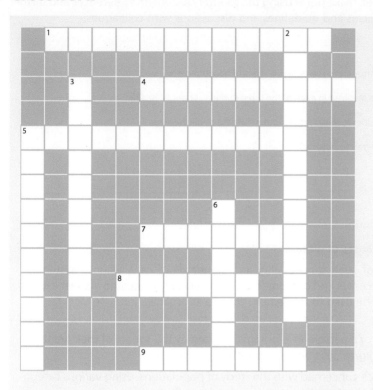

Across

1. Following health, describes the wider societal disadvantage that has a negative impact on the wellness of populations
4. Death
5. When linked to health, means providing the right information, at the right time, in the right place to inform decision-making and action-taking for people's wellbeing
7. A legal beverage which is a teratogen; when consumed in moderate or heavy quantities it is linked to a recognised spectrum disorder in the infant
8. An opiate drug which may be snorted, smoked or injected and is illegal in the United Kingdom
9. A body mass index of 30 or more kilogrammes per metre squared (kg/m^2)

Down

2. The study of the spread and causes disease and ill health in populations of people
3. The state of being ill or having a disease
5. When a child born from the 24th completed week of gestation, shows no signs of life
6. Describes something considered extremely unpleasant or harmful

Find out more

Below is a list of things you can find out about to enhance your knowledge of the issues and topics covered in this chapter. Make notes using the chapter content, the references and further reading identified, local policies and guidelines and discussions with colleagues.

1. What is the remit of public health?

2. List ways in which the midwife contributes to the different styles of health promotion.

3. Give examples of how midwives are involved in each of the three domains of public health.

4. What is health inequality and how does it contribute to understanding public health?

5. How might maternal obesity, be related to poverty?

Glossary of terms

Aetiological   Relating to the causes of diseases.

Audit/clinical audit   Process of evaluating quality and standards of care, using a systematic review. Aspects of structure, processes and outcomes are systematically evaluated against explicit criteria. The results of audit can be used to implement change at organisational, service, team or individual level.

Body Mass Index   The weight of a person (in kilograms) divided by the square of their height (in metres), the units are therefore kg/m^2 also written as $kg.m^{-2}$.

Demography   Statistical science concerned with the study of populations, using various categories such as area (local, region and national), age-group, gender and migration.

Endemic   The habitual presence or frequent occurrence of a disease within a particular location, or population.

Epidemic   Occurrence, or outbreak, of a given disease, or group of similar illnesses in a population, or region vastly exceeding usual prevalence, affecting large proportions of the population.

Epidemiology   Study of the distribution of factors which determine health and disease in populations.

Immunisation   Artificial production of immunity, by use of a vaccine or passive introduction of an immunoglobulin.

Intrauterine growth restriction (IUGR)   Where a fetus has failed to achieve its growth potential, resulting in the birth of a baby whose birth weight is abnormally low in relation to gestational age.

Macrosomia   Abnormally large for gestational age.

Morbidity   The state of being ill or having a disease.

Mortality   Death.

Obesity   Condition in which excess fat has accumulated in the body, mostly in the subcutaneous tissues.

Obstetrics   Branch of medicine that attends to the care of childbearing women during pregnancy, childbirth and the puerperium, particularly concerned with deviations from the norm.

Pandemic A worldwide epidemic (e.g. bubonic plague in 14th century Europe, or the AIDS pandemic).

Pathogen Parasite causing disease, usually a microorganism.

Pre-clinical (disease) The stage of a disease after the infected individual is not displaying clinical signs or symptoms, which will ultimately progress to clinical disease.

Puerperal Pertaining to the period after childbirth (the puerperium).

Puerperium The six to eight week period following childbirth, during which the mother's body returns to its pre-pregnant state, with the uterus returning to its normal size.

Sub-clinical (disease) A disease or condition, which is not clinically apparent, and is not destined to become so.

Vaccine A special preparation of antigenic (cell surface recognition molecules, which initiate immunity) material that can be used to stimulate the development of antibodies and thus confer active immunity against a specific disease or a number of diseases. Many are derived from culturing bacteria or viruses in such a way to remove their infectivity.

(Thain and Hickman 2004; Gordis 2009; Porth 2009; Tiran 2008; Martin 2010.)

References

Abortion Act (1967) Ch. 8. London: The Stationary Office.

Acheson, D. (1998) Independent Inquiry into Inequalities in Health Report, [Online], Available: http://www.archive.official-documents.co.uk/document/doh/ih/contents.htm

Bailey, B. (2013) Using expired air carbon monoxide to determine smoking status during pregnancy: Preliminary identification of an appropriately sensitive and specific cut-point. *Addictive Behaviors* 38 (10), pp. 2547–2550.

Baird, K., Salmon, D., White, P. (2011) *A five year follow up study of the Bristol Pregnancy and Domestic Violence Programme (BPDVP) to promote routine antenatal enquiry for domestic violence at North Bristol Trust. Project Report*. [Online], Available: http://eprints.uwe.ac.uk/15424/

Barker, D.J.P. (2001) Fetal and infant origins of adult disease. *Monatschrift Kinderheilkunder* Supplement 1, pp. S2–S6.

Barker, D.J.P. (1989) (ed.) *Fetal and Infant Origins of Adult Disease*. London: British Medical Journal.

Barker, D.J.P. (1997) Maternal nutrition, fetal nutrition, and disease in later life. *Nutrition* 13 (9), pp. 807–813.

Black, D. (1980) *Inequalities in Health. Report of a Research Working Group*. [Online], Manchester: Socialist Health Association. http://www.sochealth.co.uk/public-health-and-wellbeing/poverty-and-inequality/the-black-report-1980/

Beldon, A., Crozier, S. (2005) Health promotion in pregnancy: the role of the midwife. *Journal of the Royal Society for the Promotion of Health* 125 (5), pp. 216–220.

Bowden, J. (2006) Health Promotion and the Midwife. In: *Health Promotion in Midwifery* (eds J. Bowden, V. Manning), 2nd edn, pp. 13–24. London: Hodder Arnold.

Bowling, I. (2009) *Research Methods in Health: Investigating Health and Health Services*, 3rd edn. Maidenhead: Open University Press.

British Medical Association (BMA) Board of Science (2007) Domestic *abuse. A report from the BMA Board of Science*, [Online], Available: http://www.bma.org.uk/images/Domestic%20Abuse_tcm41-183509.pdf

Bull, L. (2007) Smoking cessation intervention with pregnant women and new parents (part two): a focus group study of health visitors and midwives working in the UK. *Journal of Neonatal Nursing* 13, 5, pp. 179–185.

Cancer Research UK (2011) *Smoking Statistics*, [Online], Available: http://info.cancerresearchuk.org/cancerstats/types/lung/smoking/#socio

Carr, S., Unwin, N., Pless-Mulloli,T., Unwin, N. (2007) *An Introduction to Public Health and Epidemiology*, 2nd edn. Maidenhead: Open University Press.

261

Centre for Maternal and Child Enquiries (CMACE) (2011) Saving Mothers' Lives: reviewing maternal deaths to make motherhood safer: 2006–08. The Eighth Report on Confidential Enquiries into Maternal Deaths in the United Kingdom. *British Journal of Obstetrics and Gynaecology* 118 (S.1), pp. 1–203.

Centre for Maternal and Child Enquiries/Royal College of Obstetricians & Gynaecologists (2010) *Management of Women with Obesity in Pregnancy*. [Online] Available: http://www.hqip.org.uk/assets/NCAPOP-Library/CMACE-Reports/15.-March-2010-Management-of-Women-with-Obesity-in-Pregnancy-Guidance.pdf

Chamberlain, M., Gallop, J. (1988) The disabled living centre: What does it do? *British Medical Journal* 297, pp. 1523–1526.

Clarke, A. (2011) *The Sociology of Healthcare*, 2nd edn. Harlow: Pearson Education.

Commissioning Board Chief Nursing Officer and DH Chief Nursing Adviser (2012) *Compassion in Practice*. [Online], Available: http://www.england.nhs.uk/wp-content/uploads/2012/12/compassion-in-practice.pdf.

Dahlgren, G., Whitehead, M. (1992) *Policies and strategies to promote equity in health*. Copenhagen: World Health Organization.

Department of Health (2000) *The NHS Plan*. London: DH.

De Angelis, L. and Robinson, F. (2010) *Clinical pathway for weight management in pregnancy*. Hull, Hull and East Yorkshire Women's and Children's Hospital.

Department of Health (2004) *National Service Framework for Children, Young People and Maternity Services: The mental health and psychological wellbeing of children and young people*. [Online] Available: https://www.gov.uk/government/uploads/system/uploads/attachment_data/file/199952/National_Service_Framework_for_Children_Young_People_and_Maternity_Services_-_Core_Standards.pdf

Department of Health (DH) (2005) *Responding to Domestic Abuse*. [Online], Available: http://www.dh.gov.uk/prod_consum_dh/groups/dh_digitalassets/@dh/@en/documents/digitalasset/dh_4126619.pdf

Department of Health (DH) (2007a) *Tackling health inequalities: 2007 status report on the Programme of Action*. [Online], Available: http://www.bris.ac.uk/poverty/downloads/keyofficialdocuments/Tackling%20Health%20Inequalities.2007status.pdf

Department of Health (2007b) *Maternity Matters*. London: DH.

Department of Health (2010a) *Healthy Lives, Healthy People: Our strategy for public health in England*. [Online], Available: http://www.dh.gov.uk/prod_consum_dh/groups/dh_digitalassets/documents/digitalasset/dh_127424.pdf

Department of Health, Department of Health Safety and Social Services, Welsh Assembly Government, Scottish Government (2010b) *Midwifery 2020 Delivering expectations*. [Online]. Available: http://www.dhsspsni.gov.uk/midwifery_2020_report.pdf

Department of Health (2011) *Public Health England's Operating Model*, [Online], Available: https://www.gov.uk/government/uploads/system/uploads/attachment_data/file/216716/dh_131892.pdf

Department of Health (DH) (2012) *Temporary programme of pertussis (whooping cough) vaccination of pregnant women*. [Online], Available: https://www.gov.uk/government/uploads/system/uploads/attachment_data/file/212947/CMO-Pertussis-27-09-2012-FINAL.pdf

Department of Health (2013a) *Public Health Surveillance: Towards a Public Health Surveillance Strategy for England*. [Online]. Available https://www.gov.uk/government/uploads/system/uploads/attachment_data/file/127475/Towards-a-Public-Health-Surveillance-Strategy.pdf

Department of Health (2013b) Nursing and midwifery actions at the three levels of public health practice Improving health and wellbeing at individual, community and population levels. [Online]. Available: https://www.gov.uk/government/uploads/system/uploads/attachment_data/file/208814/3_Levels.pdf.

Delpisheh, A., Topping, J., Tang, A., Brabin, B.J. (2007) Smoking exposure in pregnancy: use of salivary cotinine in monitoring. *British Journal of Midwifery* 15 (4), pp. 216–220.

Dunn, P. (1996) Florence Nightingale (1820–1910): maternal mortality and the training of midwives. *Archives of Disease in Childhood: Fetal and Neonatal* 74 (3), pp. F219–F220.

European Foundation for the Improvement of Living and Working Conditions (2003) *Illness, disability and social inclusion*. Luxembourg: Official Publications of the European Communities.

Farmer, R., Lawrenson, R. (2004) *Epidemiology and Public Health Medicine*, 5th edn. Oxford: Blackwell Publishing.

Furber, C.M. (2000) An exploration of midwives' attitudes to health promotion. *Midwifery* 16 (4), pp. 314–322.

García-Algar, O. (2008) Nicotine withdrawal symptoms in newborns. *Archivos de bronconeumología* 44 (10), pp. 509–511.

Goldsmith, C. (2004) Fetal alcohol syndrome: a preventable tragedy. *Access* May–June, pp. 34–38.

Gordis, L. (2009) *Epidemiology*, 4th edn. Philadelphia: Elsevier Saunders.

Green, J.H. (2007) Fetal alcohol spectrum disorders: understanding the effects of prenatal alcohol exposure and supporting students. *Journal of School Health* 77 (3), pp. 103–108.

Stillbirth definition Act (1992) Ch. 29. London: The Stationary Office.

Green, A., Ward, S. (2010) Domestic violence. *Obstetrics, Gynaecology and Reproductive Medicine* 20 (4), pp. 121–124.

Greener, J., Douglas, F., Teijlingen, E.V. (2010) More of the same? Conflicting perspectives of obesity causation and intervention amongst overweight people health professionals and policy makers. *Social Science and Medicine* 70 (7), pp. 1042–1049.

Griffiths, S., Jewell, T., Donnelly, P. (2005) Public health in practice: the three domains of public health. *Public Health* 119 (10), pp. 907–913.

Guttmacher, S. (1979) Whole in body, mind and spirit: holistic health and the limits of medicine. *The Hastings Center Report* 9 (2), pp. 15–21.

Hales, C.N., Barker, D.J.P. (2001) The thrifty phenotype hypothesis. *British Medical Bulletin* 60, pp. 5–20.

Hansson, L.M., Rasmussen, F., Ahlstrom, G.I. (2011) General Practitioners' and district nurses' conceptions of the encounter with obese patients in primary healthcare. *BMC Family Practice* 12 (7), pp. 1–10.

Health and Social Care Act (2012) Ch. 7. London: The Stationary Office.

Health Protection Agency (2013) Health Protection Report. [Online], Available: http://www.hpa.org.uk/hpr/archives/2013/hpr14-1713.pdf

Health Protection Agency (2010) *List of Notifiable Diseases*. [Online], Available: http://www.hpa.org.uk/Topics/InfectiousDiseases/InfectionsAZ/NotificationsOfInfectiousDiseases/ListOfNotifiableDiseases/

Healthy Start (no date). *Healthy Start*. [Online], Available: http://www.healthystart.nhs.uk/

Herzig, K., Danley, D., Jackson, R., Petersen, R., Chamberlain, L., Gerbert, B. (2006) Seizing the 9-month moment: Addressing behavioral risks in prenatal patients. *Patient Education and Counseling* 61 (2), pp. 228–235.

Huizink, A.C., Mulder, E.J.H. (2005) Maternal smoking, drinking or cannabis use during pregnancy and neurobehavioural and cognitive functioning in human offspring. *Neuroscience and Biobehavioral Reviews* 30, pp. 24–41.

Hull Clinical Commissioning Group (2013) *Maternity Services Commissioning Strategy 2013–2018*. Hull: NHS Hull.

Hutson, J.R., Stade, B., Lehotay, D., Collier., P., Kapur, B. (2012) Folic acid transport to the human fetus is decreased in pregnancies with chronic alcohol exposure. *PLoS ONE* 7 (5), pp. 1–6.

International Confederation of Midwives (2011) *ICM International Definition of the Midwife* [Online], Available: http://www.internationalmidwives.org/who-we-are/policy-and-practice/icm-international-definition-of-the-midwife/

Jewell, K. (2005) The public health divide. *RCM Midwives* 8 (7), pp. 318–319.

Kee, W.D. (2005) Confidential Enquiries into Maternal Deaths: 50 years of closing the loop. *British Journal of Anaesthesia* 94 (4), pp. 413–416.

Lewis, A. (1953) Health as a social concept. *British Journal of Sociology* 4 (2), pp. 109–124.

Lewis, G. (ed.) (2007) *The Confidential Enquiry into Maternal and Child Health (CEMACH). Saving Mothers' Lives: reviewing maternal deaths to make motherhood safer- 2003–2005*. The Seventh Report on Confidential Enquiries into Maternal Deaths in the United Kingdom. [Online], Available: http://www.hqip.org.uk/assets/NCAPOP-Library/CMACE-Reports/21.-December-2007-Saving-Mothers-Lives-reviewing-maternal-deaths-to-make-motherhood-safer-2003-2005.pdf

Local Government Association (2014) *Health and Wellbeing Boards (HWB) Leadership Offer* [Online] Available: http://www.local.gov.uk/health/-/journal_content/56/10180/3510973/ARTICLE

Lucchese, A., Merola, A., Caruso, A. (2004) Risk of drug-induced congenital defects. *European Journal of Obstetrics & Gynecology and Reproductive Biology* 117 (1), pp. 10–19.

Marmot, M., Allen, J., Goldblatt, P., Boyce, T., McLeish, D., Grady, M., Geddes, I. (2010) *Post-2010 strategic review of health inequalities (the Marmot Review)*. [Online]. Available: http://www.instituteofhealthequity.org/projects/fair-society-healthy-lives-the-marmot-review

Martin, E.A. (2010) *Concise Oxford Colour Medical Dictionary*. Oxford: Oxford University Press.

McCormick, A. (1993) The notification of infectious diseases in England and Wales. *Communicable Disease Report*. 3 (2), pp. R19–R34.

263

McLeod, D., Bennf, C., Pullonb, S., Viccars, A., White, S., Cooksond, T., Dowelle, A. (2003) The midwife's role in facilitating smoking behaviour change during pregnancy. *Midwifery* 19 (4), pp. 285–297.

Mold, F., Forbes, A. (2011) Patients' and professionals' experiences and perspectives of obesity in health-care settings: a synthesis of current research. *Health Expectations* 16, pp. 119–132.

Mordacci, R., Sobel, R. (1998) Health: a comprehensive concept. *Hastings Center Report* 28 (1), pp. 34–37.

Morley, R. (2006) Fetal origins of adult disease. [Online], *Seminars in Fetal and Neonatal Medicine* 11 (2), pp. 73–78.

National Health Service Act (1977) ch. 49. London: The Stationary Office.

National Institute for Health and Care Excellence (2013a) *Who we are?* [Online], Available: http://www.nice.org.uk/aboutnice/whoweare/who_we_are.jsp

National Institute for Health and Care Excellence (2013b) *Diabetes in pregnancy overview – NICE pathways*, [Online], Available: http://pathways.nice.org.uk/pathways/diabetes-in-pregnancy#content=view-node%3Anodes-neonatal-care-for-babies-of-mothers-with-diabetes.

National Institute for Health and Clinical Excellence (2011) *'The Monday Clinic'; Implementing a maternal obesity service.* [Online], Available: http://www.nice.org.uk/usingguidance/sharedlearningimplementing niceguidance/examplesofimplementation/eximpresults.jsp?o=410

National Institute for Health and Clinical Excellence (2010a) *Pregnancy and complex social factors.* [Online], Available: http://publications.nice.org.uk/pregnancy-and-complex-social-factors-cg110

National Institute for Health and Clinical Excellence (2010b) *Quitting smoking in pregnancy and following childbirth.* [Online], Available: http://guidance.nice.org.uk/PH26/Guidance/pdf/English

National Institute for Health and Clinical Excellence (NICE) (2008) *Antenatal care: Routine care for the healthy pregnant woman.* [Online], Available: http://www.nice.org.uk/nicemedia/live/11947/40115/40115.pdf

National Statistics & National Health Service Information Centre for Health & Social Care (2010) *Infant Feeding Survey: Early Results.* [Online], Available. https://catalogue.ic.nhs.uk/publications/public-health/surveys/infant-feed-surv-2010/ifs-uk-2010-chap3-feed-meths.pdf

Nightingale, F. (1871) *Introductory notes on Lying-in Hospitals.* [Online], Available: http://archive.org/details/introductorynot00nighgoog

Nursing and Midwifery Council (NMC) (2008) *The Code: Standards of conduct, performance and ethics for nurses and midwives*, [Online], Available: http://www.nmc-uk.org/Publications/Standards/The-code/Introduction/ [24 Mar 2013].

Office for National Statistics (ONS) (2012a) *Childbearing Among UK Born and Non-UK Born Women Living in the UK.* [Online], Available: http://www.ons.gov.uk/ons/dcp171766_283876.pdf

Office for National Statistics (ONS) (2012b) *Births and Deaths in England and Wales, 2011 (Final).* [Online], Available: http://www.ons.gov.uk/ons/dcp171778_279934.pdf

Office for National Statistics (ONS) (2012c) *Births Tables: Metadata 2011.* [Online], Available: http://www.ons.gov.uk/ons/guide-method/user-guidance/health-and-life-events/births-metadata.pdf

Office for National Statistics (2013) Chapter 1 – Smoking (General Lifestyle Survey Overview – a report on the 2011 General Lifestyle Survey). [Online], Available: http://www.ons.gov.uk/ons/dcp171776_302558.pdf

Oliver, M. (1983) *Social Work with Disabled People.* London: Macmillan Press.

Oken, E., Taveras, E.M. Kleinman, K., Rich-Edwards, J.W., Gillman, M.W. (2007) Gestational weight gain and child adiposity at age 3 years. *American Journal of Obstetrics and Gynecology* 196 (4), pp. 322.e1–322.e8.

Omran, A. (2005) The epidemiologic transition: a theory of the epidemiology of population change. *The Milbank Quarterly* 83 (4), pp. 731–757.

Ornoy, A., Tenenbaum, A. (2006) Pregnancy outcome following infections by coxsackie, echo, measles, mumps, hepatitis, polio and encephalitis viruses. *Reproductive Technology* 21, pp. 447–457.

Osmond, C., Barker, D.J.P., Slattery, J.M. (1989) Risk of death from cardiovascular disease and chronic bronchitis determined by place of birth in England and Wales. In: *Fetal and Infant Origins of Adult Disease* (ed. D.J.P. Barker). London: British Medical Journal.

Piper, S. (2005) Health promotion: a practice framework for midwives. *British Journal of Midwifery* 13 (6), pp. 284–288.

Porth, C. (2009) Concepts of health and disease. In: *Pathophysiology: Concepts of Altered Health States* (eds C. Porth, G. Matfin), 8th edn, pp. 1–9. Philadelphia: Lippincott and Williams.

Price, S., Baird, K., Salmon, D. (2007) Routine antenatal enquiry lead to an increased rate of disclosure of domestic abuse? Findings from the Bristol Pregnancy and Domestic Violence Programme. *Evidence Based Midwifery* 5 (3), pp. 100–106.

264

Hussein Rassool, G., Villar-Luís, M. (2006) Reproductive risks of alcohol and illicit drugs: an overview. *Journal of Addictions Nursing* 17 (4), pp. 211–213.

Royal College of Midwives (2012) *Seasonal Flu Programme Winter 2012/2013*. [Online], Available: http://www.rcm.org.uk/college/policy-practice/flu-programme-2012/

Royal College of Midwives (2011) *Response to the Public Health White Paper – Healthy Lives, Healthy People*. [Online], Available: http://community.rcm.org.uk/files/rcm/2010-129%20Public%20Health%20White%20Paper%20RCM%20Reponse.doc

Royal College of Midwives (2001) *Position Paper 24: The Midwife's Role in Public Health*. [Online], Available: http://maternalhealthtaskforce.org/component/docman/doc_view/698-position-paper-no-24-the-midwife-s-role-in-public-health?Itemid=220.

Royal College of Obstetrics and Gynaecology (2006) *Alcohol and pregnancy – information for you*, [Online], Available: http://www.rcog.org.uk/womens-health/clinical-guidance/alcohol-and-pregnancy-information-you.

Sargent, S., Clayton, M. (2010) Liver disease in women: Examining prevalence and complications. *Gastrointestinal Nursing* 8 (4), pp. 30–37.

Schmied, V.A., Duff. M., Dahlen, H.G., Mills, A.E., Kolt, G.S. (2011) 'Not waving but drowning': a study of the experiences and concerns of midwives and other health professionals caring for obese childbearing women. *Midwifery* 27, pp. 424–430.

Stroud, L., Paster, R., Goodwin, M.S., Shenassa, E., Buka, S., Niaura, R., Rosenblith, J., Lipsitt, L. (2009) Maternal smoking during pregnancy and neonatal behavior: a large-scale community study. *Pediatrics* 123 (5), pp. e842–e848.

Sidebotham, M., Walsh, T. (2011) Epidemiology. In: *Mayes Midwifery* (eds S. MacDonald, J. Macgill-Cuerden), 14th edn. Edinburgh: Balliere-Tindall.

Soanes, C., Hawker, S., Elliott, J. (2005) *Pocket Oxford English Dictionary*, 10th edn. Oxford: Oxford University Press.

Sydenstricker, E. (1935) The Changing Concept of Public Health. [Online]. Available: http://www.jstor.org/stable/3347855

Taskforce on the Health Aspects of Violence Against Women and Children (2010) *Responding to violence against women and children – the role of the NHS*. [Online], Available: http://www.health.org.uk/media_manager/public/75/external-publications/Responding-to-violence-against-women-and-children%E2%80%93the-role-of-the-NHS.pdf

Thain, M., Hickman, M. (2004) *Dictionary of Biology*, 11th edn. London: Penguin Books.

Thorne, C., Newell, M.L. (2008) HIV, hepatitis and pregnancy. *Women's Health and Medicine* 2 (2), pp. 40–43.

Thorpe, A., Griffiths, S., Jewell, T., Adshead, F. (2008) The three domains of public health: An internationally relevant basis for public health education? *Public Health* 122 (2), pp. 201–210.

Tiran, D. (2008) *Baillière's Midwives' Dictionary*, 11th edn. Edinburgh: Baillière Tindall.

Tripp, S. (1997) What contribution, if any, can social construction theories make to understanding the experience of disabling conditions? *Journal of Orthopaedic Nursing* 1, pp. 17–20.

United Kingdom's Faculty of Public Health (2010) What is Public Health? [Online], Available: http://www.fph.org.uk/what_is_public_health

Wanless, D. (2003) *Securing Good Health for the Whole Population: Population Health Trends*. Norwich: HMSO.

Weindling, A.M. (2003) The Confidential Enquiry into Maternal and Child Health (CEMACH). *Archives of Disease in Childhood* 88 (12), pp. 1034–1037.

Whitehead, D. (2003) Health promotion and health education viewed as symbiotic paradigms: bridging the theory and practice gap between them. *Journal of Clinical Nursing* 12 (6), pp. 796–805.

Wood, A. (1957) The Role of the Midwife in Public Health. [Online], Available: http://whqlibdoc.who.int/php/WHO_PHP_4.pdf

World Health Organization (WHO) (1948) *WHO Definition of Health*. [Online], Available: http://www.who.int/about/definition/en/print.html

World Health Organization (2013) *Maternal mortality ratio (per 100 000 live births*. [Online], Available: http://www.who.int/healthinfo/statistics/indmaternalmortality/en/

Chapter 12

Contraception and family planning

Liz Smith
University of Hull, Hull, UK

Sarah Wise
Diana Princess of Wales Hospital, Grimsby, UK

Learning outcomes

By the end of this chapter the reader will be able to:

- discuss the meaning of family planning
- explain the influences on women's choices in relation to contraception
- describe the methods of contraception available
- recognise the need for sensitive and individualised information and advice.

Introduction

Midwives are in an ideal position to offer information and advice with regard to contraception and family planning, but often lack confidence to do so. Since ovulation can re-commence as early as 25 days post-delivery it is important that women have sound information about their contraceptive options particularly as these may be limited by the woman's general health, breastfeeding or religious and cultural beliefs. Contraception can be a difficult topic to discuss for both women and midwives, but if it is approached with sensitivity the advice provided can empower women and allow them to make choices best suited to their individual needs.

This chapter aims to provide an overview of contraception and family planning with guidance for further reading to support development of knowledge and understanding.

What is meant by 'family planning'?

Contraception and family planning are often used by both healthcare professionals and lay people interchangeably and are generally perceived to be used to define the prevention of

Fundamentals of Midwifery: A Textbook for Students, First Edition. Edited by Louise Lewis.
© 2015 John Wiley & Sons, Ltd. Published 2015 by John Wiley & Sons, Ltd.
Companion website: www.wileyfundamentalseries.com/midwifery

pregnancy or control over fertility. Whilst this perception has some truth within it, family planning can have a much more literal meaning, i.e. a plan for the number and spacing of children within the family. This is an important issue when discussing contraception as some women may be put off discussing the prevention of pregnancy if they feel it is not placed in the context of future children. For some women religious or cultural beliefs may mean that contraception is not an option, but this does not mean they do not need advice about sex and fertility after childbirth. The National Institute for Health and Care Excellence (NICE) (2006) guidance on postnatal care states that contraception should be discussed within the first week following birth; however to fully meet women's needs midwives should be responding to individual need and ensuring that women are fully informed about sex and sexuality, contraception and plans for further pregnancy.

Appropriate timing of advice

There is a strong association between transfer from hospital to community care and discussion about contraception, but it is also provided on transfer from midwifery care to the health visitor or even left until the six week postnatal examination (Hall 2005). A review of the evidence by Hiller et al. (2002) failed to identify which timing is best. The hospital transfer appears to be the most common time, but this often means that it is rushed and women may feel overloaded with information as other health and safety advice is offered at the same time. Norris (2006) suggests that not only is information often rushed, it is also provided in an environment that offers very little privacy for such an intimate and personal discussion. She also recommends that privacy and confidentiality are of vital importance not least because some women may choose to use contraceptive measures in secret (Figure 12.1). Hall (2005) concurs with the importance of privacy and suggests that the principles of woman-centred care require that women should be asked if they want to discuss family planning and their wishes respected. This approach would give the opportunity for a discussion at a time which was best suited to the needs of the woman whether this is in the antenatal period, prior to postnatal transfer from hospital or on the community. What is essential is that this is not a topic that is simply glossed over because midwives find it a difficult subject or not something that they see as a priority. Research suggests that

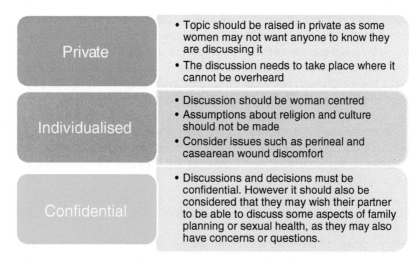

Figure 12.1 Priorities for family planning discussions.

menstruation returns around 69 days following birth on average (Hall 2005) but some women may ovulate at around 25 days (Queenan 2004) so midwifery advice regarding contraception and family planning could be beneficial in preventing unwanted pregnancies.

Psychosexual issues

Hall (2005) emphasises the need to approach any discussion about family planning and contraception with sensitivity. It is important to discuss the resumption of sexual intimacy which may be affected by a range of issues. The most obvious influence is pain from any perineal or vaginal wall trauma and this is not necessarily related to the severity of the trauma; the pain from grazes and minor tears can be significant and have a lasting effect on the woman. Similarly caesarean section wounds can remain sore for some time following delivery and this, in addition to the fatigue associated with major surgery, can result in a delay in wanting to be sexually active. Simply having a new baby and the disruption in the previous routine will be both tiring and have a constraining effect on intimacy.

The impact of childbirth on sexual relationships is not only something experienced by women. Men who have witnessed the birth may feel reluctant to cause any pain or discomfort or may worry about the risk of further pregnancy particularly if there were problems during labour or the birth.

Both women and midwives need to be able to discuss these issues. It is helpful for women to know that it is safe to resume sex when they feel ready but that they should not feel pressured into it.

Cultural aspects

The increase in global travel and movement has resulted in most nations being culturally diverse and it is therefore important that midwives have some understanding of the influence culture and religion can have on family planning and contraceptive choices. Equally, it is essential that assumptions are not made regarding an individual's beliefs and as a consequence the advice and care provided not meeting an individual's needs. Just because a woman identifies herself as being a member of a particular culture or religion does not mean that she agrees with all its associated beliefs. It is also true that many religions are sub-divided into groups that have differing interpretations of the overall teachings. In relation to family planning and contraceptive advice there is a need to be sensitive to potential cultural and religious beliefs whilst at the same time treating each woman as a unique individual. Table 12.1 provides a generalised and brief overview of the mainstream religious attitudes to contraception based on a Canadian study by Srikanthan and Reid (2008). The key to providing culturally competent care is avoiding stereotypical assumptions; recognising that all women do not necessarily share the same values and beliefs as their peers whether or not they describe themselves as having a particular cultural or religious background. For example, it may be important for some women to experience regular bleeding whilst using contraception whether or not they are adherents of those religions that value the monthly cycle.

Providing advice

As already emphasised all information and advice provided to women should be tailored to their individual needs. As well as accounting for their cultural and/or religious preferences it is also important to consider the health issues that may impact on their options. In order to do

Table 12.1   Mainstream religious attitudes to contraception

Religion	
Christian: Roman Catholic	Contraception goes against the purpose of marriage. Unnatural methods of contraception are banned – this includes barrier or chemical methods (i.e. condoms, diaphragms and spermicides). Abstinence and the rhythm method can be used for birth spacing.
Christian: Eastern Orthodox	Strict adherents permit only abstinence. More liberal adherents allow the use of contraception that does not destroy the products of conception (some IUDs and emergency contraception) for birth spacing. Monthly menstruation may be valued; therefore some methods may not be acceptable on this basis. Permanent methods, i.e. sterilisation or vasectomy are not generally acceptable.
Christian: Protestant	Some Evangelical and Fundamental Protestants may disapprove of contraception. Most however do not object to contraception in marriage.
Jewish faith	Orthodox Jews do not generally approve of contraception. Generally husbands must approve the use of contraception. Condoms, coitus interruptus and any other means of male contraception are not approved of. The rhythm method and abstinence are also not generally acceptable. Female oral contraception is permissible, but IUDs that prevent implantation are not. Some women will value monthly menstruation, and therefore methods that stop monthly bleeding would not be acceptable to them.
Islam	Contraception can be viewed as not being permitted, permitted but not approved of, or permitted and acceptable within groups. Irreversible methods and methods which are seen as inducing abortion (therefore including some IUDs) are not permitted and contraception should only be used within marriage. Monthly menstruation may be valued by some women so continuous methods would not be acceptable.
Hindu	There are no expressed prohibitions where contraception does not cause any moral or spiritual harm. Some women will not be educated about contraception until after the birth of the first child and in some families, permission should be obtained from the husband to discuss contraception.
Buddhist	Generally acceptable if preventing conception, but less acceptable if it works by stopping the development or implantation of a fertilised egg. Therefore IUDs are not acceptable. Abstinence may be the method of choice.
Chinese religions	Taoism and Confucianism permit contraceptive use, but natural methods such as withdrawal and rhythm methods may be preferred.

269

this it is essential that the woman's medical and obstetric history is known. Some contraceptive methods are not appropriate if breastfeeding because the oestrogen content negatively affects lactation.

Box 12.1 lists the essential information and includes consideration of the woman's knowledge of the menstrual cycle. Understanding the menstrual cycle is important in relation to understanding how each method works and also to women understanding why they may become pregnant before their first period. Women should have the opportunity to discuss issues that

Box 12.1   Information essential to effective contraceptive advice

- Age of the woman
- General health, including weight and Body Mass Index (BMI)
- Medical history
- Gynaecological history, including previous menstrual problems/cycles
- Obstetric history
- Lifestyle, including smoking habits and health beliefs and religion
- Family history in relation to any cardiovascular disease or breast cancer
- Previous contraceptive use including any contraception failure

Additionally it is important to consider:

- The woman's knowledge of her menstrual cycle
- Any issues that are important to the woman and her partner

are relevant to them; the midwife should therefore allow time for questions and discussion. Listening to the woman is vital to a more individualised approach to advice.

Methods of contraception
Barrier methods
Male condoms

This is the only method of contraception that provides protection against sexually transmitted infections (STI) and used correctly are very reliable (98% effective). Condoms can be obtained free of charge from a range of venues including some General Practitioner (GP) surgeries and Family Planning/Sexual Health clinics. They can also be purchased from chemists and supermarkets and many outlets have condom vending machines. Condoms must be used every time, at the right time and fitted correctly to be effective. They can split or rupture if not used correctly.

Condoms avoid the use of hormone-based contraceptives for those women who are conscious of weight gain and the effects of hormones on the body. Condoms can be used as soon as required following the birth; however the use of a water-based lubricant may be necessary if the women feels dry or sore from having sutures at delivery (see Figure 12.2).

Female condoms

These are often referred to as a 'femidom'. (Femidom was the original British brand name for the product.) They can also be obtained from Family Planning and Sexual Health Clinics; although they are not quite as freely available as the male condom. The female condom is also made of latex and is placed inside the vagina. It is also a barrier method of contraception, but is slightly less effective than the male condom (95%). Reliability is dependent on being used correctly and in particular the 'femidom' needs to fit properly otherwise it can be pushed aside during sexual intercourse. The clear advantage of this method is that it can be put in place before any sexual activity has started and therefore reduces interruption and also allows the women to be in control (see Figure 12.3).

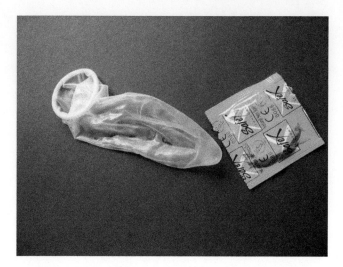

Figure 12.2   Male condoms.

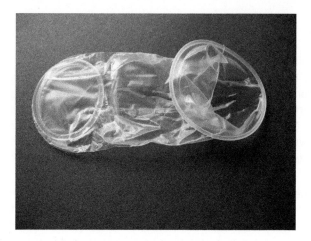

Figure 12.3   Female condom.

Diaphragms/caps

There are a variety of different types of caps and diaphragms. They work by being fitted into the vagina and covering the cervix. To be most effective (92–96%) the use of a spermicide is also encouraged which can be considered to be less desirable. This method avoids the use of hormones and it does have the advantage of not interrupting sex. Diaphragms and caps need to be fitted by a doctor or specialist nurse to ensure the right size is obtained. The cap/diaphragm needs to be in place each time the woman has sex; however it can be put in place before sexual activity starts. If the woman has previously used the cap/diaphragm before becoming pregnant she needs to be made aware that she may require a different size postpartum for it to be effective. This is considered to be a useful method of contraception for those women who wish to avoid hormone-based contraceptives (see Figure 12.4).

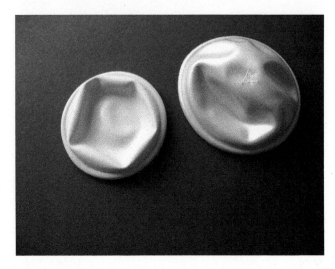

Figure 12.4   Diaphragms/caps.

Hormonal contraceptives
Combined pill

The combined pill is a very effective method of contraception (99%) if taken consistently. There are wide variety of combined pills taken daily for 21 days with a 7-day pill-free week. The pill contains two hormones progesterone and oestrogen. This method can commence on day 21 following the birth, it is *not* however recommended for those mothers who choose to breast-feed, as it has an effect on milk supply. The combined pill needs to be used with caution in those women who have a raised Body Mass Index (BMI) and who also who smoke as it increases the risk of thromboembolism.

Progesterone only pill

The progesterone only pill (POP) works slightly differently from the combined pill and there are two types of POP. One works mainly by preventing ovulation and has a 12-hour window in which it can be taken and therefore it is very effective (99%). The other works mainly by preventing the sperm entering the cervix, but it must be taken within 3 hours to be effective (96%). POP methods can result in amenorrhoea or changes in menstrual pattern. There is also the possibility that they can increase appetite levels resulting in increased weight in some cases. The POP can be commenced at 21 days following the birth and is the most appropriate pill for breastfeeding women. It is a more suitable method for those women who have an increased BMI, or suffer from migraines, and for women who would not be suitable for use of the combined pill particu-larly if they are over 35 years and smoke (see Figure 12.5).

Contraceptive patch

The patch is 99% effective when used correctly. It consists of an adhesive patch applied to the upper arm, body or buttock which releases oestrogen and progesterone into the bloodstream. This is applied once a week for 3 weeks with a patch-free week to allow for a breakthrough bleed. A major advantage of this method over oral contraceptives is that its effectiveness is not affected by any diarrhoea or vomiting. This method is ideal for women who have problems with compliance with oral contraception. It is not however suitable for women who have

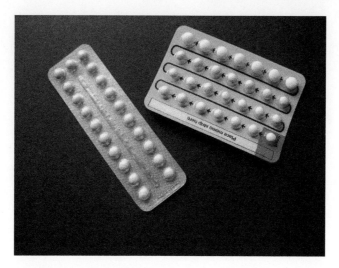

Figure 12.5   Different types of contraceptive pill.

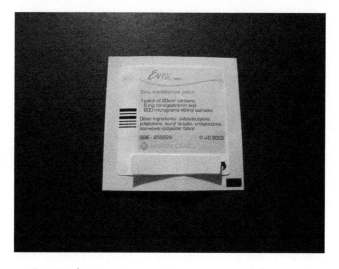

Figure 12.6   Contraceptive patch.

hypertension or high BMI and those who smoke, due to the increased risk of thromboembolism. The patch can also be used from day 21 following the birth, but is not suitable for those women who are breastfeeding due to the oestrogen content (Figure 12.6).

Contraceptive ring

This is a plastic ring inserted into the vagina that releases oestrogen and progesterone. It is 99% effective when used correctly. The ring is left in the vagina for 3 weeks and then removed for a ring free week in which a withdrawal bleed may occur. This method offers good menstrual cycle control and has a lower daily oestrogen dose than the patch and combined pill. The ring can be used from day 21 following the birth, but is not suitable for those women who are

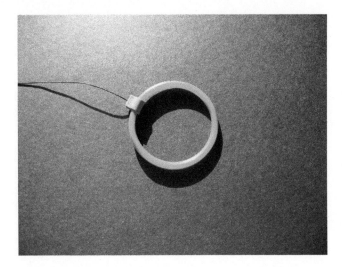

Figure 12.7   Contraceptive ring.

breastfeeding or whose vaginal muscles cannot hold the vaginal ring in place. Its effectiveness is not affected by diarrhoea or vomiting (see Figure 12.7).

Long-acting methods

Implant

An implant is a small flexible rod which remains under the skin surface and slowly releases progesterone. This method is 99% effective and the contraceptive effect is rapidly reversed on removal. An implant is used for 3 years and ideal for those women who have problems with taking a pill daily. It can be fitted from day 21 following the birth and can be used by breastfeeding women. An implant does requiring fitting and removal by a trained health professional. A disadvantage can be an associated change in menstrual pattern; this problem can be corrected with the use of oestrogen pills if these are not contraindicated.

Injection

This method is over 99% effective and contains progesterone which prevents ovulation. The injection is usually given every 12 weeks and is useful for those women who do not take the pill reliably. It can be given from day 21 following the birth, but waiting until 6 weeks is more appropriate, as irregular/heavy bleeding can occur if given earlier. This method does not affect breastfeeding, but can cause amenorrhoea or changes in menstrual pattern in some women. It cannot be immediately reversed in the event of side effects and it can take some time for fertility to return to normal. Therefore, it is not a suitable method for those women planning a shorter gap between children (see Figure 12.8).

Intrauterine device (IUD/coil)

This is a copper and plastic device which is inserted into the uterus. Essentially it works by causing an increase in the white blood cells in the cervix which prevents sperm entering. This method is 98–99% effective and can last between 5–10 years dependent on the type of coil inserted. It is an ideal method for women not wanting to use hormones, those who are considering having a wider gap between children or where the family may be complete. The IUD can also be used as a form of emergency contraception and can be fitted up to 5 days after

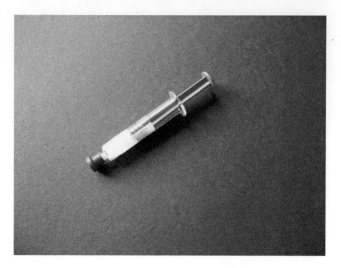

Figure 12.8   Contraceptive injection.

unprotected sex; in some cases it can then be left in situ as a long-term form of contraception. Periods can become heavier, longer and more painful initially but this should soon settle. Women are advised to feel for the threads of the coil after each period to ensure it remains in situ and has not been expelled during a heavy period. A coil can be fitted after 4–6 weeks following the birth regardless if the woman has had a vaginal or caesarean section birth. A coil requires fitting and removal by a trained health professional.

Intrauterine system (IUS)

This is a T-shaped device that is placed in the uterus and releases progesterone hormone. It lasts up to 5 years and is a rapidly reversible method of contraception. It is therefore recommended instead of sterilisation as it allows women change their mind. This method can cause amenorrhoea and changes in the menstrual cycle. It can be fitted from 4–6 weeks following the birth and does not have any effect on breastfeeding. The IUS must be fitted and removed by a trained healthcare professional (see Figure 12.9).

Natural methods

Rhythm method

This method involves recognising the fertile and infertile times of the menstrual cycle to plan when to avoid sex. This method requires the monitoring of body temperature, cervical mucus and menstrual cycle length. It avoids the use devices or hormones and can be used at all stages of reproductive life. It can take up to 6 months to learn effectively; however times of stress or illness can make the method unreliable. This method is more difficult to use after childbirth as fertility signs are harder to interpret.

Lactational amenorrhoea method

This method is 98% effective before periods return and when totally or very nearly totally breastfeeding a baby under 6 months (Szarewski and Guillebaud 2000; Van der Wijden and Kleinen 2003). Midwives often view this as an unreliable method of contraception (Jackson 2005) but the evidence does refute this belief where breastfeeding is undertaken day and night

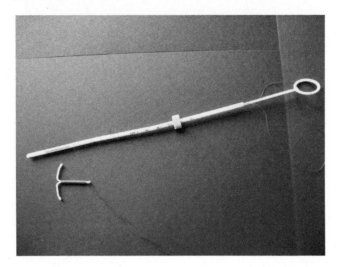

Figure 12.9   IUS and introducer.

with little or no supplementation. As with all methods the woman has a right to make an informed choice.

Emergency contraception

This method is used to help prevent an unwanted pregnancy if a contraceptive method fails or if no contraception is used. It needs to be given as soon as possible after unprotected sex or a failure of a contraceptive method. Emergency contraception should only be used as an occasional method and does not prevent a pregnancy every time it is taken. It can be obtained from pharmacies and outpatients departments in hospitals. Some accident and emergency and minor injury departments may also provide this service. There are two types: emergency contraception pills, which are thought to work by inhibiting or delaying ovulation; and an IUD, which reduces the viability of the ovum and the ability of the sperm to fertilise the ovum. If the IUD is inserted after fertilisation has occurred, then it is thought that it acts by inhibiting implantation. However, this process is not fully understood.

Sterilisation

Male sterilisation – vasectomy

Vasectomy is when the vas deferens that carry sperm from the testicles to the penis are cut, sealed or blocked. This procedure is usually done under local anaesthetic and can be done as an outpatient, or some GP practices provide this service. Male sterilisation is not effective immediately and semen tests need to be carried out as some sperm can remain in the tubal area for some time. It cannot be considered to be effective until the semen test is proven negative which can take up to 8 weeks. It is 99% effective and considered as a permanent method of contraception and cannot be easily reversed. There needs to be careful counselling before the decision to have a vasectomy is made as requests for reversal are becoming more frequent; due to the financial restraints on local health services these requests are not always available and can be expensive to obtain privately.

Female sterilisation

The uterine tubes are cut, sealed or blocked by an operation. This prevents the egg and sperm meeting and therefore fertilisation. The procedure is carried out by laparoscopy or in some cases mini-laparotomy. Usually a general anaesthetic is used or on occasions a local anaesthetic may be considered. Sterilisation is rarely considered at the time of Caesarean section any more, due to the fact that it has an increased failure rate when done at this time. Alternatives to sterilisation, such as long-acting methods, are often offered as this is preferable to a surgical procedure. It is also not advised for younger women as many regret their decision to have sterilisation, particularly if they start a new relationship. Reversal is not always possible or successful.

Further advice and treatment

An important element of the provision of contraception and family planning advice is information about where to seek further advice and treatment. A common approach to this is to recommend that the woman sees her GP; however this is not always the best source of advice as in many GP practices this role is carried out by a specialist nurse rather than the doctor, and trying to see the GP can delay access to contraception. Centres for Sexual Health also provide family planning services and have the advantage that they can also provide sexual health screening at the same time if required.

It may be appropriate to offer some women advice about where they can seek credible web-based information about family planning and contraception. The Family Planning Association have long been an organisation that has provided information, advice and treatment for women in relation to contraception and sexual health. Their website can be found at www.fpa.org.uk, and this has plenty of user-friendly information including a confidential helpline number and the addresses of the nearest clinics. The Brook organisation is also a useful source of information and advice particularly for younger women; their website is available at www.brook.org.uk

Key points

- Family planning is not just about preventing future pregnancy; it is also about spacing and planning for future children.
- Family planning advice needs to be individualised and sensitive to women's needs and given without judgement or assumptions.
- Knowledge of both contraceptive methods and local services is essential to the provision of effective care.

Conclusion

This chapter has provided an overview of the topic of contraception and family planning. Sensitive communication is essential to effective care in this area as discussions must allow for privacy and confidentiality whilst eliciting sufficient information to enable the midwife to provide appropriate and individualised advice. Midwives should have a working knowledge of available contraceptive methods as early advice is central to avoiding unplanned, and sometimes unwanted, pregnancies; they should also know where to direct women for further advice and treatment.

Midwives may find giving advice or discussing sex and sexual health difficult as it is a very intimate and sensitive subject for them as well as for the women in their care. It is important that midwives have a good knowledge of contraceptive methods and of the issues that concern women, but it is also essential that any personal embarrassment is put aside to ensure that women are provided with appropriate advice and information. Recognising this as a part of midwifery care that can make a real difference to women and their health is helpful in this regard. Midwives have a unique relationship with women and this provides them with an opportunity to be able to discuss very personal issues.

End of chapter activities
Crossword

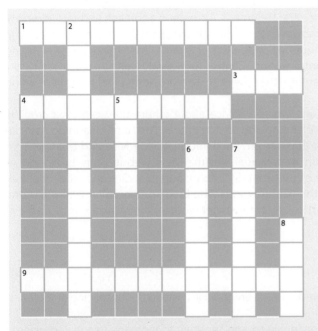

Across

1. This is essential when taking oral contraception
3. Lactational amenorrhoea is effective until the baby is this number of months old
4. Male sterilisation
9. A hormone that it is possible to take when breast feeding

Down

2. What monthly event may be important for some women when taking contraception?
5. An intrauterine device is also known as this
6. These methods include condoms
7. Another name for the female condom
8. A contraceptive patch should be changed every …?

Find out more

Below is a list of things you can find out about to enhance your knowledge of the issues and topics covered in this chapter. Make notes using the chapter content, the references and further reading identified, local policies and guidelines and discussions with colleagues.

1. When is contraception or family planning discussed in your clinical area?

2. What other advice is offered at the same time as contraception and family planning?

3. What services are available for further advice and treatment in your local area?

Glossary of terms

Barrier methods   Contraceptive devices that form a barrier between the male sperm and the female reproductive system.

Condom   A sheath placed over the penis to prevent sperm entering the vagina during intercourse.

Contraception   The prevention of conception.

Contraceptive ring   A plastic ring inserted into the vagina that releases oestrogen and progesterone.

Diaphragm   A cap which fits over the external cervical os to prevent sperm passing through the cervix.

Emergency contraception   Hormone treatment taken after intercourse to prevent pregnancy. This treatment must be taken within 72 hours of intercourse.

Family planning   Planning the number and spacing of children within the family.

Female condom   A sheath placed inside the vagina to prevent sperm entering the vagina during intercourse.

Hormonal contraception   Prescription treatments to prevent conception by means of hormones. These can be administered in the form of tablets (contraceptive pill), implants, patches, internal devices or injection.

Implant   A small flexible rod which remains under the skin surface and slowly releases progesterone.

Intrauterine device (IUD)   A copper and plastic device which is inserted into the uterus which works by causing an increase in the white blood cells in the cervix which prevents sperm entering.

Intrauterine system (IUS)   A T-shaped device that is placed in the uterus and releases progesterone.

Lactational amenorrhoea method   A natural method of contraception in the first 6 months following birth where breastfeeding is undertaken day and night with little or no supplementation.

Natural methods   Methods that attempt to prevent conception by means other than contraceptive devices or drugs, e.g. male withdrawal prior to ejaculation.

279

Rhythm method   Involves recognising the fertile and infertile times of the menstrual cycle to plan when to avoid sex and requires the monitoring of body temperature, cervical mucus and menstrual cycle length.

Sterilisation   Surgical intervention to prevent conception either by preventing passage of ova from the ovaries to the uterus (tubal ligation) or by preventing sperm travelling from the testes to the penis (vasectomy).

References

Hall, J. (2005) Postnatal fertility control advice. *The Practising Midwife* 8 (5), pp. 39–43.

Hiller, J.E., Griffith, E., Jenner, F. (2002) Education for contraceptive use by women after childbirth. *The Cochrane Database of Systematic Reviews* 3 (2).

Jackson, K. (2005) Lactational amenorrhoea method as a contraceptive. *British Journal of Midwifery* 13 (4), pp. 229–231.

NICE (2006) *Routine postnatal care of women and their babies. CG37*. London: NICE.

Norris, S. (2006) Is there a role for midwives in family planning? *British Journal of Midwifery* 14 (12), p. 701.

Queenan, J. (2004) Contraception and breastfeeding. *Clinical Obstetrics and Gynecology* 47(3), pp. 734–739.

Srikanthan, A., Reid, R.L. (2008) Religious and cultural influences on contraception. *JOGC* February, pp. 129–137.

Szarewski, A., Guillebaud, J. (2000) *Contraception: A User's Guide*. Oxford: Oxford University Press.

Van der Wijden, C., Kleinen, J. (2003) Lactational amenorrhoea for family planning (Cochrane Review). *The Cochrane Library* Issue 4.

Chapter 13

Perinatal mental health

Julie Jomeen
University of Hull, Hull, UK

Nicky Clark
University of Hull, Hull, UK

Learning outcomes

By the end of this chapter the reader will be able to:

* recognise why perinatal mental health is important for mother and baby as well as the wider family
* explain the policy context and national guidance related to perinatal mental health
* recognise the risk factors and consequences associated with perinatal mental illness
* recognise and differentiate the signs and symptoms of normal versus abnormal emotional adjustment across the perinatal period
* explain how healthcare professionals should identify and assess women's perinatal mental health and some of the associated challenges
* recognise why good pathways of care are essential to support women with perinatal mental illness.

Introduction

Perinatal mental illness (PMI) was raised to public attention following the Confidential Enquiry in Maternal and Child Health report published in 2004; for the first time psychiatric illness was the largest cause of maternal deaths. This chapter will explore why healthcare practitioners need to understand and consider PMI. It will identify risk factors and the signs and symptoms of PMI and promote consideration of normal versus abnormal emotional adaptation of the mother across the perinatal period. It will identify the health professional's role and responsibilities in identifying and assessing perinatal mental illness and offer considerations for appropriate management and referral processes, with the aim of improving outcomes for childbearing women.

Fundamentals of Midwifery: A Textbook for Students, First Edition. Edited by Louise Lewis.
© 2015 John Wiley & Sons, Ltd. Published 2015 by John Wiley & Sons, Ltd.
Companion website: www.wileyfundamentalseries.com/midwifery

The importance of mental health in a maternity context

Mental health problems which are present during pregnancy and the postnatal period (perinatal mental health problems [PMHP]) are not uncommon and can have serious consequences. In high-income countries, 10% of pregnant women and 13% of mothers of infants have significant mental health problems, depression and anxiety being the most common (O'Hara and Swain 1996; Fisher et al. 2010). Considering that in England 700,000 women give birth each year, this suggests that approximately 70,000 women will be affected antenatally and 91,000 postnatally, with rates much higher in resource-constrained countries (Fisher et al. 2010). Whilst the focus within the literature is on depression, historically on postnatal depression (PND) and more recently, antenatal depression (AND), PMI is a spectrum of conditions, varying in severity from adjustment disorders and distress, through mild to moderate depressive illness and anxiety states, severe depressive illness and post-traumatic stress disorder, to chronic serious mental illness and postpartum psychosis. Specifically, these may include generalised anxiety disorder (GAD), panic disorder (PD) post-traumatic stress disorder (PTSD), phobias and obsessive compulsive disorder (OCD) as well as the more severe conditions such as bipolar disorder, schizophrenia and personality disorders.

PMHP affect women from across the population and can have a significant impact upon the healthy functioning of the women and her long-term mental health, obstetric outcomes, her partner, the quality of family relationships, as well as on the wellbeing of the fetus and a child's development in the short and the long term. The burden of PMI in individual, societal and economic terms must not be underestimated. Childbirth provides a clear window of opportunity for professionals who come into contact with women to make a positive impact on adverse obstetric and mental health outcomes related to PMI (Alderdice et al. 2013). This, however, requires awareness and understanding of common mental health problems, as well the confidence to make enquiries of women about their mental health status. This is an area that has been traditionally identified as problematic for midwives (Ross-Davie et al. 2006; Jomeen et al. 2009), health visitors (Morrell et al. 2009; Jomeen et al. 2013), as well as health professionals generally (NSPCC 2013). It is essential that practitioners effectively assess and recognise PMI to underpin appropriate and proactive referral and care decisions, which assure the necessary support that women and their families need.

Putting PMI into perspective

Maternal mortality and morbidity

Public attention on PMI followed the Confidential Enquiries in Maternal and Child Health (CEMACH) report published in 2004. For the first time deaths from psychiatric causes were reported and identified as the overall leading cause of maternal mortality in the years from 1998–2001 (CEMACH 2004). These maternal mortality reports lucidly highlighted PMI as an issue of concern and one requiring greater attention, catapulting PMI firmly onto the maternity public health agenda. Subsequent reports (CEMACH 2007; Centre for Maternal and Child Enquiries (CMACE) 2011), have continued to evidence psychiatric disorders as a significant cause of death in both pregnant and postnatal women and highlight no decrease in suicide rates in this group.

Maternal deaths

Maternal deaths from psychiatric causes are deaths arising directly from a psychiatric condition, suicide or accidental overdose of drugs misuse. Deaths from medical and other causes are

282

Table 13.1   Causes of death in the perinatal period, due to, or associated with, a psychiatric disorder

Cause of deaths reported	Suicide Substance misuse Violence Accidents Medical conditions being aggravated by a psychiatric disorder
Main psychiatric diagnoses made on those who died	Psychosis Severe depressive illness Anxiety/depressive adjustment Alcohol dependence Drug dependence Personality disorder
Medical conditions aggravated by a psychiatric disorder	Infection Pancreatitis Incorrect diagnosis of a medical disorder delaying appropriate management Incorrect diagnosis of a psychiatric disorder delaying appropriate management

283

associated with psychiatric causes if they are the physical consequences of substance misuse. Delays in the diagnosis and treatment of other life-threatening conditions because of the presence of a psychiatric illness are also included. In the years 2003–2005, a total of 104 women died due to, or associated with, a psychiatric disorder (CEMACH 2007) and between 2006 and 2008 a total of 79 women died (CMACE 2011) (see Table 13.1).

Most psychiatric causes of maternal mortality are classed as indirect causes. Indirect causes are deaths that occur as a result of previously existing disease or disease that develops during pregnancy. This exacerbation or development of disease is not due to obstetric causes but by aggravation of the physiological effects of pregnancy.

The development of a psychiatric disorder during pregnancy and following delivery is common. Pregnancy, until recently was thought to have a 'protective effect'; unfortunately the rising suicide rate challenges this belief, with many deaths occurring in the antenatal period, or very shortly after. Additionally those women with pre-existing serious mental disorder evidence a heightened risk of relapse in pregnancy, yet paradoxically the risk of developing a serious mental disorder is significantly elevated following childbirth. This is particularly so in the first 3 months and furthermore a family history of bipolar disorder increases this risk to 50%.

PMH is a potentially preventable cause of perinatal mortality (Department of Health (DH) 2002). Disturbingly, an important feature of many of these 'indirect deaths' was considered to be the lack of coordinated multidisciplinary care (CEMACH 2004; 2007; CMACE 2011). Recommendations from these reports strongly emphasise that all professionals involved with women throughout childbirth should be alert to the possibility of sudden deteriorations and escalations. Questions about mental ill-health (see Box 13.1) should be made routinely in antenatal clinics, with effective communication between services and professionals, particularly the psychiatric, maternity, mental health and child protection services and those working within them.

CMACE is no longer commissioned to produce these reports, with MBRRACE-UK being the collaboration now appointed by the Healthcare Quality Improvement Partnership to continue with the Confidential Enquiry into Maternal Deaths (CEMD) as part of its programme of work. This work commenced on 1 January 2013. MBRRACE-UK is anxious to safeguard the continuity

Box 13.1 Identifying and assessing PMI

Prediction and detection questions (National Institute for Health and Care Excellence (NICE) 2007)
Prediction questions
At the woman's first contact with services during pregnancy and the postnatal period, healthcare professionals (including midwives, obstetricians, health visitors and General Practitioners (GPs)), should ask about:

1. Past or present severe mental illness, including schizophrenia, bipolar disorder, psychosis in the postnatal period and severe depression
2. Previous treatment by a psychiatrist/specialist mental health team, including inpatient care
3. Family history of perinatal mental illness.

Do not use other specific predictors, such as poor relationships with her partner, routinely to predict development of a mental disorder.

Detection questions (Whooley questions)
At the woman's first contact with primary care, at her booking visit and postnatally (usually at 4 to 6 weeks and 3 to 4 months), healthcare professionals (including midwives, obstetricians, health visitors and GPs) should ask two questions to identify possible depression.

1. During the past month, have you often been bothered by feeling down, depressed or hopeless?
2. During the past month, have you often been bothered by having little interest or pleasure in doing things?

If the woman answers 'yes' to either of the initial questions, also ask:
3. Is this something you feel you need or want help with?

As part of a subsequent assessment or for routine monitoring of outcomes, consider using self-report measures such as the Edinburgh Postnatal Depression Scale (EPDS), Hospital Anxiety and Depression Scale (HADS) or Patient Health Questionnaire 9 (PHQ9).

of CEMD, giving it the highest priority. MBRRACE-UK's programme of work will also include a series of themed topic-based confidential clinical reviews of serious maternal morbidity, with near-misses and cases of serious morbidity being more numerous than deaths. Women who are at high risk of major postpartum mental illness in pregnancy and who subsequently develop a postpartum psychosis requiring psychiatric admission is a topic selected to be carried out in 2014 and 2015.

Policy context

Since 2004 there has been an increasing focus on PMI in UK maternity policy (DH 2004) and national maternity guidelines (NICE 2003; 2006) which ultimately culminated in the publication in the UK of the NICE guidelines for antenatal and postnatal mental health (NICE 2007). These guidelines set out key priorities for PMH, emphasising that women with PMI must be recognised early, have access to effective treatment and be supported by services to promote optimal recovery. These guidelines gave all healthcare professionals working with pregnant and post-natal women, a clearly defined remit for prediction of the current disorder, detection of risk factors, familiarity with the signs and symptoms of mental health disorders and referral through clearly identified pathways and involvement in a multidisciplinary approach to care.

Identification and assessment

Through early identification and the provision of professional care and treatment options, the onset of such illnesses can often be prevented or the severity significantly lessened. As such, it has been identified that effective prevention, detection, and treatment of PMI could have posi-tive impact on those suffering from these conditions, and improve the health and wellbeing of children and families across the UK (NSPCC 2013). The need for specialist psychiatric services where pregnant and postpartum women can be referred, via rapid access pathways is empha-sised in all the confidential enquiry reports and is indeed clearly mandated in the NICE guidance (NICE 2007).

Worthy of consideration for practitioners, however, is that whilst short self-report measures are undoubtedly attractive for use in clinical practice due to their ease of use (as in the Whooley questions) and potential cut-off scores (as for the EPDS) which help facilitate practitioner judge-ments (Alderdice et al. 2013); measures are not without their problems. They are not diagnostic in nature and a score on a screening tool only serves to highlight possible or probable PMI. Issues have been raised in relation to both embedded anxiety items within the EPDS with impli-cations for threshold scores (Jomeen and Martin 2005) and the validity of the Hospital Anxiety Depression Scale (HADS) in a childbearing population (Jomeen and Martin 2004). Authors have also recommended differing thresholds for antenatal and postnatal use of measures such as the EPDS (Matthey et al. 2006), which have not necessarily translated into practice. A good screen-ing test should reflect both reliability and validity, and the National Screening Committee have expressed concerns about the widespread implementation of the EPDS in particular as a screen-ing tool (Raynor and England 2010). Indeed while tools might be useful in underpinning mood assessment, they should not be considered a replacement for clinical skills and expertise, but as part of a broader assessment and decision-making process (Jomeen 2012).

Further reading activity

For further short reading on the issues related to measures and assessment see the following editorial:

Jomeen, J. (2013) Women's psychological status in pregnancy and childbirth – measuring or understanding? *Journal of Reproductive and Infant Psychology* 30 (4), pp. 337–340.

Identifying risk factors

The successive confidential enquiry reports all highlight the difficulties with identifying the risk, as well as managing the risk appropriately. Risk factors are best described as vulnerability or adverse factors or characteristics that are present in a person's life and hence put them at greater risk of developing PMI (Raynor and England 2010; see Box 13.2).

Box 13.2   Potential risk factors for PMI (WHO 2004; CEMACH 2004, 2007; CMACE 2011)

- Previous psychiatric disorder
- Family history of serious mental ill-health
- Social disadvantage and isolation
- Poverty
- Minority ethnic group
- Asylum seekers and refugees
- Late bookers and those who repeatedly miss appointments
- Domestic violence
- Substance misuse
- Known to child protection services
- Employment status
- Physical ill health
- Life events
- Lack of support

Box 13.3   Predictors of PND (Beck 2001)

- Antenatal depression
- Antenatal anxiety
- Marital relationship
- Maternity blues
- Unplanned pregnancy
- Self-esteem
- Life stress
- History of depression
- Marital status
- Childcare stress
- Social support
- Infant temperament
- Socio-economic status

Other authors have identified risk factors as significant in the development of PND in particular (for examples see O'Hara and Swain 1996; Beck 2001). No consistently reliable risk factors have emerged for predicting the onset of mental disorders during pregnancy and the postnatal period. Hence, risk factors, as independent causal variables, cannot be recommended to predict AND or PND (NICE 2007). This is because risk factors are not necessarily causal, that is, their presence will not necessarily result in PMI. Presence of risk factors may well, however, increase an individual's vulnerability, particularly if the individual is subject to 'a cluster of these adverse factors' (Raynor and England 2010, p.55). The presence of risk factors may also support midwives and healthcare professionals in sketching out profiles of vulnerable women; profiles which can be considered when assessing a woman's needs across the perinatal period (see Box 13.3 for predictors of postnatal depression).

Antenatal, postnatal or a continuum

Activity 13.1   Antenatal or postnatal?

Reflect on how many of Beck's predictors of PND could equally apply to the antenatal period.

Box 13.4   Common false beliefs related to PND

- Its symptoms and effects are less severe.
- It goes away by itself.
- It is somehow associated with whether or not the woman is breastfeeding.
- It is all due to hormones.
- It has no risk of non-puerperal recurrence.
- It carries an inevitable risk of future postnatal recurrence.
- Depression is less common antenatally.
- Depression which is already present before birth is not the same thing.

There has been concern that misuse of the term (PND) is widespread with potentially serious negative consequences. These include its use in clinical situations as a label for any mental illness occurring postnatally (NICE 2007) and a traditional tendency to have a preoccupation with PND to the exclusion of other aspects of mental health. This reinforces a view that PND is somehow different from depression at other times. (Box 13.4 summarises some of the false beliefs relating to PND.)

Individual women will demonstrate wide variation in their emotional status, from a minor transient experience such as baby blues to severe mental illness (SMI), such as puerperal psychosis (PP). Whilst the range and type of PMI might vary, they form part of a continuum. All PMI can present across the perinatal period. Practitioners will see both women with existing mental health disorder who become pregnant, as well as women who develop PMHP when they have previously been well.

Activity 13.2

Consider some of the potential stressors that might be associated with pregnancy that might affect a woman's emotional state during:

- antenatal period
- intrapartum period
- postnatal period

Prevalence and incidence

Psychiatric conditions are prevalent in the general population, with over 20% of individuals affected (ONS 2002). A large proportion of those will be mild to moderate anxiety and depression and often those conditions can be co-morbid (Teixeira et al. 2009), a profile which is reflected in the pregnant population (Oates 2006). The incidence of mild–moderate affective states such as depression and anxiety in the perinatal period are approximately 10–15%, with higher figures quoted in some studies (Jomeen and Martin 2008). The prevalence of AND is at least as high of that of PND and rates have been demonstrated to be higher in late pregnancy than postnatal (Evans et al. 2001; Jomeen and Martin 2008), with a similar profile identified for anxiety (Jomeen and Martin 2008). Approximately 3% of women will suffer from a more severe depression (Joint Commissioning Panel for Mental Health 2012); one to two of every 1000 women with a live birth will develop puerperal psychosis (PP) (Brockington 1996; Munk-Olsen et al. 2006). PTSD occurs in 3% of all maternities and in 6% of women following an emergency caesarean section (Joint Commissioning Panel for Mental Health 2012). Clearly pregnancy is a more vulnerable time for the inception of PMI than at other times in a woman's life even though the level of risk is broadly similar to the general population. The risk of being admitted to hospital with an SMI following childbirth is significantly increased compared to the general population (Oates 1996). New cases of SMI are more likely to occur in the postnatal rather than antenatal periods. However, for certain SMIs such as severe depressive illnesses, schizophrenia and bipolar disorder, the risk of reoccurrence of relapse can be increased in pregnancy, particularly if medication is stopped (Joint Commissioning Panel for Mental Health 2012).

Categories of PMI

Oates and Raynor (2009) suggest six categories of PMI (see Table 13.2).

Further categories within which women might present

- **Organic disorders** which would include infections, anaemia, nutritional deficiencies (for example, Vitamin D), stroke, endocrine problems (hypo/hyperthyroidism).
- **Medically unexplained symptoms** which might include unexplained chest pain, abdominal pain, gynaecological problems, pseudo-pregnancy, hypochondriasis, Munchausen syndrome or Munchausen by proxy.

Table 13.2   Categories of PMI

Category	Associated conditions
Severe (psychotic disorders)	Schizophrenia, bipolar disorder, severe depression and other psychotic conditions.
Mild to moderate (neurotic disorders)	Mild–moderate depression (non-psychotic), mixed anxiety and depression, panic disorder, anxiety disorders such as OCD, PTSD and panic disorder.
Adjustment reactions	Distressing reactions to life events such as bereavement or social adversity.
Substance misuse	Those who misuse or are dependent on substances such as alcohol and legal or illegal drugs.
Personality disorder	Individuals who have persistent and severe problems throughout their adult life in dealing with the stresses of normal life. As a consequence they demonstrate difficulty in areas such as controlling their behaviour, maintaining satisfactory relationships, causing distress to others and acting irresponsibly with no insight into the consequences of their actions.
Learning disability	Individuals with intellectual or cognitive impairment.

Depression

As already stated, depression is one of the most prevalent conditions across the perinatal period. A number of studies have identified that women with PND also had AND and could have been identified antenatally (NSPCC 2013). Approximately 10% of women will, however, develop a new episode of depressive illness (Raynor and England 2010), which may vary in level of severity. Whilst risk factors have been identified, as outlined earlier, their predictive value is unclear. One of the challenges of identifying depression can be the overlap with symptoms of pregnancy and the effects of early motherhood, fatigue and sleeplessness being good examples, which also highlights the importance of not over-pathologising women's emotional status. The weeks and months after giving birth have been identified as time of considerable stress (Glazener 2005a; Glazener 2005b), which has led to a focus in the international literature (Yelland et al. 2009) and policy on postpartum psychological morbidity (CMACE 2011). Yet, some emotional lability and even some depressive type symptoms may just be part of the adaptation to pregnancy and the mothering role (Raynor and England 2010). It is therefore crucial that practitioners are familiar with the signs and symptoms of depression, levels of severity and can recognise how women might present (see Figure 13.1). This is important, firstly to avoid the dangers of over-diagnosing PMI, but also to be able to create a context from which women feel able to disclose; women are unlikely to do so if they feel stigmatized and judged by revealing a SMI in either in pregnancy or postnatally.

Cognitive symptoms might be reflected in the kind of things that women say.

Uselessness: 'I'm a useless mother.'
Worthlessness: 'I'm good for nothing and burden on the family.'
Hopelessness: 'Nothing is going to get better, no light at the end of tunnel.'
Guilt: 'I feel miserable for neglecting my baby's and family's need.'
Failing: 'People look at me and think that I'm failing.'
Death wishes: 'There is no point in carrying on … I wish I don't wake-up the next day.'
Suicidal thoughts: 'I feel like ending it all', 'the children will be better off without me.'
Extended suicide: 'No future for the kids without me, so better I take them with me.'

Mild to moderate depression

The majority of depressive illness in the perinatal period will be mild to moderate as defined in Table 13.3. The word mild is perhaps deceiving as this level of PMI can still cause significant distress to women. If left untreated there are implications for the fetus, obstetric outcomes and effects on the development of the child in the short and long term. Depression during late pregnancy is associated with a significant increase in the use of epidural analgesia, caesarean section, instrumental deliveries and increased rates of admission for the neonate to intensive care (Chung et al. 2001). Apart from inflicting distress on the mother, depression undermines the marital relationship and an association between a mother's depression and the subsequent report of depression in her partner have been demonstrated (Scottish Intercollegiate Guidelines Network [SIGN] 2002). Further maternal depressive symptomology at any time, but particularly antenatally, has been identified as a risk factor for a child's wellbeing (Louma et al. 2001) in both emotional and cognitive terms (Hay and Kumar 1995; Murray et al. 1991), particularly when associated with other risk factors such as poverty (Murray and Cooper 1997). NICE (2007) recommends psychological therapies managed within a primary care setting, for the management of

289

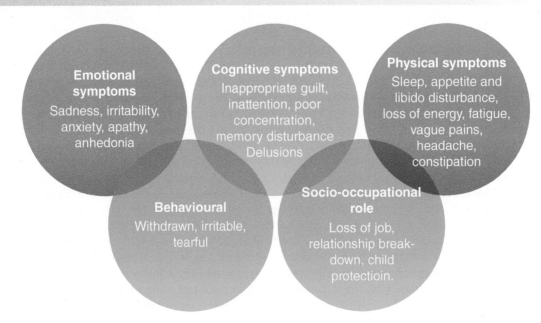

Figure 13.1   Key symptoms of depression.

Table 13.3   Symptoms of the different levels of depression

Classification	Symptoms
Mild	Low mood, tearfulness, reduced interest or enjoyment but able to function.
Moderate	A number of depressive symptoms and difficulty in functioning.
Severe	All the above, along with early morning waking, feeling worse in the morning, significant weight/appetite loss, marked disinterest in life, suicidal thoughts other risk issues.
Depression with psychotic symptoms	Severe depression with hallucinations, delusions or other psychotic experiences.

mild to moderate depression with generally good results observed. Pharmacological treatments should obviously be used with caution due to potential effects on both mother and the developing fetus.

Severe depression

Major depressive illness is more likely to occur in the postnatal period, but clearly can have a significant impact on a woman, her baby and her wider family during a major life transition. Onset can be as early as 2–4 weeks and be clearly evident by 4–6 weeks postnatally. However for the majority of cases presentation usually occurs between 8 and 12 weeks postnatally and can be enduring. Some women who develop this condition will have no previous history. However, there is an identified increased risk from women with a previous personal or family history of severe depression, either during or outside the perinatal period. Women with a known history have a significant risk of reoccurrence in subsequent pregnancies. Treatment for severe depression is no different to treatment outside of the perinatal period, but speedy resolution is clearly important to optimise maternal recovery and promote the cognitive, emotional and social development of the child. Treatment often consists of antidepressant therapy combined with psychotherapy as recommended by NICE (2007), which if timely can enable a full recovery. Women who suffer severe depression are, however, at increased risk of suffering depression, outside of the childbearing context.

Anxiety disorders

Anxiety can have a negative effect on pregnancy; including a higher incidence of obstetric complications including placental abruption, premature labour, low Apgar score and low birth weight (Crandon 1979, Cohen et al. 1989), with pregnancy specific anxieties linked to an increased risk of spontaneous abortion (Neugebauer et al. 1996). Antenatal stress and anxiety has also been demonstrated to have a programming effect on the fetus with enduring effects until at least middle childhood, that may well persist into adulthood (O'Connor et al. 2002). A level of anxiety is of course normal in pregnancy and as with depression there are physical symptoms of pregnancy that may mimic those of anxiety (Hadwin 2007). For healthcare professionals, what is important is to differentiate between pathological anxiety and normal anxiety. Whilst some concerns about the health of the baby, her own health and adaptation to parenthood are essentially normal; generalised thoughts of anxiety about other aspects of life may not be so (Hadwin 2007). Assessment needs to also consider whether the experience outweighs the woman's coping strategies and whether such symptoms are unusual (Hadwin 2007). See Figure 13.2 for symptoms of generalised anxiety disorder (GAD).

The question whether anxiety and depressive orders are separate entities has been a controversial issue (Gorman 1997). Clark and Watson (1991) introduced the idea that anxiety and depression each have distinct features but also share a common dimension, called general distress or negative effect. This co-morbid relationship between anxiety and depression in pregnant women has been demonstrated (Da Costa et al. 2000) and recognition of mixed

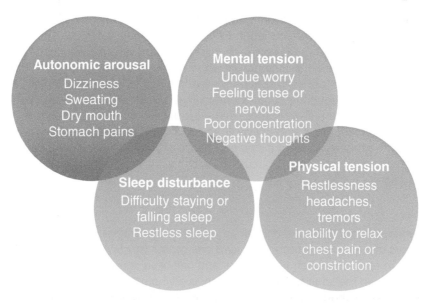

Figure 13.2   Symptoms of generalised anxiety disorder (Hadwin 2007).

anxiety and depression is important as this is thought to be one of the most common presentations both generally (Tyrer 2001) and in maternity (Raynor and England 2010). More so than the presentation of anxiety and depression individually and Hadwin (2007) suggests that health professionals need to bear this in mind when women present with symptoms that do not necessarily meet the diagnostic criteria of an individual condition. What is important is not necessarily diagnosis *per se* but recognition of the signs and symptoms a woman is experiencing and appropriate response.

Panic disorders

Panic attacks may sometimes happen with GAD, but normally would manifest in individuals experiencing generalized arousal (Hadwin 2007). An increase in panic attacks following birth has been demonstrated (Cohen and Noncas 2005). However, some authors feel it is the severity of symptoms that are more significant (Hadwin 2007). Symptoms of panic disorder include intermittent episodes of panic or anxiety where the individual take action to avoid these feelings. These spontaneous episodes start suddenly, rise rapidly and can last from minutes to up to an hour. Physical symptoms include palpitations, cheat pain, sense of choking, churning stomach, dizziness, feelings of unreality, detachment from oneself and fear of impending disaster (WHO 2004). Women may seek to avoid the places where attacks have occurred, which may be significant if attacks have occurred in care settings. Support is therefore critical and healthcare professionals need to promote both self-confidence and self-efficacy to manage symptoms. It is worthy of note that some physical factors may aggravate panic disorder including hyperthyroidism, hyperventilation, sleep deprivation, caffeine, alcohol, cannabis and chest pain (March and Yonkers 2001).

Obsessive compulsive disorder (OCD)

The onset of OCD or the worsening of symptoms has been associated with childbirth (NSPCC 2013), and pregnancy is a recognised risk factor for triggering OCD (Abramowitz 2003; Kalra et al. 2005). The prevalence of perinatal OCD is not well-defined, and some authors suggest that the relationship between OCD and pregnancy is coincidental, although it can be common with other disorders such as depression (Hadwin 2007), with the concomitant risk of misdiagnosis. Studies have suggested it affects around 3% of new mothers (NSPCC 2013). Possible explanations are hormonal and stress-related and whilst symptoms vary in the perinatal period, women's obsessions and compulsions are more likely to focus on the baby (NSPCC 2013; Hadwin 2007). Often thoughts focus on fears of harming the baby which may lead to excessive checking; however morbid thoughts are not uncommon in early motherhood and form part of the transition to motherhood. It is also accepted that most people will experience obsessive or intrusive thoughts at different times in their lives (Hadwin 2007). Clearly, however OCD can significantly interfere with women's wellbeing, their experience of pregnancy, and parenting and healthcare professionals can recognise and discuss these behaviours to promote appropriate referral and care packages.

Post-traumatic stress disorder (PTSD)

PTSD emerges from the experience of an exceptionally distressing event and is defined by 3 key factors that are experienced for at least one month (see Box 13.5).

PTSD can recur or worsen in childbirth and has been shown to be higher in the pregnant population than the adult female population as a whole (Seng et al. 2009). The experience of being pregnant is thought to trigger symptoms of these disorders, in vulnerable women such as those who have experienced childhood abuse (NSPCC 2013) or following a previous stillbirth

Box 13.5   Signs of PTSD

1. Intrusion of thoughts, memories, flashbacks in which the person seems to re-experience the distressing event and nightmares.
2. Avoidance of reminders, situations or events, emotional numbness or blunting, detachment.
3. Increased arousal, for example hypervigilance, irritability, insomnia, impaired concentration.

Box 13.6   Women at risk of serious mental illness

- Women who have a previous history of bipolar illness or a psychotic episode in early life, who are well and not in contact with psychiatric services. They may not be at risk in pregnancy, but are at an increased risk postpartum. Requires a proactive management plan and awareness of early risk and identification.
- Women who have had a previous or recent episode and are stable but are medicated. There is risk of relapse in pregnancy if women stop their medication. Expert advice on medication and a proactive management plan is essential.
- Women with a chronic SMI with complex social needs, symptomatic and medicated. Usually these women will be in contact with psychiatric services. Effective multidisciplinary joined-up working is critical to ensure effective care planning.

293

(Turton et al. 2001). It is thought that PTSD can also be triggered by childbirth with links posited between a traumatic birth and PTSD, with women particularly at risk after an emergency caesarean section or admission of their baby to NICU (Joint Commissioning Panel for Mental Health 2012).

Serious mental illness (SMI)

Schizophrenia and bipolar disorder affect only a small proportion of the general population which is reflected in the perinatal population, with risk being most elevated in the postnatal period (Raynor and England 2010). Oates describes three groups of women (Raynor and England 2010; Box 13.6).

Pre-pregnancy counselling can be extremely helpful, but is clearly challenging when many pregnancies are unplanned. It should not be assumed that women with an SMI will be easier to identify and sensitive questioning is key to identification, assessment and effective referral.

Puerperal psychosis (PP)

Whilst the numbers of women suffering puerperal psychosis (PP) are relatively small, the consequences can be a devastating for women and their families, including suicide, infanticide (Spinelli 2004) and subsequent puerperal and non-puerperal psychiatric episodes (Robertson et al. 2005). PP has an acute onset, within the first four weeks after giving birth (Cantwell and Cox 2006) and is characterised by delusions, hallucinations, bizarre behaviour and mood lability (Heron et al. 2008).

Women who have a history of bipolar disorder have been identified as particularly vulnerable (Brockington 1996; Jones and Craddock, 2001). Familial factors play an additional role (Jones

Box 13.7   Other identified risk factors for PP

- Poor socioeconomic circumstances
- Pregnancy complications/shorter gestation
- Birth complications/caesarean section
- Female baby
- Marital status
- Stillbirth
- Longer labour with associated sleep deprivation/night-time birth

and Craddock 2001; 2002). A personal history of PP predisposes approximately 57% of women to experience another episode after a subsequent pregnancy (Robertson et al. 2005). However, primipara women are consistently reported to be at greater risk of experiencing PP than multiparous (Blackmore et al. 2006), with some suggestion that older first time mothers might be at greater risk (Nager et al. 2005). Childbirth itself is a risk factor for PP, albeit a small one (Nager et al. 2005) and episodes can occur 'out of the blue' to women without previous psychiatric history (Heron et al. 2012). Box 13.7 highlights other risk factors for PP.

The key theoretical explanations for the aetiology of PP remain genetic, biochemical and endocrine (NICE 2007). The presentation of PP is acute, florid and women deteriorate rapidly, hence hospitalisation is often required (Doucet et al. 2011) and recommended (NICE 2007). Early recognition and prompt treatment can facilitate the resolution of the florid features of PP, but risk of relapse remains high in the early weeks. Whilst there is often a perception that women with PP present a risk to their baby, this is more likely to be through neglect rather than active harm to the baby. The mother–baby interaction will improve as the mother recovers (Raynor and England 2010). Longer term prognosis is good, although women often pass through a period of depression and anxiety during recovery. There is a risk of relapse in a subsequent pregnancy and outside the puerperium. Recent exploratory work highlights that symptoms of stress–vulnerability experienced during pregnancy and/or birth and aspects which might influence those symptoms, such as a woman's early environment and experienced levels of expressed emotion may facilitate consideration of a psychological account of the development of PP. This may present future opportunities to develop antenatal interventions (Glover et al. 2014).

Care provision

Effective service provision for PMI, requires joint working between mental health services, midwifery and obstetrics, acute care, primary care, children's services, paediatrics and the voluntary sector (NSPCC 2013). Joint working within or across organisations must be facilitated by effective communication and provide a seamless perspective to care. It is noteworthy that despite a 7-year time-lag since publication of the NICE (2007) guidelines, support for women with PMI remains spasmodic and lacking across the UK and it remains a lottery whether women get access to services and the right help (Jomeen and Martin 2014). Whilst some areas have specialist services, mental health specialist midwives and voluntary sector services; the Patients' Association (2011), reported that 64% of local authorities do not have a PMH commissioning strategy, highlighting this as a critical issue. The government has recently pledged to ensure specialist midwives in each trust to deal with PMI; however unless this is supported by adequate services the risk of the service users 'dropping out' through gaps in the system will remain a reality. Local strategies need to prioritise the development of pathways of care for women with PMI at all levels, which are critical to optimise care for women and their families, but are also essential to support practitioners to confidently and proactively identify and assess women's PMHP and needs (Jomeen et al. 2013).

Further reading activity

For further reading on what a good service looks like see the following report:

Joint Commissioning Panel for Mental Health (2012) *Guidance for commissioners of perinatal mental health services.* JCP-MH: London [available online] http://www.jcpmh.info/good-services/perinatal-mental-health-services

Key points

- PMI is a key public health issue.
- PMI can occur at any point across the childbearing spectrum.
- Healthcare practitioners need to accurately identify and effectively assess women's mental health status using the NICE guidelines, underpinned by an awareness of risk factors, sensitive questioning, effective listening and communication skills.
- It is the ability to define normal and abnormal adjustment that is important.
- Whilst it is critical to accurately assess women's mental health status and needs, it is equally important to avoid over-pathologising women's emotional status in the perinatal period.
- If these vulnerable women are identified, healthcare practitioners are ethically bound to ensure that adequate pathways for care are available.

Conclusion

PMH has been thrust into the social spotlight since its lucid relationship with maternal mortality was identified. The impact of PMI is significant for the mother, baby and family as well as having wider public health consequences, yet detection and management are often sporadic and inequitable. The intensification of national policies and guidelines signal a drive and commitment from government to ensure that healthcare professionals address the issue of PMI. Accruing evidence highlights the support women and their families living with PMI require and deserve. The overarching aim of policy, national guidelines and research endeavour in this area is to better equip healthcare workers with the knowledge and skills to underpin accurate identification of PMHP across the maternity spectrum, undertake appropriate assessment and effectively promote adequate, appropriate and available care pathways for women.

Further reading activity

Martin, C.R. (2012) *Perinatal Mental Health: A Clinical Guide.* Keswick: M&K Publishing.

Henshaw, C., Cox J., Barton, J. (2009) *Modern Management of Perinatal Psychiatric Disorders.* London: RCoP Press.

End of chapter activities
Crossword

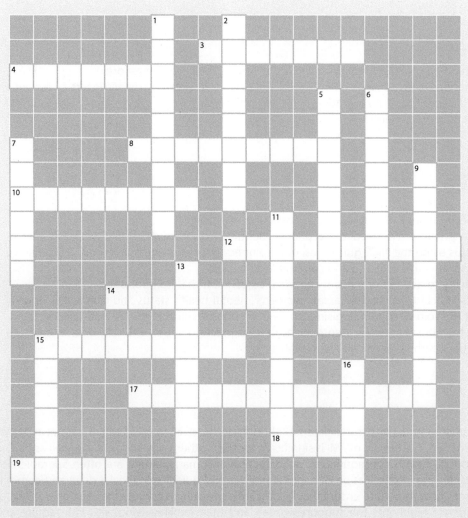

Across

3. Mental or emotional strain
4. A feeling of unease
8. The state of being diseased or unhealthy within a population
10. A relatively mild personality disorder
12. Occurrence at any given time

14. Lack of order or regular arrangement
15. The period surrounding birth
17. Where a person hears, sees (and in some cases smells) things that are not really there; a common hallucination is when people hear voices in their

Down

1. A word used to describe mental health problems that stops the person from thinking clearly, telling the difference between reality

and their imagination, and acting in a normal way.
2. A false belief or opinion

5. The medical specialty devoted to the study, diagnosis, treatment, and prevention of mental disorders
6. The act of intentionally ending your life
7. Aspects or things relating to the mind

9. A syndrome which is a serious perinatal mental health issue, with medically unexplained symptoms

Find out more

Below is a list of things you can find out about to enhance your knowledge of the issues and topics covered in this chapter. Make notes using the chapter content, the references and further reading identified, local policies and guidelines and discussions with colleagues.

- Read the Guidelines for Antenatal and Postnatal Mental Health (NICE 2007).
- Find out what screening tools are used to assess perinatal mental health in the clinical area.
- Consider what might affect a woman's mood in pregnancy and the postnatal period.
- Map out an ideal service model for perinatal mental health for women with existing mental health problems and women who develop psychological mental health problems in pregnancy.

Consider the following:
- Referral processes
- Management guidelines
- Pathways of care
- Initial care
- Defined roles of staff
- Communication networks, systems and methods
- Services and access.
- What voluntary organisations offer support to women with mental health illness?

Glossary of terms

Affect   Refers to the experience of feeling or emotion

AND   Antenatal depression

BPD   Bipolar disorder

CEMACH   Confidential Enquiry into Maternal and Child Health

CEMD   Confidential Enquiry into Maternal Deaths

CMACE   Centre for Maternal and Child Enquiries

Co-morbid   A medical condition that co-occurs with another

Delusion   A false belief or impression maintained despite being contradicted by reality or rational argument

DH   Department of Health

EPDS   Edinburgh Postnatal Depression Scale

GAD   Generalised anxiety disorder

HADS   Hospital Anxiety and Depression Scale

Hallucination   A sensory experience of something that does not exist

Incidence   The number of new cases per population at risk in a given time period

MBRRACE – UK   Mothers and Babies: Reducing the Risk through Audits and Confidential Enquiries across the UK

Morbidity   The state of being diseased or unhealthy within a population

Mortality   The incidence of death or the number of deaths in a population

NICE   National Institute for Health and Clinical Excellence

NICU   Neonatal Intensive Care Unit

NSC   National Screening Committee

NSPCC   National Society for the Prevention of Cruelty to Children

OCD   Obsessive compulsive disorder

ONS   Office of National Statistics

Perinatal   Describes the period surrounding birth, and traditionally includes the time from fetal viability from about 24 weeks of pregnancy up to either 7 or 28 days of life but can be up to 2 years

PHQ9   Patient Health Questionnaire 9

PMHP   Perinatal mental health problems

PMI   Perinatal mental illness

PND   Postnatal depression

PP   Puerperal psychosis

Prevalence   The proportion of cases in the population at a given time, rather than rate of occurrence of new cases

Psychiatric disorder   A mental or behavioural pattern or anomaly that causes distress or disability, and which is not developmentally or socially normative

Psychological   Related to the mental and emotional state of a person

PTSD   Post-traumatic stress disorder

RCOG   Royal College of Obstetrics and Gynaecologists

SIGN   Scottish Intercollegiate Guidelines Network

SMI   Serious mental illness

UK   United Kingdom

WHO   World Health Organization

References

Alderdice, F., McNeill, J., Lynn F. (2013) A systematic review of systematic reviews of interventions to improve maternal mental health and well-being. *Midwifery* 29 (4), pp. 389–399.

Abramowitz J.S., Schwartz S.A., Moore K.M., Luenzmann K.R. (2003) Obsessive-compulsive symptoms in pregnancy and the puerperium: A review of the literature. *Journal of Anxiety Disorders* 17, pp. 461–478.

Beck, C.T. (2001) Predictors of postpartum depression: an update. *Nursing Research* 50 (5), pp. 275–285.

Blackmore, E.R., Jones, I., Doshi, M., Haque, S., Holder, R., Brockington, I., Craddock, N. (2006) Obstetric variables associated with bipolar affective puerperal psychosis. *British Journal of Psychiatry* 188, pp. 32–36.

Brockington, I.F. (1996) *Motherhood and Mental Health*. Oxford: Oxford University Press.

Cantwell, R. Cox, J.L. (2006) Psychiatric disorders in pregnancy and the puerperium. *Current Obstetrics and Gynaecology* 13, pp. 7–13.

Cohen, L.S., Noncas, R.M. (2005). *Mood and Anxiety Disorder during Pregnancy and Postpartum*. Washington, DC: American Psychiatric Publishing.

Confidential Enquiry into Maternal and Child Health. (2004) *Why mothers die (2000–2002)*. London: RCOG.

Confidential Enquiry into Maternal and Child Health (2007) *Saving Mothers Lives: Reviewing Maternal Deaths to Make Motherhood Safer (2003–2005)*. London: RCOG.

Centre for Maternal and Child Enquiries (2011) Saving Mothers' Lives: reviewing maternal deaths 2006–2008. *British Journal of Obstetrics and Gynaecology* 118 (Suppl. 1), pp. 1–203.

Cohen, .LS., Rosenbaum, J.F., Hleer, V.L. (1989) Panic-attack associated placental abruption: case report. *Journal of Clinical Psychiatry* 50, pp. 266–267.

Chung, T.K., Lau, T.K., Yip, A.S., Chiu, H.F., Lee, D.T. (2001) Antepartum depressive symptomology is associated with adverse obstetric and neonatal outcomes. *Psychosomatic Medicine* 63, pp. 830–834.

Clark, L.A., Watson, D. (1991). Tripartite model of anxiety and depression: Psychometric evidence and taxonomic implications. *Journal of Abnormal Psychology* 100, pp. 316–336.

Crandon, A.J. (1979) Maternal anxiety and obstetric complications. *Psychosomatic Research* 23, pp. 109–111.

Da Costa, D., Larouche, M.P., Drista, M., Bender, W. (2000) Psychosocial correlates of prepartum and postpartum depressed mood. *Journal of Affective Disorders* 59 (1), pp. 31–40.

Department of Health (2002) *Women's Mental Health: Into the Mainstream*. London: Department of Health.

Department of Health, & Department of Education and Skills (2004) *National Service Framework for Children, Young People and Maternity Services: Maternity Services*. London: Department of Health.

Doucet, S., Jones, I., Letourneau, N., Dennis, C., Blackmore, E.R. (2011) Interventions for the prevention and treatment of postpartum psychosis: A systematic review. *Archives of Women's Mental Health* 14 (2), pp. 89–98.

Evans, J., Heron, J., Francomb, H., Oke, S., Golding, J. (2001) Cohort study of depressed mood during pregnancy and after childbirth. *British Medical Journal* 323, pp. 257–260.

Fisher, J., de Mello, M., Patel, V., Rahman, A., Tran, T., Holton, S., Holmes, W. (2010) Prevalence and determinants of common perinatal mental disorders in women in low- and lower-middle-income countries: a systematic review. *Bulletin of the World Health Organization* 90, pp. 139–149H. Available from http://www.who.int/bulletin/volumes/90/2/11-091850/en/

Glazener, C.M.A. (2005a) Parental perceptions and adaptation to parenthood. *British Journal of Midwifery* 13 (9), pp. 578–583.

Glazener, C.M.A. (2005b) Women's Health after Childbirth. In: C. Henderson, D. Bick (eds) *Perineal Care: An International Issue*. London: Quay Books Division, pp. 11–17.

Glover, L., Jomeen J., Urquhart, T., Martin, C.R. (2014) Puerperal Psychosis – A qualitative study of women's experiences. *Journal of Reproductive and Infant Psychology* http://www.tandfonline.com/doi/full/10.1080/02646838.2014.883597

Gorman, J.M. (1997) Comorbid depression and anxiety spectrum disorders [Review]. *Depression and Anxiety* 4 (4), pp. 160–168.

Hadwin, P. (2007) Common mental health disorders. In: S. Price (ed.) *Mental Health in Pregnancy and Childbirth*. Philadelphia: Elsevier, pp. 79–103.

Hay, D.F., Kumar, R. (1995) Interpreting the effects of mother's postnatal depression on children's intelligence: a critique and reanalysis. *Child Psychiatry and Human Development* 25, pp. 165–181.

Heron, J., McGuinness, M., Blackmore, E.R., Craddock, N., Jones, I. (2008) Early postpartum symptoms in puerperal psychosis. *International Journal of Obstetrics and Gynaecology* 115 (3), pp. 348–353.

Heron, J., Gilbert, N., Dolman, C., Shah, S., Beare, I., Dearden, S., Muckelroy, N., Jones, I. Ives, J. (2012) Information and support needs during recovery from postpartum psychosis. *Archives of Women's Mental Health* 15 (3), pp. 155–165.

Joint Commissioning Panel for Mental Health (2012) *Guidance for Commissioners of Perinatal Mental Health Services*. London: JCP-MH.

Jomeen, J., Martin, C.R. (2004) Is the Hospital Anxiety and Depression Scale (HADS) a reliable screening tool in early pregnancy? *Psychology and Health* 19 (6), pp. 787–800.

Jomeen, J., Martin, C.R. (2005) Confirmation of an occluded anxiety component within the Edinburgh Postnatal Depression Scale (EPDS) during early pregnancy. *Journal of Reproductive and Infant Psychology* 23 (2), pp. 143–154.

299

Jomeen, J., Martin, C.R. (2008) The impact of choice of maternity care on psychological health outcomes for women during pregnancy and the postnatal period. *Journal of Evaluation in Clinical Practice* 14 (3), pp. 391–398.

Jomeen J., Glover, L.F., Davis, S. (2009) Midwives' illness perceptions of antenatal depression. *British Journal of Midwifery* 17 (5), pp. 296–303.

Jomeen, J. (2012) Women's psychological status in pregnancy and childbirth – measuring or understanding? *Journal of Reproductive and Infant Psychology* 30 (4), pp. 337–340.

Jomeen, J., Glover, L., Jones, C., Garg, D., Marshall, C. (2013) Assessing women's perinatal psychological health: Exploring the experiences of Health Visitors. *Journal of Reproductive and Infant Psychology* 31 (5), pp. 479–489.

Jomeen, J., Martin C.R. (2014) Developing specialist perinatal mental health services. *Practising Midwife* 17 (3), pp. 18–21.

Jones, I., Craddock, N. (2001) Familiality of the puerperal trigger in bipolar disorder: Results of a family study. *American Journal of Psychiatry* 158 (6), pp. 913–917.

Jones, I., Craddock, N. (2002) Do puerperal psychotic episodes identify a more familial subtype of bipolar disorder? Results of a family history study. *Psychiatric Genetics* 12 (3), pp. 177–180.

Kalra, H., Tandon, R., Trivedi, J.K., Janca, A. (2005) Pregnancy induced obsessive compulsive disorder: A case report. *Annals of General Psychiatry* 4, 12. Available from http://www.ncbi.nlm.nih.gov/pmc/articles/PMC1164400/#B4

Louma, I., Tamminen, T., Kaukonen, P., Laippala, P., Puura, K., Samelin, R., Alomqvist, F. (2001) Longtitudinal study of maternal depressive symptoms and child wellbeing. *Journal of American Academy of Child and Adolescent Psychiatry* 40, pp. 1376–1374.

March, D., Yonkers K.A. (2001) Panic disorder. In: K.A. Yonkers, B. Little (eds) *Management of Psychiatric Disorders in Pregnancy*. London: Arnold, pp. 134–148.

Matthey, S., Henshaw, C., Elliott, S., Barnett, B., (2006) Variability in use of cut-off scores and formats on the Edinburgh Postnatal Depression Scale – implications for clinical and research practice. *Archives of Women's Mental Health* 9 (6), pp. 309–315.

MBRRACE-UK [online] Available: https://www.npeu.ox.ac.uk/mbrrace-uk

Morrell, C.J., Slade, P., Warner, R., Paley, G., Dixon, S., Walters, S.J., Brugha, T., Barkham, M., Parry G.J., Nicholl, J. (2009) Clinical effectiveness of health visitor training in psychologically informed approaches for depression in postnatal women: pragmatic cluster randomised trial in primary care. *British Medical Journal* Available online at http://www.bmj.com/content/338/bmj.a3045.pdf%2Bhtml.

Munk-Olsen, T., Laursen, T. M., Pedersen, C. B., Mors, O., Mortensen, P.B. (2006) New parents and mental disorders: a population-based register study. *Journal of the American Medical Association* 296, pp. 2582–2589.

Murray, L., Cooper, P.J., Stein, A. (1991) Postnatal depression and infant development. *British Medical Journal* 302, pp. 978–979.

Murray, L., Cooper, L. (1997) Postpartum depression and child development. *Psychological Medicine* 27 (2), pp. 253–260.

Nager, A., Johansson, L. M., Sundquist, K. (2005) Are sociodemographic factors and year of delivery associated with hospital admission for postpartum psychosis? A study of 500,000 first-time mothers. *Acta Psychiatrica Scandinavica* 112 (1), pp. 47–53.

National Institute for Clinical Excellence (2003) *Clinical Guidelines for Antenatal Care: routine antenatal care*. London: Department of Health.

National Institute for Clinical Excellence (2006) *Postnatal Care Guideline*. London: Department of Health.

National Institute for Clinical Excellence (2007) *Antenatal and Postnatal Mental Health; Clinical Management and Service Guidance*. London: Department of Health.

Neugebauer, R., Kline, J., Stein, Z., Shrout, D., Warburton, D., Susser, M. (1996) Association of stressful life events with chromosomally normal spontaneous abortion. *American Journal of Epidemiology* 143, pp. 588–596.

NSPCC (2013) *Prevention in Mind. All Babies Count: Spotlight on Perinatal Mental Health*. Available from: http://www.nspcc.org.uk/Inform/resourcesforprofessionals/underones/spotlight-mental-health-landing_wda96578.html

Oates, M. (1996) Psychiatric services for women following childbirth. *International Review of Psychiatry* 8, pp. 87–98.

Oates, M. (2006) Perinatal psychiatric syndromes: clinical features. *Psychiatry* 5 (1), pp. 5–9.

Oates, M., Raynor, M.D. (2009) Perinatal mental health. Part B: Perinatal psychiatric disorders. In: D.M. Fraser and M.A. Cooper (eds). *Myles Textbook for Midwives*, 15th edn. Edinburgh: Churchill Livingstone, pp. 686–704.

O'Connor, T.G., Heron, J., Golding, J., Beveridge, M., Glover, V. (2002) Maternal antenatal anxiety and children's behavioural/emotional problems at 4 years: report from the Avon Longtitudinal Study of Parents and Children. *British Journal of Psychiatry* 180, pp. 502–508.

O'Hara, M.W., Swain, A.M. (1996) Rates and Risks of postpartum depression – a meta-analysis. *International Review of Psychiatry* 8, pp. 37–54.

Office for National Statistics (2002) *Living in Britain, General Household Survey No 31*. London: ONS.

Patients' Association, (2011) *Postnatal Depression Services: An Investigation into NHS Services*. Available from http://patients-association.com/Portals/0/Public/Files/ResearchPublications/Postnatal/depression.pdf

Raynor, M., England, C. (2010) *Psychology for midwives: pregnancy, childbirth and puerperium*. Maidenhead: Open University Press.

Robertson, E., Jones, I., Haque, S., Holder, R., Craddock, N. (2005) Risk of puerperal and non-puerperal recurrence of illness following bipolar affective puerperal (post-partum) psychosis. *British Journal of Psychiatry* 186, pp. 258–259.

Ross-Davie, M., Elliot, S., Sarkar, A., Green, L. (2006) A public health role in primary mental health: are midwives ready? *British Journal of Midwifery* 14 (6), pp. 330–334.

Scottish Intercollegiate Guidelines Network (SIGN: 2002) *Postnatal Depression and Puerperal Psychosis. A National Clinical Guideline (Vol. 1)*. Edinburgh: SIGN Executive.

Seng, J.S., Low, L.M.K., Sperlicj, M., Ronis, D.L., Liberzon, I. (2009) Prevalence, trauma, history and risk for post-traumatic stress disorder among nulliparous women in maternity care. *Obstetrics and Gynaecology* 114 (4), pp. 839–847.

Spinelli, M. (2004) Maternal infanticide associated with mental illness: prevention and the promise of saved lives. *American Journal of Psychiatry* 161, pp. 1548–1557.

Teixeira, C., Figueiredo, B., Conde, A., Pacheco, A., Costa, R. (2009) Anxiety and depression during pregnancy in women and men. *Journal of Affective Disorders* 119 (3), pp. 9–18

Turton, P., Hughes, P., Evans, C.D,H., Fainman, D. (2001) Incidence, correlates, and predictors of post-traumatic stress disorder in the pregnancy and stillbirth. *British Journal of Psychiatry* 178, pp. 556–560.

Tyrer, P. (2001) The case for cothymia: mixed anxiety and depression as a single diagnosis. *British Journal of Psychiatry* 179, pp. 191–193.

Yelland, J.S., Sutherland, G.S., Wiebe, J.L., Brown, S.J. (2009) A national approach to perinatal mental health in Australia: exercising caution in the roll-out of a public health initiative. *The Medical Journal of Australia* Available online at https://www.mja.com.au/journal/2009/191/5/national-approach-perinatal-mental-health-australia-exercising-caution-roll-out?0=ip_login_no_cache%3D6fe312ac9a2778613dded80e26bfbcdf#9.

World Health Organization (2004) *WHO Guide to Mental and Neurological Health in Primary Care: A guide to mental and neurological ill health in adults, adolescents and children*, 2nd edn. London: Royal Society of Medicine Press.

301

Chapter 14

Complementary and alternative medicines applied to maternity care

Catriona Jones
University of Hull, Hull, UK

Jane Marsh
Hull and East Yorkshire Community Acupuncture, Cottingham, UK

Learning outcomes

By the end of this chapter the reader will be able to:

- understand the broad characteristics of the group of healing systems known as complementary and alternative medicines (CAM)
- identify the different categories of complementary and alternative medicines
- understand the philosophy which underpins complementary and alternative medicines
- identify some of the issues in relation to research and evidence of the safety and efficacy of complementary and alternative medicines
- discuss the role of the midwife in the context of complementary and alternative medicines.

Introduction

Complementary and alternative medicines (CAM) have been reportedly popular among child-bearing women for many years, and yet many CAM treatments reside in the margins of main-stream maternity provision, and do not form any part of routine National Health Service (NHS) care. This chapter attempts to define and categorise CAM, and to identify how it differs from Western medicine. CAM provision will be discussed, the growth of CAM will be explored, and finally this chapter will also address aspects relevant to respecting women's rights to self-administer CAM products. The clinical effectiveness and safety, using the best available evidence to underpin practice, and working within, and being guided by, relevant policies, protocols and professional requirements, will also be examined.

Fundamentals of Midwifery: A Textbook for Students, First Edition. Edited by Louise Lewis.
© 2015 John Wiley & Sons, Ltd. Published 2015 by John Wiley & Sons, Ltd.
Companion website: www.wileyfundamentalseries.com/midwifery

Definition of complementary and alternative medicines (CAM)

First, it is important to define CAM and to understand how it differs from other medicines. CAM is a term used to describe a wide range of healing systems that are not considered part of mainstream or conventional Western medicine. Western medicine is the term used for the products and treatments that are provided predominantly within mainstream health care in the United Kingdom (UK). Western medicine is focused upon addressing and trying to prevent disease, through diet, exercise, prescription drugs and surgery.

A variety of definitions of CAM exist across the literature. For the purposes of this chapter the overarching term CAM is used to capture all of the complementary and alternative systems and processes which are associated with healing. Although the word medicine is used within the CAM acronym, the term CAM itself refers to treatments, therapies and products, as well as medicines.

It is helpful to be able to see some of the differences between the two approaches to healing (CAM and Westernised medicine). In Table 14.1, the Western and the Eastern approaches are identified.

Although the acronym CAM is used regularly, and the terms complementary and alternative are often used together; *'complementary'* and *'alternative'* have different meanings in the context of the role they play in healing. It is important to have a general understanding of the terms, and how they exist within a Western medicine framework. An *alternative* medicine or therapy

303

Table 14.1   Western and Eastern approaches to healing (Adapted from 'Eastern Medicine versus Western Medicine' Vaxa [online] Available: http://www.vaxa.com/eastern-medicine-vs-western -medicine.cfm)

Eastern medicine	Western medicine
Health is a balance between mind, body, and spirit	Health is the absence of pain, symptoms, and physical or mental defects
Being unhealthy is an imbalance or disharmony of the natural body energy *(qi)*	Being unhealthy means there is a defect of the bodily structure with a cause and symptoms
Symptoms are the body's way of showing that it is healing	Symptoms are a sign of illness and must be eliminated or suppressed
The cause of an illness is any action that will cause disharmony of the *qi*	The cause of an illness is a foreign pathogen or force from outside the body
The patient's responsibility is to prevent illness and live a healthy, harmonious lifestyle	Personal lifestyle and living conditions don't play as much of a role, as more of an emphasis is put on healing vs. staying well
The role of the doctor is as an assistant, to help people stay well instead of fixing them once they become ill	The role of the physician is that of a mechanic, to fix what is broken and find things that are wrong
The goal of treatment is to restore balance through lifestyle changes and other natural means	The goal of treatment is to suppress symptoms, usually through drugs or surgery
The main strength of Eastern medicine is that it focuses on prevention and management of chronic illness, and the recognition of the importance of lifestyle and the mind/body connection	The main strength of Western medicine is that it is able to treat structural trauma and defects, as well as address life-threatening illnesses that require medical or surgical intervention

would be one which is used as a separate and different approach to healing, different from one which is generally accepted in Western medicine as appropriate for relieving uncomfortable symptoms of a bodily defect (for example if acupuncture is used to alleviate or cure back pain instead of 'routine' analgesia). A *complementary* medicine or therapy is used in addition to or alongside a conventional approach (for example if acupuncture is used alongside analgesia to alleviate or cure back pain).

The field of CAM

The field of CAM is very broad and constantly changing. The systems that exist within CAM are diverse. For those who have an emerging understanding of CAM, it is perhaps easier to group CAM practices into categories, and whilst these categories may not always be formally defined, establishing and acknowledging CAM within three broad groups, may be a useful way of facilitating the development of a knowledgebase for students and those new to CAM. In 2000, an enquiry into the regulation of, evidence for, accessibility of information about, the training of practitioners, and NHS provision of CAM, was undertaken by The Science and Technology Committee of the House of Lords. At the time of the enquiry, the Committee identified a detailed list of CAM therapies which they admitted is *'not all-inclusive'*; however, it does provides an indication and framework of the main types of therapies considered within the broad definitions of CAM. For someone with an emerging interest in CAM, this may be a helpful categorisation of CAM and its associated practices. Table 14.2 outlines the House of Lords Scientific and Technology Categorisation of CAM.

Table 14.2　Short and simplified descriptions of CAM disciplines: Science and Technology Committee of the House of Lords

(i) Group 1: Professionally Organised Alternative Therapies	
Therapy	**Description**
Acupuncture	Originating from China, acupuncture involves inserting small needles into various points in the body to stimulate nerve impulses. Traditional Chinese acupuncture is based on the idea of 'qi' (vital energy) which is said to travel around the body along 'meridians' which the acupuncture points affect. Western Acupuncture uses the same needling technique but is based on affecting nerve impulses and the central nervous system; acupuncture may be used in the West as an anaesthetic agent and also as an analgesic.
Chiropractic	Used almost entirely to treat musculoskeletal complaints through adjusting muscles, tendons and joints and using manipulation and massage techniques. Diagnostic procedures include case histories, conventional clinical examination and x-rays. Chiropractic was originally based on the idea that 'reduced nerve flow' led to disease.
Herbal medicine	A system of medicine which uses various remedies derived from plants and plant extracts to treat disorders and maintain good health. Another term for this type of treatment is phytotherapy.
Homeopathy	A therapy based on the theory of treating like with like. Homeopathic remedies use highly diluted substances that if given in higher doses to a healthy person would produce the symptoms that the dilutions are being given to treat. In assessing the patient homeopaths often take into account a range of physical, emotional and lifestyle factors which contribute to the diagnosis.

Table 14.2 (*Continued*)

(i) Group 1: Professionally Organised Alternative Therapies	
Therapy	**Description**
Osteopathy	A system of diagnosis and treatment, usually by manipulation, that mainly focuses on musculo-skeletal problems, but a few schools claim benefits across a wider spectrum of disorders. Historically differs from chiropractic in its underlying theory that it is impairment of blood supply and not nerve supply that leads to problems. However in practice there is less difference than might be assumed. Mainstream osteopathy focuses on musculo-skeletal problems; but prior to osteopathy gaining statutory protection of title, other branches of this therapy purported to diagnose and treat a range of disorders. One such branch is now known as cranio-sacral therapy, which should be considered as a distinct therapy which would fall into Group 3.

(ii) Group 2: Complementary Therapies	
Therapy	**Description**
Alexander technique	Based on a theory that the way a person uses their body affects their general health. This technique encourages people to optimise their health by teaching them to stand, sit and move according to the body's 'natural design and function'. This is, in essence, a taught technique, rather than a therapy.
Aromatherapy	Use of plant extract essential oils inhaled, used as a massage oil, or occasionally ingested. Common in France but practised there by medical doctors only. Can be used to alleviate specific symptoms or as a relaxant.
Bach and other flower remedies	The theory behind flower remedies is that flowers contain the life force of the plant and this is imprinted into water through sun infusion which is used to make the flower remedy. Flower remedies are often used to help patients let go of negative thoughts; usually flower remedies are ingested.
Body work therapies, including massage	Therapies that use rubbing, kneading and the application of pressure to address aches, pains and musculo-skeletal problems. Often used as a relaxant.
Counselling stress therapy	A series of psychical therapies that attempt to help patients to work through their thoughts and to reflect on their lives so as to maximise wellbeing.
Hypnotherapy	The use of hypnosis in treating behavioural disease and dysfunction, principally mental disorders.
Meditation	A series of techniques used to relax a patient to facilitate deep reflection and a clearing of the mind (see Maharishi Ayurvedic medicine below).
Reflexology	A system of massage of the feet based on the idea that there are invisible zones running vertically through the body, so that each organ has a corresponding location in the foot. It has also been claimed to stimulate blood supply and relieve tension.
Shiatsu	A type of massage originating from Japan which aims to stimulate the body's healing ability by applying light pressure to points across the body. Relies on the meridian system of 'qi' in a similar way to traditional Chinese medicine and acupuncture.
Healing	A system of spiritual healing, sometimes based on prayer and religious beliefs, that attempts to tackle illness through non-physical means, usually by directing thoughts towards an individual. Often involves 'the laying on of hands'.

305

(Continued)

Table 14.2 *(Continued)*

(iii) Group 2: Complementary Therapies (Continued)	
Therapy	**Description**
Maharishi Ayurvedic medicine*	A system which promotes transcendental meditation, derived from the Vedic tradition in India. Recommends the use of herbal preparations similar to those used in Ayurvedic medicine (see below) and Traditional Chinese medicine (see below).
Nutritional medicine	A term used to cover the use of nutritional methods to address and prevent disease. Uses diets and nutritional supplements. Often used to address allergies and chronic digestive problems. The difference between nutritional medicine and dietetics is that nutritional therapists work independently in accordance with naturopathic principles and focus on disorders which they believe can be attributed to nutritional deficiency, food intolerance or toxic overload. They believe these three factors are involved in a wide range of health problems. Dieticians usually work under medical supervision, using diets to encourage healthy eating and tackle a narrower range of diseases. Nutritional therapists often use exclusion diets and herbal remedies to tackle patients' problems.
Yoga	A system of adopting postures with related exercises designed to promote spiritual and physical well-being.

(iv) Group 3 (a): Alternative Disciplines: Long Established and Traditional Systems of Healthcare	
Therapy	**Description**
Anthroposophical medicine	'Anthroposophy' describes people in terms of their physicality, their soul and their spirit. Anthroposophical medicine aims to stimulate a person's natural healing forces through studying the influence of their soul and spirit on their physical body.
Ayurvedic medicine	An ancient discipline, originating in India, based upon the principle of mind-spirit-body interaction and employing natural herbs, usually mixtures, in treatment.
Chinese herbal medicine*	(See Traditional Chinese medicine below). A tradition of medicine used for thousands of years in China, which has its own system of diagnosis. Uses combinations of herbs to address a wide range of health problems.
Eastern medicine (Tibb)*	Tibb is a tradition which synthesises elements of health philosophy from Egypt, India, China and classical Greece. It literally means 'nature'. The concept of wholeness and balance permeates the principle of Tibb. Imbalance is thought to cause disease. It is thought to occur on four levels: physical, emotional, mental and spiritual. Tibb uses a range of treatments including massage, manipulation, dietary advice and herbal medicine, and a psychotherapeutic approach to restore imbalances which are considered the cause of disease.
Naturopathy	A method of treatment based on the principle that the natural laws of life apply inside the body as well as outside. Uses a range of natural approaches including diet and herbs and encourages exposure to sun and fresh air to maximise the body's natural responses.
Traditional Chinese medicine	The theory behind Traditional Chinese medicine is that the body is a dynamic energy system. There are two types of energy - Yin qi and Yang qi – and it is thought if there is an imbalance in Yin and Yang qi then symptoms occur. Traditional Chinese medicine uses a number of treatment methods to restore the balance of Yin and Yang qi; these include acupuncture, herbal medicine, massage and the exercise technique Qigong.

Table 14.2 *(Continued)*

(v) Group 3 (b): Other Alternative Disciplines	
Therapy	**Description**
Crystal therapy	Based on the idea that crystals can absorb and transmit energy and that the body has a continuing fluctuating energy which the crystal helps to tune. Crystals are often placed in patterns around the patient's body to produce an energy network to adjust the patient's energy field or 'aura'.
Dowsing	Traditionally used as a way to identify water sources underground. Is not itself a therapy but is used by a range of other disciplines to answer questions through intuitive skills. Often used in conjunction with Radionics.
Iridology	A method of diagnosing problems and assessing health status that relies on studying the iris of the eye and noting marks and changes.
Kinesiology	A manipulative therapy by which a patient's physical, chemical, emotional and nutritional imbalances are assessed by a system of muscle testing. The measurement of variation in stress resistance of groups of muscles is said to identify deficiencies and imbalances, thus enabling diagnosis and treatments by techniques which usually involve strengthening the body's energy through acupressure points.
Radionics	A type of instrument-assisted healing which attempts to detect disease before it has physically manifested itself. It is based on the belief that everyone is surrounded by an invisible energy field which the practitioner tunes into and then attempts to correct problems which have been identified. Practitioners believe it can be done over long distances. Instruments are a focus of the healer's intent and include sugar tablets which carry the healing 'idea'.

*We received evidence about these therapies, although they were not included in our original Call for Evidence.

307

Alternatively, for the purposes of discussing CAM, the United States Department of Health and Human Services, suggest the useful categorisations outlined in Table 14.3.

Why is CAM important to know about?

Reports of increasing consumer demand for CAM by pregnant women and new mothers are well-documented in studies and discussion papers (Jones 2012). Anecdotal evidence suggests that childbearing women reportedly pursue and use CAM before, during and after birth (Tiran 1996; Tiran 2003; Tiran and Chummun 2004; Tiran 2006a; Mitchell et al. 2006; Mitchell and Williams 2007; Evans 2009; Kenyon 2009; Mousley 2010; Cant et al. 2011; Tiran 2006b; Tiran 2006c; Mitchell and Williams 2006). It is not entirely clear if large numbers of childbearing women are actually engaging with CAM as the literature would suggest, as there have been very few primary studies which involve data collection directly from women in the UK (Jones 2012).

A recent report on the frequency of CAM use by a population of pregnant women in the former county of Avon in South West England, revealed that 26.7% (n = 3774) had used CAM at least once in pregnancy, the use rising from 6% in the first trimester to 12.4% in the second trimester, to 26.3% in the third trimester, with herbal teas being the most commonly reported CAM at any time (Bishop et al. 2011). Surveys undertaken in the United States by Gibson et al. (2001) and Ranzini et al. (2001) suggest that approximately one in three people have used CAM, two-thirds of them being women, and a recent study in Australia reported that almost 50% of a large nationally representative sample of Australian women consult a CAM practitioner during

Table 14.3 United States Department of Health and Human Services suggest these useful categorisations of CAM (US Department of Health and Human Services 2008)

Group 1: Natural products
Herbal medicines (botanicals)
Vitamins and minerals
Group 2: Mind and body medicine
Meditation
Yoga
Acupuncture
Deep breathing exercises
Guided imagery
Hypnotherapy
Progressive relaxation
Qi gong
Tai Chi
Group 3: Manipulative and body-based practices
Spinal manipulation (Including chiropractors, osteopath practitioners, naturopathic physicians)
Massage therapy
Group 4: Other CAM practices
Whole medical systems
Ayurvedic medicine
Traditional Chinese medicine
Homeopathy
Naturopathy

pregnancy and birth (Steel et al. 2012). Given these figures, it is likely that student midwives and midwives may be involved in discussions with women on the subject of CAM and therefore it is helpful to be informed about this continually evolving aspect of healthcare. Hall et al. (2011) reports a significant challenge when interpreting the literature on the prevalence of CAM use by pregnant women; this results from a lack of information about the instruments used for data collection, and differences between how CAM has been defined for each study. Indeed, it has to be said that research into CAM is complex, and aspects such as safety, effectiveness and satisfaction are difficult to explore for a number of reasons. Hall et al. (2011) highlight the lack of clarity in relation to data collection and definitions of CAM can further complicate some of the research issues.

The CAM philosophy

The ideas, the principles, and the way in which users and practitioners consider CAM are often referred to as the 'CAM philosophy'; which underpins practice. The term philosophy in this sense relates to the fundamental theories which contribute to the effectiveness of CAM. The philosophy is one which acknowledges the successes of the CAM intervention based on the links between the mind, the body, and spirit, alongside the relationship between the therapist and the individual who is engaging in the treatment. As identified earlier, health and disease are believed to involve a complex interaction of physical, spiritual, mental, emotional, genetic, environmental, and social factors (University of Maryland Medical Centre [UMMC] 2011). It would make sense then, that during consultations, CAM practitioners often search for emotional, physiological, psychological, spiritual and environmental factors which may be affecting someone's health. Box 14.1 is an example treatment for back pain with acupuncture, where the interplay of mind-body, and external factors are given due consideration to the healing approach.

Box 14.1   Clinical consideration: acupuncture and a back problem

The practitioner will consider the lifestyle of the patient as well as their general health and wellbeing. The lower back is where the kidney Qi is stored, considered in Traditional Chinese Medicine (TCM) to be the source of original (inherited) Qi. TCM attributes emotions to the different energy systems as well as physical functions. The emotion associated with the kidneys is fear. Pregnancy and childbirth are very taxing on kidney Qi and anxiety about the forthcoming birth and parenthood is common in late pregnancy. Exposure to environmental factors such as cold (due to inappropriate clothing in winter) can lead to stagnation of Qi in the lower back also resulting in pain. An acupuncturist would therefore work on introducing heat where there is cold, supporting kidney Qi and alleviating anxiety when treating back pain during pregnancy as well as assessing any muscular-skeletal problems.

The growth of interest in CAM

So far in this chapter, it is recognised that there are limited UK reports of CAM use in pregnant women; however, the data which is currently available does indicate that a proportion of pregnant women may be interested in adopting some non-biomedical approaches to healthcare during the course of their childbearing episode. Of those patients/consumers who have used CAM in the past, much of the evidence given by the Consumers' Association and the Patients' Association in relation to CAM treatment suggests that patient satisfaction is high (House of Lords 2000), and this is likely to account in part for a significant proportion of CAM use generally, certainly among those who have previously engaged with CAM.

It remains unclear what is responsible for the growth of interest in the general population. Suggestions that overall trust in medical care has declined and efforts to portray CAM use as a means of increasing the amount of control a patient has over their care have not been consistently supported with research; however these factors may contribute to patients becoming more engaged with, and proactive in, managing their health. There is some evidence to suggest that the general popularity of CAM in Europe, Australia and North America is reportedly linked with a number of factors including disappointment with biomedical healthcare alongside the rise of chronic health complaints (Nissen 2011).

A generation ago, healthcare appeared to be based on the notion that doctors were the 'sole gatekeepers' to medical and healthcare information; however within contemporary healthcare, patients now have access to unlimited medical knowledge and insights. Today, the internet provides access to a wealth of information and research, with health professionals increasingly caring for a new generation of well-informed patients. Information technology increases patient involvement in healthcare management and evidence suggests that a growing number of people are shifting away from being the dependant patients of old (Accenture 2010). Patients have significantly more information available to them; at times, expectations may differ from what the NHS or 'state funded' healthcare can provide. A 2010 survey of over 12,000 people across 12 countries showed that nearly two-thirds (64%) of people who use the internet to research health do so to check up on their medicines, or evaluate alternatives (Park and MacDaid 2011). With consideration given to the unlimited access patients have to information about their health and healthcare, the growth of CAM could be representative of a major transformation of the relationship between doctors and their patients and doctors and the larger community (Turner 2004).

CAM and patient satisfaction

Whilst the holistic approach of CAM and the individual emphasis are considered to be relatively appealing to patients, it is also the consultation style of CAM practitioners that is believed to be an important aspect of its popularity (House of Lords 2000). It is worthwhile discussing what is known about the differences between the approaches of the practitioners, and the differences of the consumer experiences of Eastern and Western medicine. This should provide some context to the claims of high patient satisfaction.

Goldner (2004) suggests that a patient's relationship with a CAM practitioner is different because of the expectation that consumers will take individual responsibility for their health, and thus become empowered, and most, if not all CAM practitioners would support this claim. Whilst little is known about the mechanisms which facilitate patient empowerment in the context of CAM activity, it is generally recognised that CAM use is considered an empowering experience for people, in comparison to their experiences within a conventional healthcare system. In support of this, a study by Barrett et al. (2003) revealed that patients using CAM perceived themselves to be empowered in their healthcare decision processes. The qualitative accounts from patients illustrated the concept of empowerment through narratives of being *'put in the driver's seat'* by the practitioner, in contrast to conventional medicine, where they often felt disempowered by their perceptions of being *'a cog on the machine'* (Barrett et al. 2003). The benefits of a healthcare approach where individuals are expected to take personal respon-sibility, as opposed to society taking responsibility for health, are currently being debated across both the fields of academia and practice; there appears to be a growing body of evidence sup-porting the importance of individual responsibility for health, suggesting that this concept has benefits for some members of society. Warriner et al. (2013) conclude that the notion of wellbe-ing encapsulates a demand for being recognised as an active, empowered and knowledgeable agent on the part of those using CAM, and there is anecdotal evidence to suggest that there is an association between an individual sourcing and taking steps to provide their own form of treatment, and consequently feeling responsible for bringing about their own 'healing', recovery and wellbeing.

In the UK, whilst a growing number of patients opt to have some or all of their investigations and treatment privately, healthcare and medical consultations are dealt with predominantly through the NHS. A recent Department of Health (DH) initiative in which NHS patients in England have formal rights to make choices about their General Practitioner (GP) surgery and GP (DH 2013), demonstrates that steps are being taken to provide greater flexibility and choice, which may enhance the concept of empowerment for some patients.

Women, midwifery and CAM

The reported growth of interest in the use of CAM by pregnant women is thought in part to be due to a desire to regain control over a normal life process which has become ever-more technological and medically dominated (Tiran 2007). The integrated approach of mind–body and healthcare with which CAM practice is associated, appears to have strong links with the concept of achieving 'normality' within childbirth. Interview data from pregnant women in an Australian antenatal clinic suggests that CAM use is a reflection of women's health beliefs, and amongst this population of women, CAM use did not appear to reflect dissatisfaction with conventional care or medicine (Gaffney and Smith 2004). Hall et al. (2011) identifies in a literature review on the use of CAM by pregnant women, that there is limited data on the motivations for CAM usage; however a belief that CAM offers a safer alternative than pharmaceuticals was highlighted in one study (Hall et al. 2011). Alongside this is the notion that CAM therapies give pregnant women more control and satisfaction in childbirth (Gaffney and Smith 2004; Mitchell and Williams 2007). Choice and control featured as a theme in a study by Warriner et al. (2013), aimed at exploring the nature of CAM use in a sample of pregnant women. Women in this sample viewed CAM as outside of biomedicine and part of an approach to health and wellbeing over which they are able to maintain personal control, instead of being told what they should do by doctors and midwives (Warriner et al. 2013).

The demand for advice on non-pharmacological means of managing with symptoms of pregnancy, pain in labour and postnatal discomforts, parallels the rise of the movement away from what many view as the medicalisation of childbirth (Warriner et al. 2013). Increased job satisfaction, fulfilment of the midwifery role, and added individual enthusiasm were found to be associated with CAM use by midwives within a number of studies, which allude to a consumer-driven demand (Tiran 1996; Mitchell et al. 2006; Mitchell and Williams 2007). Furthermore, empirical evidence drawn from two qualitative studies supports the concept of midwives experiencing informal rewards, such as the extension of occupational roles, and enhanced relationships with women (Mitchell and Williams, 2007; Cant et al. 2011). In a qualitative study exploring CAM in hospital midwifery in Australia, Adams (2006) highlight that CAM integration is far from a clinical issue. There is a suggestion that the promotion of CAM by midwives feeds into 'wider professional boundary and power struggles inherent in the hospital care of pregnancy and birthing' (Adams 2006). Interview data from midwives demonstrates that midwifery is considered distinct from, what is known as the 'medical model' and obstetrics, and Adams (2006) suggest that the integration of CAM equips midwives with a resource for challenging the dominance of the medical model. Included in the discussion of this study is an acknowledgement of CAM providing an additional range of treatment options to childbearing women, a fact that is less acknowledged in the CAM literature, as much of the research which is currently ongoing in this field of healthcare focuses on the sociological and professional issues, which, whilst very important, have the potential to render the other aspects of CAM use less significant.

311

Promoting normality and reducing unnecessary intervention

The internet is replete with websites providing information about the use of CAM for pregnancy and labour. The discourse is largely focused on promoting the use of CAM for relaxation or pain relief, and facilitating a normal birthing experience. Whilst there is a limited scientific evidence base for the effectiveness of many forms of CAM used in pregnancy and labour, there is widespread belief and acknowledgement that the incorporation of aspects of CAM into the birthing experience by the attending midwife, in particular, those aspects which are aimed at promoting relaxation, for example, massage therapy and aromatherapy, may be one way in which a midwife can assist women to avoid unnecessary medical intervention, and experience spontaneous vaginal birth. This may account for some of the reported increase in interest in CAM use by pregnant women in the third trimester, identified in the study by Bishop et al. (2011). As some women approach their expected date of birth they may be more engaged in discussions with midwives about the strategies they should adopt to induce labour and to avoid medical intervention during labour and birth. It is important that midwives who are advising on, administering, or involved in administering, any form of CAM have the knowledge base, and have achieved the appropriate training requirements of the organisation within which they practice. The 2013 Cochrane review by Sandall et al. (2013), of midwifery-led models of care in developed countries, concluded that women attended by midwives were consistently more likely to labour without major intervention and analgesia and more likely to experience a spontaneous vaginal birth. The results from Cochrane may be used to explore the potential for midwives incorporating CAM into their practice in an attempt to avoid unnecessary intervention and facilitate normal birth.

Among the indications given to pregnant women for the use of CAM in maternity care are outlined in Box 14.2.

The Information presented in Box 14.2, accessible by pregnant women via the internet and patient leaflets, is often based on a degree of what is called anecdotal evidence. 'Anecdotes' are best defined as interesting accounts or stories of an individual's experience of something, and there are mixed views about the reliability this type of evidence. The National Institute for Health and Care Excellence (NICE) has the responsibility of evaluating the evidence for different NHS treatments, and expresses concern about the validity of anecdotal evidence. Whilst anecdotal

Box 14.2   Indications given to women for the use of CAM in maternity services

- To provide relaxation, for the relief of anxiety, fear, tension and stress in pregnancy, labour or early postnatal period.
- To offer alternative options for helping mothers to cope with pain and discomfort in late pregnancy and labour, including contractions, backache, nausea, tiredness and constipation.
- To provide additional choice for situations that may require medical intervention or attempt to prevent the need for medical intervention, such as induction of labour.
- To aid recovery from birth and adaptation to parenthood, to relieve pain and discomfort, stress and tension in order to facilitate breastfeeding and reduce the impact of postnatal depression.

evidence may not have been acquired through rigorous scientific research, there may be elements of truth within the accounts, and sometimes this type of evidence can be a useful point of reference in lieu of more reliable information.

When examining the concept of relaxation, it is helpful to consider the mechanisms of the relaxation response, a term first used by Herbert Benson in 1975, in response to observations of physiological changes which occur during transcendental meditation. It is defined as a natural innate protective mechanism which facilitates the removal of harmful effects from stress through changes that decrease heart rate, lower metabolism, decrease rate of breathing, and bring the body back into a healthier balance (Benson and Klipper 2000).

Proving 'relaxation' by scientific means, that is measuring and demonstrating that a relaxation response has occurred, within the context of a scientific research study, is complex and involves the observation of a number of activities. Roche (2011) identifies the following as eliciting the relaxation response:

- Your metabolism decreases.
- Your heart beats slower and your muscles relax.
- Your breathing becomes slower.
- Your blood pressure decreases.
- Your levels of nitric oxide are increased.

313

At the time of writing this chapter, no evidence could be found of any research studies that have successfully scientifically observed and measured a relaxation response during labour and birth when a form of CAM has been incorporated; therefore at present, the claims of increased measurable relaxation in the context of labour and childbirth can not be substantiated with any other form of evidence other than that of anecdote.

It is important to bear in mind that whilst a wide range of pain management methods are available to women during childbirth, including both pharmacological and non-pharmacological interventions, little evidence is currently available which facilitates assessing the effectiveness of CAM. A 2006 Cochrane review of evidence for complementary and alternative therapies for pain management in labour concluded that acupuncture and hypnosis may be beneficial for the management of pain; however, the number of women studied was small. In addition to these findings, the review further concluded that few other complementary therapies have been subjected to rigours scientific study (Smith et al. 2006).

Evidence for the safety and efficacy of CAM

Despite its rising popularity over the last two decades, CAM remains in the margins of NHS care. It is necessary to understand the general state of the CAM evidence base, in order to consider the reasons. CAM has been criticised by some for not having scientific evidence to back its claims, and some CAM practitioners openly admit to not adopting a 'scientific approach' to treatment. The scientific approach may be described as a body of techniques for undertaking research investigations. Many conventional medicines have been proven to be safe and effective as a result of a research which has taken a scientific approach, and the use of the randomised controlled trials (RCT) is one way in which treatments are tested for their safety and efficacy. An RCT is defined by NICE (2013) as:

> ...A study in which a number of similar people are randomly assigned to two (or more) groups to test a specific drug or treatment. One group (the experimental group) receives the treatment being tested; the other (the comparison or control group) receives an alternative

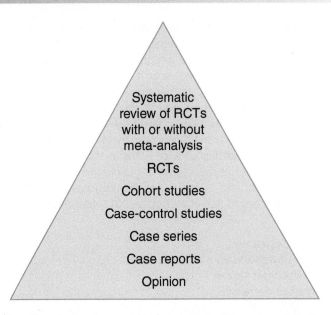

Figure 14.1   Hierarchy of evidence. Source: Akobeng 2005, Figure 1, p. 841. Reproduced with permission of the BMJ Publishing Group.

treatment, a dummy treatment (placebo) or no treatment at all. The groups are followed up to see how effective the experimental treatment was. Outcomes are measured at specific times and any difference in response between the groups is assessed statistically. This method is also used to reduce bias…

It is recognised that some research designs are better than others in their ability to answer research questions about safety and effectiveness. Akobeng (2005) highlights that this notion gives rise to what is known as a 'hierarchy of evidence' (see Figure 14.1).

The ranking has an evolutionary order, moving from simple observational methods at the bottom, through to increasingly rigorous methodologies (Akobeng 2005). The RCT is considered to provide the most reliable evidence on the effectiveness of interventions because the processes used minimise the risk of 'confounding factors' (aspects of the study situation that distort the association between the intervention and the participants), influencing the results. Evans (2003), states that the findings generated by RCTs are likely to be closer to the true effect than the findings generated by other research methods. RCTs have become the underlying basis for evidence-based medicine (Stolberg et al. 2004); however the relevance of the RCT to CAM research is continually being debated and discussed among researchers, academics and practitioners. There is some dissatisfaction of the concept of EBM. Aickin (2010) points out the failing of RCTs are that they focus exclusively on the treatment of groups of patients, and usually discourage the extension of findings to subgroups, never recommending extending the findings to individuals.

Although many scientists see RCTs as the ultimate analytical tool, RCTs may not fully embrace the CAM philosophy. So, for example, one aspect of the philosophy relies on the fact that the success of the treatment is based upon the positive relationship between the therapist and the individual who is engaging in the treatment. However, the randomisation and control processes of an RCT will in most cases prevent that relationship being based on an individualised and personal approach. Some CAM practitioners suggest that RCTs cannot do justice to the individualised, person-centred approach of therapies (House of Lords 2000). Comparative effectiveness research (CER) is a method which may be considered more appropriate; the core question in CER being which treatment works best, for whom, and under what circumstances? However, CER has at present, very limited recognition as a reliable and methodologically rigorous research design. Clearly, CAM and research evidence is an evolving area, and there is ongoing debate about the most appropriate research methods for establishing safety and efficacy. This controversial absence of a scientific evidence base for the safety and efficacy of those more widely used therapies by childbearing women has the potential to impact upon the midwifery role and responsibilities.

The role of the midwife in CAM administration

Whilst there are a wealth of statements within Nursing and Midwifery Council (NMC) documentation (NMC 2008; NMC 2012) about midwives' responsibilities in the context of CAM use, these do's and don'ts offer very little to midwives in relation to managing difficult discussions with women when they choose to adopt an aspect of CAM into their care which has not been fully recognised and acknowledged as being safe. Maternity Matters (DH, 2007) set out a strategy that placed women and their partners at the centre of maternity provision, with a commitment to women having opportunities to make well-informed decisions about their care throughout pregnancy, birth and postnatally (DH 2007). The legacy of Government policy in relation to choice and decision-making means that midwives should support women and remain committed to maintaining strong, positive relationships, whilst having to negotiate difficult situations, for example, when women make decisions about their care which may not always be the safest or the most sensible. Sometimes, due to the lack of evidence for safety and efficacy of certain CAM treatments, midwives may have to engage in difficult discussions with women and they may feel that they are unprepared for this challenging aspect of their role. The midwife has to somehow find the correct balance between not appearing to be overly authoritative, whilst ensuring that the wellbeing of the woman and the fetus or baby remain central to her role. However, if women feel that they are not full partners in decision-making; this could increase their anxiety during pregnancy and affect how they labour (Hall et al. 2011). It is likely that some midwives encounter anxieties and may feel insufficiently skilled to challenge women if their choices appear to border on being unsuitable in the CAM context. Whilst most midwives aim to provide excellent care; both from a clinical, and a public health perspective, they need to feel empowered to discuss such aspects of care confidently. As a result of the Government pledge to providing women with increased choice and decision-making, there is a growing need for midwives to become confident and equipped with the skills to support women in their choices and expectations; however midwives can often feel under prepared for this aspect of their role. It is important, as a student midwife and a midwife, that the relationship between you and the women in your care, and her partner, remain positive. It is vital that women do not feel inadequate as a result of these discussions; moreover, the outcome of any discussions such as those mentioned above will be very dependant on good communication and interpersonal skills on behalf of the midwife. Sometimes the involvement of a third party can be helpful, for example a Supervisor of Midwives or a midwifery manager. At all times however, the midwife should be guided by the relative NMC documentation as detailed below.

The NMC (2012), state that the system of regulation and registration of complementary therapists in the UK is voluntary self-regulation through the Complementary and Natural Healthcare Council (CNHC). Whilst the CNHC has been set up with Government support to establish and maintain a national register for practitioners, the NMC regulates the

315

practice of nurses and midwives who practice complementary and alternative therapies (NMC 2012).

The NMC information for midwives practising CAM is clear and concise. Midwives practising CAM are accountable through The Code: standards of conduct, performance and ethics for nurses and midwives (NMC 2008). The NMC urges practitioners to:

Ensure that the use of CAM is safe and in the best interests of those in your care.

(NMC 2008)

Furthermore, Standard 23 in the Standards for Medicines Management states that:

Registrants must have successfully undertaken training and be competent to practise the administration of complementary and alternative therapies.

(NMC 2012)

For those midwives who are not practising CAM, the advice in The Midwives Rule and Standards (NMC 2012) states that:

You must only supply and administer those medicines for which you have received training as to use, dosage and methods of administration.

(NMC 2012)

As we have previously established, the definition of CAM is broad and constantly changing, and therefore the use of the term 'medicine' may be unclear in the context of some forms of CAM, for example, essential oils and aromatherapy. Midwives and student midwives are encouraged to refer to the protocols, policies and guidelines of the organisations within which they practice for further clarification in relation to their role in the supply and administration of CAM.

Regulation

In the UK, with the exception of osteopathy and chiropractic, there is no statutory professional regulation of CAM. This means that anyone in the UK can legally call themselves a CAM practitioner, and practise on patients, even if they have no training or experience, and this can create a number of challenges for midwives when women seek advice about the use of CAM. The range of training and educational courses in complementary and alternative health is vast, and midwives should not be expected to have unlimited knowledge about such matters; therefore when advising women on the use of CAM through a practitioner, midwives should refer women to an appropriate resource in relation to the type of therapy under discussion. There are a number of regulatory bodies which may be useful for student midwives and midwives to be aware of.

The key purpose of regulatory bodies is to act in the public interest and enable proper public accountability of the complementary therapists that it registers. These voluntary regulators have a key function to enhance public protection, and strongly encourage complementary therapists on its register to be a member of a relevant professional association. Their registers are designed to enhance public safety, by giving the general public access to a list of complementary therapy practitioners who have been assessed as meeting national standards of competence and practice. Typically, practitioners can only join these associations or registers if they hold certain qualifications, and agree to adhere to certain standards of practice. However, there is no legal requirement to join and practitioners can still offer services without being a member of any organisation. The Department of Health recommends that where people are looking for complementary healthcare therapists, they use someone who is registered. Midwives aren't expected to have complete knowledge of every aspect of CAM practice, and therefore, women should be encouraged to make the use of professional bodies and voluntary registers relevant to the discipline for which they are enquiring, such as the Complementary and Natural Health-care Council (CNHC), or the British Acupuncture Council to help them find a practitioner.

Key points

- Complementary and alternative medicine (CAM) is a term used to describe a wide range of healing systems that are not considered part of mainstream or conventional Western medicine.
- A complementary medicine or therapy is used in addition to, or alongside a conventional approach, and an alternative medicine or therapy would be one which is used as a separate and different approach to healing, different from one which is generally accepted in Western medicine.
- Whilst there are many references to consumer demand for CAM from childbearing women in the UK, it is not entirely clear if large numbers of childbearing women are engaging with CAM as the literature would suggest, as there have been very few primary studies which involve data collection directly from women themselves.
- CAM and research evidence is an evolving area, and there is ongoing debate about the most appropriate research methods for establishing safety and efficacy. The absence of a 'scientific' evidence base for the safety and efficacy of those more widely used therapies by childbearing women has the potential to impact upon the midwifery role and responsibilities.
- Midwives and student midwives are encouraged to refer to the protocols, policies and guidelines of the organisations within which they practice, and the regulatory body NMC for further clari-fication in relation to their role in the supply and administration of CAM.
- It is not possible for midwives (and student midwives) to have complete knowledge of every aspect of CAM practice. Therefore women should be encouraged to make use of professional bodies and voluntary registers relevant to the discipline for which they are enquiring, such as the Complementary and Natural Healthcare Council (CNHC), or the British Acupuncture Council to help them find a practitioner.

Conclusion

This chapter has outlined the fundamental aspects of CAM in the context of midwifery care. The definitions and categories of CAM may change over time as new and more interesting healing systems emerge; however the role of the midwife should remain consistent in relation to ensur-ing the provision of safe and competent care to childbearing women. As pregnant women and new mothers increasingly engage with CAM it is important that the midwifery profession con-tinues to develop their understanding of how this growing phenomenon affects the midwifery role and responsibilities. Whilst the growth of CAM has allowed for the introduction of new, exciting and rewarding ways of caring for women, this has coincided with discussions about the increasing need for midwives to maintain their autonomy, facilitate normality, and ensure that women have a safe and satisfying childbearing experience. It is important that midwives continue to seek ways of facilitating normality safely and effectively, with or without the use of CAM, so that all women can continue to make use of the range of both conventional, main-stream and CAM's available to them.

End of chapter activities
Word search

E	S	T	X	H	I	T	L	A	E	F	D	A	P	G	L	F	R	W	B
H	R	N	Y	U	W	B	W	T	X	F	M	W	B	Q	Y	Y	E	W	I
R	C	U	G	D	Z	Z	J	E	J	P	L	T	V	D	H	S	G	K	F
C	E	R	T	H	O	M	E	O	P	A	T	H	Y	P	A	A	U	M	G
J	O	L	A	C	I	B	S	I	W	Y	A	H	O	F	N	O	L	A	N
G	U	N	A	E	N	X	G	C	J	X	I	S	E	E	C	Y	A	C	V
Q	U	T	T	X	S	U	D	A	J	L	O	T	C	M	E	O	T	N	N
E	K	W	B	R	A	E	P	W	Y	L	Y	D	N	V	N	T	I	S	L
N	F	H	F	Y	O	T	R	U	I	S	O	K	Z	V	Z	M	O	M	M
E	E	W	Q	G	G	L	I	H	C	T	H	E	R	A	P	Y	N	E	R
R	T	A	F	O	N	G	P	O	E	A	E	C	N	E	D	I	V	E	L
G	G	H	J	L	I	D	V	S	N	D	K	Q	X	I	U	U	U	A	B
Y	W	F	T	O	L	L	Y	M	O	L	Y	M	W	Z	C	A	T	K	C
Z	A	V	R	X	A	S	N	K	G	R	E	I	Z	Y	Z	S	Y	D	S
H	Q	O	E	E	E	W	I	O	H	L	B	Y	K	L	Y	B	J	L	V
O	W	Z	L	L	H	O	U	U	I	D	V	U	L	R	O	F	V	V	I
O	B	M	P	F	M	M	E	C	I	O	H	C	C	A	U	S	R	I	N
Y	P	A	R	E	H	T	O	N	P	Y	H	L	S	P	T	Z	Q	I	C
M	V	A	O	R	Z	V	Q	I	Y	F	T	B	P	E	T	C	V	Q	B
G	J	J	D	P	Z	T	F	R	E	H	P	V	X	V	D	X	S	O	W

ACUPUNCTURE, REGULATION, HOMEOPATHY, HYPNOTHERAPY, NMC, PHILOSOPHY, REFLEX-OLOGY, RELAXATION, RESEARCH, SAFETY, THERAPY, ANECDOTES, BODY, CAM, CHOICE, CONTROL, CRYSTAL, ENERGY, EVIDENCE, HEALING

Find out more

Below is a list of things you can find out about to enhance your knowledge of the issues and topics covered in this chapter. Make notes using the chapter content, the references and further reading identified, local policies and guidelines and discussions with colleagues.

1. Taking medication whilst using CAM

2. Comparative effectiveness research

3. Randomised controlled trials

4. Complementary and Natural Healthcare Council (CNHC)

5. Training and educational courses on CAM

Glossary of terms

Alternative medicine   An alternative medicine or therapy would be one which is used as a separate and different approach to healing, different from one which is generally accepted in Western medicine as appropriate for relieving uncomfortable symptoms of a bodily defect (for example if acupuncture is used to alleviate or cure back pain instead of 'routine' analgesia).

Anecdote   Interesting accounts or stories of an individual's experience of something, and there are mixed views about the reliability this type of evidence.

Biomedical   Relating to both biology and medicine.

Childbearing   The process of giving birth to children.

Complementary therapy   A complementary medicine or therapy is used in addition to or alongside a conventional approach (for example if acupuncture is used alongside analgesia to alleviate or cure back pain).

Cranio-sacral   Of or associated with both the cranium (the skull) and the sacrum (a triangular bone in the lower back formed from fused vertebrae and situated between the two hip bones of the pelvis).

Empowerment   The act of someone feeling more powerful (about a specific thing) as a result of them accessing or being provided with something.

Holistic   Focusing on the whole thing or the whole person/being.

Manipulation   A therapeutic intervention performed on the specific parts of the body (joints or parts of the skeletal structure).

Meridians   The meridian system is a belief about a path, in the body, through which life energy flows.

Non-pharmacological   Refers to treatments with no direct effects on a specific biological target.

Pathogen   Something that produces disease.

Pharmacology/pharmacological   The branch of medicine and biology concerned with the study of drug action.

Philosophy   A theory or attitude that acts as a guiding principle for behaviour.

Randomised control trial   A randomized controlled trial (RCT) is a specific type of scientific experiment. RCTs are often used to test the efficacy and/or effectiveness of various types of medical intervention within a patient population.

Relaxation   Natural innate protective mechanism facilitating the removal of harmful effects from stress through physiological changes that decrease heart rate, lower metabolism, decrease rate of breathing, and bring the body back into a healthier balance.

Synthesis   The combination of components or elements to form a connected whole.

Transcendental meditation   A technique for detaching oneself from anxiety and promoting harmony and self-realization by meditation.

References

Accenture (2010) The empowered patient: the changing doctor patient relationship in the era of 'self service' health care [online] Available: http://www.accenture.com/SiteCollectionDocuments/PDF/Accenture-Empowered-Patients-Change-Traditional-Doctor-Patient-Relationship.pdf

Adams, J. (2006) An exploratory study of complementary and alternative medicine in hospital midwifery: Models of care and professional struggle'. *Complementary Therapies in Clinical Practice* 12 (1), pp. 40–47.

Aickin, M. (2010) Comparative effectiveness research and CAM. *Journal of Alternative Complementary Medicine* 16 (1), pp. 1–2 [online] Available: http://www.ncbi.nlm.nih.gov/pmc/articles/PMC3116569/

Akobeng, A.K. (2005) Understanding randomised controlled trials. *Archives of Disease in Childhood* 90, pp. 840–844 [online] Available: http://adc.bmj.com/content/90/8/840.full

Barrett, B., Marchand, L., Scheder, J., et al. (2003) Themes of holism, empowerment, access, and legitimacy define complementary, alternative, and integrative medicine in relation to conventional biomedicine, *The Journal of Complementary and Alternative Medicine* 9 (6), pp. 937–947.

Benson, H., Klipper, M.Z. (2000) *The Relaxation Response*. New York: Harper Collins.

Bishop, J.L., Northstone, K., Green, J.R., Thompson, E.A. (2011) The use of complementary and alternative medicine in pregnancy: data from the Avon Longitudinal Study of Parents and Children (ALSPAC) *Complementary Therapies in Medicine* 6, pp. 303–310.

Cant, S.L., Watts, P., Ruston, A. (2011) Negotiating competency, professionalism and risk: the integration of complementary and alternative medicine by nurses and midwives in NHS hospitals. *Social Science and Medicine* 72 (4), pp. 529–536.

Department of Health (2007) *Maternity Matters; choice, access, and continuity of care in a safe service*. London: Department of Health.

Department of Health (2013) NHS Constitution for England [Online] Available: http://www.nhs.uk/choiceintheNHS/Rightsandpledges/NHSConstitution/Documents/2013/handbook-to-the-nhs-constitution.pdf

Department of Health and Human Services (2008) *CAM Basics: What is complementary and alternative medicine?* United States (US) Department of Health and Human Services [Online] Available: http://nccam.nih.gov/health/whatiscam/

Evans, D. (2003) Hierarchy of evidence: a framework for ranking evidence evaluating healthcare interventions. *Journal of Clinical Nursing* 12, pp. 77–84.

Evans, M. (2009) Post dates pregnancy and complementary therapies. *Complementary Therapies in Clinical Practice* 15 (4), pp. 220–224.

Gaffney, L., Smith, C.A. (2004) Use of complementary therapies in pregnancy: the perceptions of obstetricians and midwives in South Australia. *Australian and New Zealand Journal of Obstetrics and Gynaecology* 44 (1), pp. 24–29.

Gibson, P.S., Powrie, R. (2001) Herbal and alternative medicine use during pregnancy: a cross sectional survey. *Obstetrics and Gynaecology* 97 (4), p. 44.

Goldner, M. (2004) Cited in: Tovey P., Easethope G., Adams, J. (2004) *The Mainstreaming of Complementary and Alternative Medicine: Studies in a Social Context*. London: Routledge.

Hall, H.G., Griffiths, D.L., McKenna, L.G. (2011) The use of complementary and alternative medicine by pregnant women: a literature review. *Midwifery* 27 (6), pp. 817–824.

House of Lords (2000) Science and Technology, Sixth report, Complementary and alternative medicine [online] Available: http://www.publications.parliament.uk/pa/ld199900/ldselect/ldsctech/123/12304.htm#a14

Jones, C. (2012) Complementary and Alternative medicine in the maternity setting. *British Journal of Midwifery* 20 (6), pp. 409–418.

Kenyon, C. (2009) Risk management standards in midwifery are no substitute for personal knowledge and accountability. *Complementary Therapies in Clinical Practice* 15 (4), pp. 209–211.

Mitchell, M., Williams, J. (2006) Integrating complementary therapies. *Practicing Midwife* 9 (3), pp. 11–16.

Mitchell, M., Williams, J. (2007) The role of midwife-complementary therapists: data from in-depth telephone interviews. *Evidence Based Midwifery* 5 (3), pp. 93–99.

Mitchell, M., Williams, J., Hobbs, E., Pollard, K. (2006) The use of complementary therapies in maternity services: A survey. *British Journal of Midwifery* 14 (10), pp. 576–582.

Mousley, S. (2010) taking the first step: a midwife's reflection on experiences as an aromatherapist in midwifery. *MIDIRS Midwifery Digest* 20 (3), pp. 395–398.

Nissen, N. (2011) Challenging perspectives: women, complementary and alternative medicine, and social change. *Interface: A Journal for and About Social Movements* 3 (2), pp. 187–212 [online] Available: http://www.interfacejournal.net/wordpress/wp-content/uploads/2011/12/Interface-3-2-Nissen.pdf

National Institute for Health and Care Excellence (NICE) (2013) Glossary [online] Available: http://www.nice.org.uk/website/glossary/glossary.jsp?alpha=R

Nursing and Midwifery Council (NMC) (2012) *Midwives Rules and Standards*. London: NMC.

Nursing and Midwifery Council (NMC) (2008) *The Code: Standards of Conduct, Performance and Ethics for Nurses and Midwives*. London: NMC.

Nursing and Midwifery Council (NMC) (2012) Complementary and alternative therapies [online] Available: http://www.nmc-uk.org/Nurses-and-midwives/Regulation-in-practice/Regulation-in-Practice-Topics/Complementary-and-alternative-therapies/

Park, A., MacDaid, D. (2011) Modelling the potential cost-effectiveness of acupressure in the treatment of chronic low back pain. *Journal of Traditional Chinese Medicine* 3 (1).

Ranzini, A., Allen, A., Lai, Y.L. (2001) Use of complementary medicines and therapies among obstetric patients. *Obstetrics and Gynaecology* 97 (4), 46s.

Roche, L. (2011) The Relaxation Response [online] Available: http://www.lorinroche.com/benefits/benefits/relaxation.html

Sandall, J., Soltani, H., Gates, S., Shennan, A., Devane, D. (2013) Midwife-led continuity models versus other models of care for childbearing women. *Cochrane Database of Systematic Reviews*, Issue 8. [Online] Available: http://summaries.cochrane.org/CD004667/midwife-led-continuity-models-versus-other-models-of-care-for-childbearing-women

Smith, C.A. ,Collins, C.T., Cyna, A.M., Crowther, C.A. (2006) Complementary and alternative therapies for pain management in labour. *Cochrane Database for Systematic Reviews* 18 (4):CD003521.

Steel, A., Adams, J., Sibbritt, D., Broom, A., Gallois, C., Frawley, J. (2012) Utilisation of complementary and alternative medicine (CAM) practitioners within maternity care provision: results from a nationally representative cohort study of 1835 pregnant women. *BMC Pregnancy and Childbirth*. [Online] Available: http://www.biomedcentral.com/content/pdf/1471-2393-12-146.pdf

Stolberg, H.O., Norman, G., Trop, I. (2004) Randomised controlled trials. *Fundamentals of Clinical Research for Radiologists* [online] Available: http://www.ajronline.org/doi/pdf/10.2214/ajr.183.6.01831539

Tiran, D. (1996) The use of complementary therapies in midwifery practice: a focus on reflexology. *Complementary Therapies in Nursing and Midwifery* 2 (2), pp. 32–37.

Tiran, D. (2003) Implementing complementary therapies into midwifery practice. *Complementary Therapies in Nursing and Midwifery* 9 (1), pp. 10–13.

Tiran, D., Chummun, H. (2004) Complementary therapies to reduce physiological stress in pregnancy. *Complementary Therapies in Nursing and Midwifery* 10 (3), pp. 162–167.

Tiran, D. (2006a) Complementary therapies in pregnancy: midwives and obstetricians appreciation of risk. *Complementary Therapies in Clinical Practice* 12 (2), pp. 126–131.

Tiran, D. (2006b) Late for a very important date. *Practicing Midwife* 9 (3), pp. 16–28.

Tiran, D. (2006c) Midwives' responsibilities when caring for women using complementary therapies during labour. *MIDIRS: Midwifery Digest* 16 (1), pp. 77–80.

Tiran, D. (2007) The importance of obstetric knowledge for complementary practitioners [online] Available: http://www.positivehealth.com/article/midwife/importance-of-obstetric-knowledge-for-complementary-practitioners

Turner, B.S. (2004) cited in Tovey, P., Easethope, G., Adams, J. (2004) *The Mainstreaming of Complementary and Alternative Medicine: Studies in a Social Context*. London: Routledge.

University of Maryland Medical Center (UMMC) (2011) An introduction to CAM [online] Available: http://www.umm.edu/altmed/articles/an-introduction-000346.htm

Warriner, S., Bryan, K., Brown, A.M. (2013) Women's attitude towards the use of complementary and alternative medicines (CAM) in pregnancy. *Midwifery* 30 (1), pp. 138–143.

Chapter 15

Pharmacology and medicines management

Mary Beadle
University of Hull, Hull, UK

Andrea Hilton
University of Hull, Hull, UK

Learning outcomes

By the end of this chapter the reader will be able to:

- describe the principles of safe administration of medicines
- list the rights of medication
- describe what to check before, during and after giving medications
- discuss what to do after a medication error
- describe the key principles of pharmacokinetics and pharmacodynamics
- identify these key principles in relation to commonly used medicines in midwifery.

Introduction

The management of medicines is one of the key skills of a midwife; it is important that midwives and student midwives have the knowledge around what they need to do in order to do this safely and to facilitate the elimination or reduction of errors. This chapter will identify this knowledge and the key points at which this needs to be applied to practice. As part of this process it is important that student midwives and midwives have the most up to date knowledge about the medicines involved. This is essential if patients are to make informed choices about whether or not they want to take the medication. The chapter also includes information about some of the key medicines used within the maternity services. This chapter will look at two important aspects in relation to midwifery practice: medicines management and pharmacology.

Fundamentals of Midwifery: A Textbook for Students, First Edition. Edited by Louise Lewis.
© 2015 John Wiley & Sons, Ltd. Published 2015 by John Wiley & Sons, Ltd.
Companion website: www.wileyfundamentalseries.com/midwifery

The term 'patient' will be used throughout the chapter as this is the one that tends to be used in pharmacology and medication texts.

Medicines management

Medicines management is *'about enabling patients to make the best possible use of medicines'* (National Prescribing Centre (NPC) 2008, p.25), making the most of any benefits and minimising any risks or harm (NPC 2008). It can encompass clinical assessment and the monitoring and review of medicines. Other key features of medicines management include ensuring cost-effective medication is prescribed for patients; guidelines and policies are reviewed and information is exchanged efficiently with both patients and carers. This is seen as an essential skill and is a theme within any pre-registration midwifery education programme (Nursing and Midwifery Council (NMC) 2009).

Midwives must use the principles of safe administration of medicines at all times. One could say that these principles are clear and simple; however, it is evident from the number of medication errors that there is more to this than just following a list of actions. The fact is that there are agreed principles around what to do and that these are enshrined in professional standards and the law, but this process also requires critical and clear thinking to underpin the practice, otherwise the process becomes routine and open to mistakes and people taking risks. These principles are generally explained as *'Rights of Medication'* (see Box 15.1) although how many of these there are does vary (Agyemang and While 2010, Alexis and Caldwell 2013; Elliott and Liu 2010).

There are also possible rights around the right form/formulation, the right duration and the right to refuse (Elliott and Liu 2010). It is important not to include too many rights, otherwise they become difficult to remember. It can help to divide the 'Rights' into the timing within the process of administration, including before, during and after administration.

What to check before administration

This would include that you have the *Right* patient; this can be done using the patient's identity (ID) bracelet (if in hospital) and asking the patient their name and date of birth. This should be checked against the patient's prescription chart or care record. This should be a simple action,

Box 15.1   *Rights* of Medication

1. The *Right* patient
2. The *Right* medication
3. The *Right* dosage
4. The *Right* route
5. The *Right* time
6. The *Right* reason
7. The *Right* documentation
8. The *Right* practitioner
9. The *Right* environment
10. The *Right* evaluation

but it has been identified that patients often do not have an ID bracelet or can have the wrong information recorded on it. This is why it is important also to ask the patient to confirm their name and date of birth.

Once it is clear that you have the *Right* patient then the next checks are related to the actual medication itself. This includes that you have the *Right* medication, and the *Right* dosage, and that you are planning to give it using the *Right* route and at the *Right* time. All this information is available via the prescription chart or patient records. This is also linked to the issue of having the *Right* documentation available prior to administration. It is essential to check that the prescription and medicine label are written clearly and there is no ambiguity. It is important to check for an expiry date.

What to know before administration

This includes that the medication is being given for the *Right* reason; in order to know this then you must have access to the patient's records and care pathway. This must include any allergies that the patient might have. The NMC (2010) identify that prior to administration of any medicine you must know the therapeutic uses of the medicine, its normal dosage, side effects, precautions and contraindications. You must be aware that the patient has the *Right* to refuse to take any medication and that you must have informed consent from a patient before administration. This means that you need to explain to the patient the reason for taking the medication and possible side effects. It is essential that you know if the patient has any allergies and if this would impact on the administration of this medication. This means that you need to know what the medication contains as it is not always clear what drugs are contained within a specific medication. Some Trusts have a policy of having special patient identity bracelets to warn of allergies, but it is always important to check that there are no allergies that the patient may not have informed staff about. Some medicines are linked to specific physiology of the patient, for example their weight, so it is essential to have an up to date weight on the patient prior to calculating the dosage. This is significant with the increasing numbers of obese women that are seen in maternity services, as well as caring for babies.

What to check during administration

That there is the *Right* environment for administering medicines; there should be no distractions and the practitioner giving the medicines is focusing solely on this task. It has been identified that this can reduce the number of medication errors. It is essential that the *Right* practitioner is involved in administering medicines. This can depend on what type of medicine is being given and to whom, for example controlled drugs require two registered practitioners. It is important to check that the patient has taken the medication, and particularly with injections and intravenous drugs that there is no immediate allergic reaction to the medicine. There are also the issues of the *Right* duration if this relates to intravenous medication. If a patient queries the medication then it is important to follow up their questions before administering the medication. Patients are often experts in their condition and medication. The Department of Health (DH; 2008) has published guidance for service users and practitioners suggesting appropriate questions.

What to do after administration

It is important that the administration of the medicine is accurately recorded in the *Right* documentation. If the medicine has not been given for some reason, for example the patient declines, then this must also be recorded. Communication around the administration of medicines is crucial and can prevent errors occurring, for example: a patient being given a medicine in error as the first practitioner did not record that it had already been given. It is important that if there is a delay in giving a medicine then this is recorded, as many medicines have specific issues about timing between doses which must be adhered to, in order to prevent toxicity or a failure of reaching a therapeutic dose (Jordan 2010). This is explained in more detail in the pharmacology section.

What to check after administration

This is in relation to the *Right* evaluation; it is important to check that the medicine is having the right effect on the patient and to observe the patient for possible side effects. This evaluation should be recorded in the *Right* documentation and any relevant changes made to the patients care pathway. There is no point in giving a medicine if there is no evaluation of its effects. If the medicine is not found to be effective, or has unacceptable side effects then the practitioner needs to discuss this with the relevant doctor or whoever prescribed the medicine. As Griffith (2013) identifies healthcare practitioners are well placed to report adverse drug reactions and it is important that they do so.

If a practitioner relates their practice to the above rights then this should reduce the possibility of errors significantly.

When and how mistakes can happen

It can be useful to review errors in care and to explore how these have happened, in order to learn lessons and prevent further mistakes (DH 2000). This can then alert health professionals involved in medicine management when and how they are at risk of making mistakes. Fry and Dacey (2007) split these incidents into different parts which are; *design, equipment, procedure, operator, supplier and environment*. These can then link into other issues such as similar packaging, similar names of drugs, problems with equipment such as infusion pumps, not following guidelines and policies, stress and poor memory of staff, distractions and excessive workload. This is in addition to poor numeracy skills and lack of knowledge around medicines (Cleary-Holdforth and Leufer (2013), inaccurate or incomplete documentation, wrong drug or the wrong dose (Cox 2008). Cleary-Holdforth and Leufer (2013) also discuss the issue of complacency with staff not keeping up to date and adhering to the guidelines and policies around medicine management. Harkanen et al. (2013) also identify errors in patient identification as a key area of concern. Tingle (2012) discusses the errors around prescribing medicines, which midwives need to be aware of. These include: incorrect medicine and dose, the medicine not being needed or appropriate, failure to prescribe, allergy or contra indication errors and poor documentation. As midwives work within a team it is their responsibility to check the prescription for such errors prior to administering any medicine.

It is important to ensure that the patient has enough information in which to make an informed decision around whether to consent to the administration of the medicine. This is also important in relation to patient compliance during self-medication. Chummun and Bolan (2013) identified that a large number of patients do not take their medication as prescribed because they do not believe that they need it and that it does not work; this they see as a breakdown in communication between the patient and the healthcare practitioner. In order to overcome this problem the patient needs to be fully involved in the decision making process around medicines.

What to do if an error is made

Medication errors are the most common mistake and reason for adverse events within the NHS and health services worldwide (Elliott and Liu 2010). An error can be related to using the wrongs of medication instead of the rights. These can be related to omission, in that the drug is not given, prescription mistakes, giving a drug that is not prescribed, wrong dose, wrong drug, wrong route, wrong form (for example tablet instead of liquid), wrong time, wrong patient. There can also be errors made in dispensing of drugs (Meetoo 2012; Tingle 2012).

It is essential that a doctor is informed so that the possible effects on the patient can be assessed. The patient should be informed and a Supervisor of Midwives should be contacted to discuss the situation with the patient. It must be recorded in the patient's notes that this error has been made. A critical incident form must be completed so the reasons behind this error can be reviewed. The medication needs to be given to the correct patient. A Supervisor of Midwives should be contacted so that the practitioner who made the error can discuss the situation with them and reflect on what happened, in order for them to learn from the situation and to support them. The National Patient Safety Agency reviews medicine errors and makes recommendations to prevent this type of error reoccurring. This is termed the *circle of safety* in which it is hoped that the whole of the Trust and NHS can learn from these mistakes and put systems in place to prevent their reoccurrence (NPSA 2004; Agyemang and While 2010).

Keeping up to date

It is always important to keep up to date with current issues around any topic in midwifery, including medicine management and pharmacology, particularly as they are key to safe practice. The British National Formulary (BNF) is aimed at health professionals involved in administering medicines and should be available in clinical areas; information can also be found on medicines compendium UK, as well as specific texts related to maternity services (Hale 2012; Jones 2013). The NMC also regularly publish standards for medicines management. By going to the NMC website you can access the most up to date information regarding medicine management (see Further Reading Activity). Other NMC documents may also have information regarding medicine management. Anyone prescribing, dispensing or administering medicines needs to be aware of the relevant legislation around this practice. The Medicines and Healthcare products Regulatory Agency (MHRA) have a role to play in safeguarding the public in relation to medicines and provide information around safety alerts and legislation related to medicines (see Further Reading Activity).

Further reading activity

For further information access the following
   [available online] http://www.medicines.org.uk/emc/.
   [available online] http://www.nmc-uk.org/Publications/Standards/.
   [available online] http://www.mhra.gov.uk/index.htm#page=DynamicListMedicines.

There are rules around what medicines student midwives can administer; all students should make sure that they are familiar with these. The NMC and MHRA give out information about this, which is available via their websites. Currently *student midwives can administer medicines on the midwives exemption list, except Controlled Drugs, under the direct supervision of a sign off midwife* (NMC 2011; MRHA 2013). The medicines contained on the midwives exemption list are identified by the NMC (2011) and MRHA (2013). Student midwives may also administer medicines if they are prescribed by a doctor; however, students must always be under the direct supervision of a sign-off midwife or nurse. There may be specific medicines that hospital Trusts do not allow students to administer so it is important that all students and qualified practitioners are aware of their drug policies. If there is any doubt about the role of students in the administration of medicines then students must discuss this with the mentor and refer to the Trust guidelines for the placement area.

Off label and unlicensed

When a medicine is licensed it means it holds a marketing authorisation. It is licensed for a particular indication(s), route, age of patient and direction. However, medicines can be prescribed and used off label. The use of medicines outside the terms of the license (i.e., 'off-label') may be judged by the prescriber to be in the best interest of the patient on the basis of available evidence. Such practice is particularly common in certain areas of medicine: for instance, in paediatrics where difficulties in the development of age-appropriate formulations means that many medicines used in children are used 'off-label' (MHRA 2009).

Unlicensed is when a medicine does not hold a marketing authorisation in this country and therefore needs to be made or imported. This should only be prescribed if the clinical need of the patient cannot be met by a licensed product or off label use. An example of unlicensed is the prescribing of two drugs for use in one syringe driver, or the prescribing of total parenteral nutrition; both of these are examples of acceptable clinical practice and recognised nationally.

Pharmacology

Ensuring the right medicine is given to the right patient at the right time is key to ensuring safe and effective practice. However, once you have administered the medication what is it actually doing for the patient? (A more in-depth analysis of pharmacology, cell structure and targets for medicines can be found in general pharmacology textbooks and are referenced at the end of this chapter.)

What is pharmacology?

Pharmacology is concerned with scientific principles which can be applied to how the body interacts with medicinal compounds (medicines) and drugs in general. As healthcare practitioners who will administer medicines, we need to know the affect that that particular medication will have in the body and also what the body (a living system) will do with that foreign substance.

Drug/medicinal compounds or medicines

Throughout this chapter, 'medicines' will be referred to when discussing a licensed medicinal compound rather than drugs. Drugs are chemical substances which interact with biological systems. Pharmacologists will be interested in drugs which will never be licensed medicines for human use. Further information can be obtained from the British Pharmacology Society [available online] http://www.bps.ac.uk/

Two important principles in pharmacology are:

* pharmacodynamics
* pharmacokinetics.

Pharmacodynamics is usually referred to as 'what the drug does to the body'. When we administer a medicine we expect there to be an effect. For example, if we have a headache and take an analgesic there is an expectation it will help the pain.

Pharmacokinetics is usually referred to as 'what the body does to the drug'. When we administer a medicine for example orally, this medicine must first be absorbed into the blood stream; it must then be distributed around the body, to the site of action to give the desired effect 'Pharmacodynamic'; the medicine will often be metabolised (chemically changed) and then excreted or eliminated out of the body.

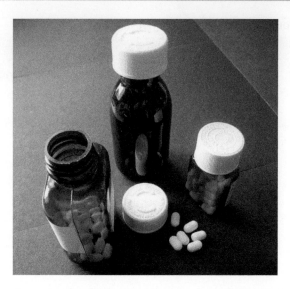

Figure 15.1   Medication for oral administration in the form of tablets and liquid.

These four principles are:

- absorption
- distribution
- metabolism
- elimination.

Prescribers will make evidence-based decisions of which treatment (often a medication) a patient receives. Clinical decision-making is discussed elsewhere, but prescribers can also make decisions about which route of administration is used. The most commonly encountered route is oral (enteral) with liquid medicines, tablets and capsules (see Figure 15.1). In midwifery, intravenous (IV) is used (into the vein, this allows for quick administration and usually a rapid effect). The IV route can be dangerous and fatalities have occurred. Other routes of administration in midwifery are identified in Table 15.1.

Pharmacokinetics – absorption

When a medicine is administered orally to a patient it is absorbed into the blood. The absorption of a medicine is dependent on the route of administration. Unless a medicine is given by the intravenous route, it will have to pass through membranes. A medicine given directly into the vein naturally reaches the blood stream immediately and has an effect sooner than oral.

When a medicine is given orally, it must pass through membranes in the intestines. It is absorbed and transported to the liver by the hepatic portal vein. From the liver it is then distributed round the body. There can be challenges to oral absorption, e.g. from digestive enzymes, pH of the stomach. Oral medication must be both enzymatic and pH stable.

The design of the medicine has been considered for its route of administration, and therefore should also be administered by the correct route, unless specific guidance has been given to change the route of administration. There have been fatalities when the wrong route of administration has been used.

Table 15.1   Different routes for medication administration

Route	Medication example
Topically (e.g. eyes, ears)	Chloramphenicol eye drops 0.5% or eye ointment 1%
Buccal	Prochlorperazine
Rectal	Diclofenac
Sub-lingual	GTN spray
Intramuscular	Pethidine
Subcutaneous	Fluids – sodium chloride 0.9%
Vaginally	Prostaglandin
Transdermal	Nicotine replacement therapy
Inhalation	Salbutamol

Activity 15.1

The dose of IV medicines are different from that of oral equivalents.
Can you think of an example of this difference?

Pharmacokinetics – distribution

Once a medicine has been absorbed, it needs to get around the body to its site of action (to have an effect). This may mean that the medicines will have to pass through membranes and barriers. Distribution can be quite complex and dedicated pharmacology textbooks will discuss this in more detail. Organs and areas of the body which have a rich blood supply (good blood perfusion) will receive medication which is administered quicker than those areas which have a less blood perfusion such as skin, fat, bone tissue.

Another aspect to consider is barriers within the body. If you wish the medicine to work within the central nervous system, then it must pass the blood–brain barrier (BBB). The BBB will only allow lipid soluble medicines through (unless there is a specific carrier/transport system). Some medicines will not routinely pass the BBB unless the barrier is inflamed such as in meningitis.

Another 'barrier' to consider is the placenta. When any medicine is administered to a pregnant woman, consideration must be given as to whether this will cross the placenta and the implications of this. For example, the medicine may not be known to be harmful, or the benefit outweighs the risk, or it should not be used in pregnancy or a particular point in the pregnancy.

Pharmacokinetics – metabolism

Metabolism is often described as how the body gets rid of the medicine which has been administered. Metabolism is actually where the chemical structure of a medicine is changed, usually from fat soluble to more water soluble. Medicines which are excreted from the kidney must be water soluble. Metabolism usually occurs in the liver, but not exclusively and not all medicines undergo metabolism.

Metabolism in the liver is an enzymatic process utilising the liver enzymes known as cytochrome P450 (CYP450). Metabolism of fat soluble compounds is often a two-stage process. Phase I involves a chemical change using involving oxidation, reduction or hydrolysis. Phase II involves conjugation with another compound, this results in a water-soluble compound which can be excreted via the kidney.

Cytochrome P450 is the main enzyme system involved in metabolism. There are many different types (isoenzymes) which are all very similar to each other. Common types involved in the metabolism of medicinal compounds include (although there are many others) are CYP 3A4 and CYP 2D6. These enzymes can be influenced by: other medication, smoking, genetic variation.

Pharmacokinetics – excretion

This simplistically is the removal or excretion out of the body. This usually happens via the kidneys, but excretion can occur via the lungs (in the case of anaesthetics and gases) or via the liver and bilary tract (into bile) for large molecular weights. Although the following routes are not routinely used to remove medicines from the body, metabolites can be found in the tears, saliva and breastmilk. Medication within breastmilk is a key consideration for midwives; consideration must include whether the medicine is presented in breastmilk, in what concentrations and whether it is known to be harmful. For example, often medicines will be present in breastmilk, but are not known to be harmful to such a degree that the mother should not breastfeed. This is when it is important to refer to specific literature (Hale 2012) and liaise with your local lactation consultant for guidance, rather than just referring to the BNF; otherwise women may be given inaccurate advice about whether or not they can continue to breastfeed when using medication.

Another aspect to consider is whether the prescribed medication actually affects breastmilk production in terms of volume. For example, knowing the pharmacodynamics of the medicine (what the medicine is doing to the body) will help this. An example is cabergoline; dostinex tablets will work on the D_2 receptor and suppress milk lactation. It is licensed for the inhibition of physiological lactation soon after delivery (eMC 2013); an example of this would be following the birth of a stillborn baby.

Pharmacodynamics

There are some terms to review in this section and again more detail will be available in a dedicated pharmacology text.

Agonist

This is a medicine (hormone; ligand) which binds to a receptor and produces a specific response. For example, when Salbutamol binds to the beta$_2$ receptors in the lungs, this produces bronchodilation and helps open up the airways, this is used for acute relief during an asthma attack.

Antagonist

This is a medicine which when bound to a receptor does not produce a response; its action is to block. Antagonists can be competitive or non-competitive, with competitive antagonists making easily reversible bonds. For example, ranitidine is an H_2 receptor antagonist; this means it blocks the H_2 receptor which is involved in stomach acid secretion and acid secretion is reduced.

Half life

The half life of a medicine is the time taken for plasma concentration to reduce by a half of its original value. It is normally taken that when a medicine is stopped it needs five half lives to be eliminated from the body. For examples, if a medicine has a half live of 24 hours and the patient stops taking it, in 5 days time it will not detected in the body. Conversely, to reach steady state, i.e. a constant level of medication in the body, it takes five half lives to reach steady state with regular administration. Some medications have a very short half life (e.g. adrenaline) and others have a very long half life (e.g. amiodarone).

First pass metabolism

When a medication is taken orally, it is absorbed and reaches the liver via the hepatic portal vein. When the medicine passes through the liver it will undergo some degree of metabolism, i.e. first pass through the liver. For some medication the degree of metabolism is extensive and the metabolite has little biological activity and therefore is rendered biological inactive. If a medicine undergoes extensive first pass metabolism then usually another route other than oral is used. An excellent clinical example is GTN; this is not given orally due to extensive first pass metabolism and is given sublingually (usually), which means it reaches the blood stream first and has a biological effect before been rendered inactive via the liver. First pass metabolism can account for the dose differences between the same medications but different routes of administration – please see the section on bioavailability.

Bioavailability

This is the proportion of an administered dose which will reach the circulation unaltered, and therefore will be able to have an effect. The IV route ensures 100% bioavailability, but the oral route can be reduced by: Gastrointestinal contents and gastric retention time; pH: First pass effect. This will often mean that the dosages given for same medication is different if given IV or oral but the manufactures have already calculated this.

Morphine 10 mg IV = 30 mg oral

We will also explore other terms encountered when administrating medicines such as adverse drug reactions and drug interactions. An adverse drug reaction has been defined by the World Health Organization (2008) as 'harmful and unintended reaction to a medicine'. Adverse drug reactions are always harmful.

Any medicines can cause a side effect. Some can be unintended such as drowsiness with codeine, but some side effects can be intended and in fact be beneficial. For example sedating antihistamines cause drowsiness as a side effect, but this can be used to aid sleep; another example is amitriptyline has the side effect of urinary retention but this can be used for nocturnal enuresis.

The following sections are summary monographs for the commonly encountered medicines you may administer. All the following information should be reviewed with the latest edition of the British National Formulary and a copy of the Summary of Product Characteristics, these explain how medicines work. The monographs have also been constructed with the latest edition of *Rang and Dale's Pharmacology* (2012).

Monographs
Medication name/Class: Antibacterial

Penicillin – Co-amoxiclav, Penicillin, Fluxcloxicillin

Licensed indication	Prescription only medicine (POM). You should refer to the latest edition of the British National Formulary.
Pharmacodynamic	Penicillins are bactericidal (kill). They affect the bacterial cell wall synthesis. Co-amoxiclav inhibit the synthesis of bacterial peptidoglycan; this weakens the cell wall; which is followed by death of the cell.
Pharmacokinetics	Generally are well absorbed when given orally. Penicillins cross the placenta and into breastmilk. There are trace amounts in breastmilk. There are excreted in the urine (kidneys).
Contraindications	Penicillin hypersensitivity. Rashes and anaphylaxis – which can be fatal. Full details will be given in the summary of product characteristics (the data sheet) for each individual medicine. The latest edition of the British National Formulary will also have a section on this. Co-amoxiclav is contraindicated with patients with jaundice or hepatic problems. Fluxcloxicillin – should not be used in patients with hepatic dysfunction, caution with hepatic impairment.
Side effects	Include: nausea, diarrhoea, vomiting. Broad spectrum penicillins can cause antibiotic-associated colitis.
Consideration for practice	Allergy status. With or after food administration. The prescribing of antibacterial medicines should follow your Trust antibacterial guidelines/ Public Health England.

333

Medication name/Class: Antibacterial

Macrolides, e.g. erythromycin

Licensed indication	Prescription only medicine (POM). You should refer to the latest edition of the British National Formulary.
Pharmacodynamic	Macrolides inhibit bacterial protein synthesis. They bind to the 50s ribosomal subunits of susceptible organisms. Action can be bactericidal or bacteriostatic.
Pharmacokinetics	Usually given orally, clarithromycin and erythromycin can be given by intravenous infusion. Diffuse readily in to most tissue, but not across the blood brain barrier. Care must be taken when these are prescribed in patients with hepatic or renal impairment. Azithromycin and clarithromycin – not suitable in pregnancy. Manufacturers advise only if no other alternatives; is present in breastmilk, use only if no other alternatives. Erythromycin not known to be harmful in pregnancy and small amounts present in breastmilk.

Contraindications	Hypersensitivity. Macrolides should be used in caution with patients with QT interval prolongation. There are several important and potentially clinically significant interactions with macrolides including: Antihistamines Calcium channel blockers Lipid-regulating drugs and several more.
Side effects	Include: Gastrointestinal – diarrhoea vomiting, nausea Hepatotoxicity Pancreatitis.
Consideration for practice	Allergy status. The prescribing of antibacterial medicines should follow your Trust antibacterial guidelines/Health Protection Agency.

334

Medication name/Class: Opioid

Codeine; Pethidine; Dihydrocodeine

Licensed indication	Usually a prescription only medicine (POM). Codeine and dihydrocodeine (at low strengths and a maximum pack size) and be brought over the counter, but with a caution for a maximum of 3 days. Opioids are usually controlled drugs, ranging from Schedule 2, 3 and 5 of the misuse of drug act regulation. Opioids are used for pain.
Pharmacodynamic	Opioid medication will bind to a variety of opioid receptors within the central nervous system and gastrointestinal system, thus helping with pain (as an agonist action). The extent of respiratory depression and constipation will depend on the individual opioid medication. The pharmacology of opioids can be complex.
Pharmacokinetics	The pharmacokinetics depends on whether the medication is administered orally or intravenously. For example codeine is a pro-drug and is metabolised to morphine and other opioids and then excreted by the kidney.
Contraindications	Opioids should be avoided in patients with acute respiratory depression and increased risk of paralytic ileus. Caution is needed in hepatic and renal impairment.
Side effects	There are many different side effects depending on which opioid medication. Common side effects include nausea and vomiting, constipation, drowsiness, rash, respiratory depression with larger doses.
Consideration for practice	Access to naloxone (opioid antagonist). Respiratory rate monitoring. Side effect monitoring.

Medication name/Class: Paracetamol

Paracetamol

Licensed indication	Can be a prescription only medication, a pharmacy (pharmacy) medicine and a general sales list (supermarket) medicine. Pain and pyrexia.
Pharmacodynamic	The full pharmacodynamics is not known. Paracetamol has analgesic properties and antipyretic effects.
Pharmacokinetics	When given orally it is well-absorbed from the GI tract. It is inactivated by the liver.
Contraindications	Hypersensitivity to the ingredients. Cautions in alcohol dependence, liver disease and renal disease.
Side effects	Rare.
Consideration for practice	Correct doses must be followed. Correct weight needed for IV paracetamol.

Medication name/Class: Non-Steroidal Anti-inflammatory Drugs (NSAIDS)

Specifically – Diclofenac (PR)

Licensed indication	Prescription only medicine (POM). Licensed for pain and inflammation.
Pharmacodynamic	Anti-inflammatory, nonsteroidal anti-inflammatory drugs (NSAIDs). Inhibits prostaglandin synthesis.
Pharmacokinetics	Absorption is rapid, reaching peak concentration one hour after administration. Is metabolised by the liver and excreted via the kidney.
Contraindications	There are several key contraindications and the British National Formulary or summary of product characteristics should be consulted. But with respect to midwifery, key contraindications are: 'During the third trimester of pregnancy, all prostaglandin synthesis inhibitors may expose the fetus to: – cardiopulmonary toxicity (with premature closure of the ductus arteriosus and pulmonary hypertension); – renal dysfunction, which may progress to renal failure with oligo-hydroamniosis. The mother and the neonate, at the end of the pregnancy, to: – possible prolongation of bleeding time, an anti-aggregating effect which may occur even at very low doses; – inhibition of uterine contractions resulting in delayed or prolonged labour. Consequently, Voltarol is contraindicated during the third trimester of pregnancy' (eMC 2013).
Side effects	Gastrointestinal, hypersensitivity reactions, headache and dizziness, vertigo, rash.
Consideration for practice	Local practice guidelines should be consulted.

Medication name/Class: Laxatives

Laxatives

Licensed indication	Most but not all can be brought over the counter. Licensed for the relief of constipation.
Pharmacodynamic	There are several different types of laxatives: Bulk forming laxatives – (e.g. ispaghula) increasing faecal mass which helps with peristalsis, useful for hard stools. Stimulant laxatives – (senna) intestinal motility is increased. Osmotic laxatives – (lactulose, macrogols) increase the amount of water in the bowel.
Pharmacokinetics	See individual drug's summary of product characteristics.
Contraindications	Bulk forming – difficulty in swallowing, intestinal obstruction, colonic atony and faecal impaction. Stimulant – acute surgical abdominal conditions, severe dehydration acute inflammatory bowel disease. Osmotic laxatives – see individual drugs.
Side effects	Bulk forming – flatulence, distension, gastrointestinal obstruction or impaction. Stimulants – nausea and vomiting, cramps. Osmotic – nausea, vomiting, pain and distension.
Consideration for practice	Involving the patient in the decision-making process with respect to the laxative of choice.

Medication name/Class: Antiemetics

e.g. Cyclizine, Metoclopramide, Prochlorperazine

Licensed indication	Prescription only medicines (POM). Used for nausea and vomiting.
Pharmacodynamic	Cyclizine – the exact mechanism is not known, it is an H1 receptor antagonist antihistamine. Metoclopramide – affects the parasympathetic nervous system and control in the gastrointestinal system and blocks the Dopamine receptor.
Pharmacokinetics	Cyclizine – well absorbed when given orally, effect within 2 hours and lasts for 4 hours. Metoclopramide – has a half live of 4–5 hours, quick onset of action, excreted in the urine.
Contraindications	Hypersensitivity. Metoclopramide – gastrointestinal obstruction, phaeochromocytoma, epilepsy.
Side effects	Cyclizine – includes rash, dryness of the mouth, blurred vision. Metoclopramide – includes extra-pyramidal side effects (EPSE), hyperprolactinaemia, anxiety, restlessness. Prochlorperazine – includes hyperprolactinaemia, insomnia, dry mouth.
Consideration for practice	Is the patient breastfeeding? (some medication needs to be avoided). Age of the patient – Metoclopramide may cause EPSE in young people (15–19 years old).

Medication name/Class: Low molecular weight heparins

e.g. Dalteparin

Licensed indication	Prescription only medicine (POM). Treatment of venous thromboembolism (VTE) presenting clinically as deep vein thrombosis (DVT), pulmonary embolism (PE) or both.
Pharmacodynamic	Inhibits Factor Xa and thrombin by antithrombin.
Pharmacokinetics	The half life following i.v. and s.c. administration is 2 hours and 3.5–4 hours respectively, twice that of unfractionated heparin (eMC 2013).
Contraindications	Includes 'history of confirmed or suspected immunologically mediated heparin induced thrombocytopenia (type II); acute gastroduodenal ulcer; cerebral haemorrhage; known haemorrhagic diathesis or other active haemorrhage; serious coagulation disorder; acute or sub-acute septic endocarditis; haemorrhagic pericardial effusion and haemorrhagic pleural effusion; injuries to and operations on the central nervous system, eyes and ears.' (eMC 2013)
Side effects	Include haemorrhage and pain on injection.
Consideration for practice	Which low molecular weight heparin your organisation uses.

Medication name/Class: Vitamin K$_1$ (phytomenadione)

Vitamin K$_1$

Licensed indication	Prescription only medicine (POM). Vitamin K deficiency bleeding.
Pharmacodynamic	'Essential for the formation within the body of prothrombin, factor VII, factor IX and factor X, and of the coagulation inhibitors, protein C and protein S.' (eMC 2013)
Pharmacokinetics	'Following oral administration vitamin K$_1$ is absorbed from the small intestine. The systemic availability following oral dosing is approximately 50%, with a wide range of interindividual variability. Absorption is limited in the absence of bile.' (eMC 2013)
Contraindications	Hypersensitivity.
Side effects	Mainly with injections.
Consideration for practice	What is your local policy? The chief medical officer and chief nursing office have recommended that all newborn babies should receive vitamin K to prevent vitamin K deficiency bleeding.

Numeracy

All nursing and midwifery students need to be numerically competent; this is part of the essential skills clusters for pre registration midwifery education. The standards for pre-registration midwifery education state that students should be able to undertake medicinal product calculations correctly and safely (NMC 2009).

There are several books on numeracy for healthcare which are included in the find out more section. However included below are some common areas which students may need to revisit.

Converting fractions into percentages

Percentages are fractions out of 100. Therefore, when converting fractions to percentages you should convert to an equivalent fraction out of 100 and the top number is the percentage.

i.e.
$$\frac{3}{4} \xrightarrow[\times 25]{\times 25} \frac{75}{100} \longrightarrow 75\%$$

Converting percentages into fractions

As before, percentages are fractions out of 100. So, to convert a percentage to a fraction, make the percentage a fraction out of 100 and then simplify to the simplest fraction.

i.e.
$$40\% \longrightarrow \frac{40}{100} \xrightarrow[\div 10]{\div 10} \frac{4}{10} \xrightarrow[\div 2]{\div 2} \frac{2}{5}$$

Converting decimals into percentages

To convert a decimal into a percentage you simply multiply by 100. This means you need to move the decimal place two spaces to the right.

i.e.
$$0.45 \longrightarrow 045. \longrightarrow 45\%$$

Converting percentages to decimals

To convert a percentage to a decimal you divide by 100. This means you need to move the decimal place two spaces to the left.

i.e.
$$32\% \longrightarrow 32. \longrightarrow 0.32$$

Converting fractions to decimals

Fractions are like division sums. Therefore, fractions can be converted to decimals by using long division.

i.e.
$$\frac{3}{5} \longrightarrow 5\overline{)3} \longrightarrow 5\overline{)30} \longrightarrow 5\overline{)30}$$
(with 0. and 0.6 shown above the division brackets)

Converting decimals to fractions

Probably the simplest way to convert a decimal to a fraction is to convert the decimal to a percentage and then convert the percentage to a fraction using the methods above.

Converting between units

Converting between units involves multiplying or dividing by 1000 or 1,000,000. This involves moving the decimal place 3 or 6 places to the right or left depending on the conversion (right for multiplying, left for dividing).

Table 15.2 Conversion table for weight (g, mg and mcg)

		To convert to		
		mcg	mg	g
To convert from	mcg		÷ 1000	÷ 1,000,000
	mg	× 1000		÷ 1000
	g	× 1,000,000	× 1000	

Table 15.3 Conversion table for volume (L and mL)

		To convert to	
		mL	L
To convert from	mL		÷ 1000
	L	× 1000	

Tables 15.2 and 15.3 show what to multiply or divide by to convert between the standard units for weight (g, mg and mcg) and volume (L and mL). Below that are some example conversions.

Example 1 – 65 milligrams to micrograms

Milligrams to micrograms is x 1000 so the decimal place needs to move 3 places to the right.

i.e.
$$65 \longrightarrow 65.000 \longrightarrow 65000. \longrightarrow 65000 \text{ mcg}$$

Example 2 – 12.5 milligrams to grams

Milligrams to grams is ÷ 1000 so the decimal place needs to move 3 places to the left.

i.e.
$$12.5 \longrightarrow 0012.5 \longrightarrow 0.0125 \longrightarrow 0.0125 \text{ g}$$

Example 3 – 250 millilitres to litres

Millilitres to litres is ÷ 1000 so the decimal place needs to move 3 places to the left.

i.e.
$$250 \longrightarrow 0250. \longrightarrow 0.250 \longrightarrow 0.25 \text{ L}$$

Example 4 – 0.3 grams to micrograms

Grams to micrograms is x 1000000 so the decimal place needs to move 6 places to the right.

i.e.

0.3 ⟶ 0.300000 ⟶ 0300000. ⟶ 300000 mcg

Top tips

- Follow the *'Rights'* of medicine management.
- Never view medicine management as 'routine'.
- Follow the NMC guidance and standards for medicine management.
- Have a good level of knowledge about the medicines to be administered.
- Obtain fully informed consent from the patient or document refusal.
- Know what to do if a medication error occurs.
- Give full attention to medicine management.
- Do not interrupt someone who is prescribing, preparing or administering a medicine.
- Make sure that all the records are readable and give an accurate reflection of the action taken.
- If in doubt seek clarification and advice before taking any action.

Key points

- Always think about the pharmacology of medication
  - What the body does to the medicine
    - Absorption
    - Distribution
    - Metabolism
    - Excretion.
- Pharmacodynamics
  - What the drugs does to the body.
- Key definitions need to be remembered:
  - Half life
  - Bioavailability
  - First pass metabolism.
- Side effects of medication.
- Issues for your practice.

Conclusion

This chapter has identified the process which students and midwives should use when managing medicines; this involves the identification of key points when great care needs to be taken. As medication errors is a key area of concern for Trusts and the Department of Health due to the number of errors which occur, this is essential information for all healthcare workers involved in prescribing or giving medication. Specific information around pharmacology has been discussed and related to some of the key medicines used within the maternity services. Students and midwives need to keep up to date in relation to medicines management and the introduction of new medicines, how this can be achieved has been explored.

End of chapter activities
Crossword

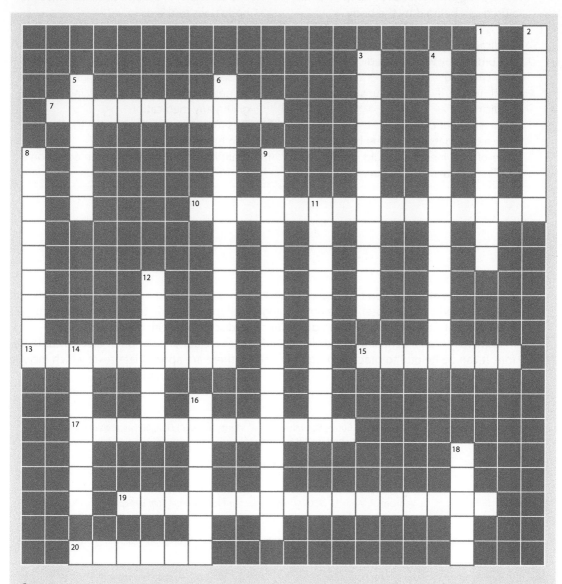

Across

7. Occurs in the liver
10. The amount of the medicine which becomes available for use
13. How the body removes the medicine from the body
15. A medicine which binds to a receptor to produce a specific response
17. What can happen after giving a drug
19. The term that is used to describe what a drug does to the body
20. There are at least 9 of these

Down

1. Something which needs to happen before a drug can be used by the body
2. This is essential to check before giving any medication.
3. The process by which a medicine is chemically changed
4. What to do if you are unsure about a medicine
5. What a patient can do
6. How a drug gets around the body
8. Type of enzymes that could present as a challenge to oral absorption of a medicine

9. The term that is used to describe what the body does to the drug
11. A medicine which binds to a receptor to block a response
12. What medicine management must never be seen as
14. Something which must be gained before giving any medication
16. This must be completed once the medication has been given
18. What is needed when giving medication

342

Find out more

Below is a list of things you can find out about to enhance your knowledge of the issues and topics covered in this chapter. Make notes using the chapter content, the references and further reading identified, local policies and guidelines and discussions with colleagues.

Numeracy is an essential skill in order to undertake safe administration of medicines. Therefore, it can be helpful to practice drug calculations, there are appropriate texts which include tests, as well as websites where this skill can be practised, as outlined below.

Access the following textbook	Chernecky, C., Butler, S., Graham, P., Infortuna, H. (2006) *Drug Calculations and Drug Administration*. London: WB Saunders.
Access the following textbook	Keogh, J. (2009) *Dosage Calculations Demystified*. London: McGraw Hill.
Access the following textbook	Lapham, R., Agar, H. (2009) *Drug Calculations for Nurses: A Step by Sept Approach*. London: Hodder Education.
Access the following textbook	McFadden, R. (2009) *Introducing Pharmacology for Nursing and Healthcare*, 2nd edn. Essex: Pearson.
Access the following textbook	Rang, H.P., Dale, M.M., Ritter, J.M., Flower, R., Henderson, G. (2012) *Rang and Dale's Pharmacology*, 7th edn. Edinburgh: Elsevier.
Access the drug calculations for health professionals website	[online] Available: http://www.testandcalc.com/
Read the NMC Guidelines	The NMC publish guidelines and standards around professional issues which include medicine management, therefore it is important to make sure that you are aware of the most up to date documents which should be referred to and these can be accessed [online] available: http://www.nmc-uk.org/.

Read the NMC circular 07/2011	This circular explains what midwifery exemptions are and the role that student midwives can take in administering these medications.
	http://www.nmc-uk.org/Documents/Circulars/2011Circulars/nmcCircular07-2011-Midwives-Exemptions.pdf
	You should make sure that this is the most up to date information available.
Access the Trust Drug Policy and Guidelines	The Trust in which you work will also have policies and procedures around medicine management and it is important to make sure you are aware of these. These can usually be found on the Trust intranet, you should discuss this with your mentor. There are certain aspects of medicine management which students are not able to take part in; this should be discussed with your programme leader or mentor. The NMC give guidance and information about this as well as the MRHA [online] Available: http://www.mhra.gov.uk/index.htm#page=DynamicListMedicines
	You should pay particular attention to the rules and regulations around midwives exemptions.
For more information visit the websites	Central Alerting System NHS https://www.cas.dh.gov.uk/Home.aspx
	EMC Medicine Guides http://www.medicines.org.uk/Guides
	Medicines and Healthcare products Regulatory Authority http://www.mhra.gov.uk/#page=DynamicListMedicines
	National Institute for Health and Social Care http://www.nice.org.uk/
	NHS Patient Safety http://www.nrls.npsa.nhs.uk/
	National Patient Safety Agency http://npsa.nhs.uk/
	Nursing and Midwifery Council http://www.nmc-uk.org/Publications-/
	British National Formulary http://www.bnf.org/bnf/index.htm

Glossary of terms

Absorption   The uptake of a substance by the tissues of the body.

Agonist   This is a medicine which binds to a receptor and produces a specific response.

Antagonist   This is a medicine which when bound to a receptor does not produce a response; its action is to block.

Bioavailability   This is the proportion of an administered dose which will reach the circulation unaltered, and therefore will be able to have an effect.

Blood–brain barrier   A structure which protects the central nervous system.

Buccal   Of or relating to the mouth cavity.

Contraindication   A reason not to give a specific drug due to something in the patient's history.

Drug   Chemical substances which interact with biological systems.

Excretion   Removal out of the body.

First pass metabolism   The amount of drug which is metabolise by the liver before reaching general circulation.

Half life   The time taken for plasma concentration to reduce by a half of its original value.

Inhalation   Breathing in.

Intramuscular   Into a muscle.

Licensed   A marketing authorisation.

Medicines management   The clinical, cost effective and safe use of medicines to ensure patients get the maximum benefit from the medicines they need, while at the same time minimising potential harm.

Metabolism   How the body gets rid of the medicine.

Off label   The use of medicines outside the terms of the license.

Pharmacodynamics   What the drug does to the body.

Pharmacology   Concerned with scientific principles which can be applied to how the body interacts with medicinal compounds (medicines) and drugs in general.

Pharmacokinetics   What the body does to the drug.

Side effect   An unwanted effect from a drug.

Subcutaneous   Beneath the skin.

Sub lingual   Under the tongue.

Therapeutic   The dose needed to affect a clinical effect.

Topical   Apply directly to area being treated, skin or membrane.

Unlicensed   When a medicine does not hold a marketing authorisation in this country.

References

Agyemang, R., While, A. (2010) Medication errors: types, causes and impact on nursing practice *British Journal of Nursing* 19 (6), pp. 380–385.

Alexis, O., Caldwell, J. (2013) Administration of medicines – the nurse role in ensuring patient safety *British Journal of Nursing* 22 (1), pp. 32–35.

Chummun, H., Bolan, D. (2013) How patient beliefs affect adherence to prescribed medicine regimens *British Journal of Nursing* 22 (5), pp. 270–276.

Cleary-Holdforth, J., Leufer, T. (2013) The strategic role of education in the prevention of medication errors in nursing: Part 2 *Nurse Education Today* 13, pp. 217–220.

Cox, K. (2008) The application of crime science to the prevention of medication errors *British Journal of Nursing* 17 (14), pp. 924–927.

Department of Health (2008) *Medicines Management: Everybody's Business*. London: DH.

Department of Health (2000) *Organisation with a Memory*. London: DH.

Elliott, M., Liu, Y. (2010) The nine rights of medication administration: an overview. *British Journal of Nursing* 19 (5), pp. 300–305.

eMC (2013) Summary of Product Characteristics – Dostinex Tablets [online] Available: http://www.medicines.org.uk/emc/medicine/10003/SPC/Dostinex+Tablets/

eMC (2013) Summary of Product Characteristics – Fragmin 12,500 IU/0.5 mL solution for injection [online] Available: http://www.medicines.org.uk/emc/medicine/26890/SPC/Fragmin+12%2c500+IU+0.5ml+solution+for+injection/

eMC (2013) Summary of Product Characteristics – Konakion [online] Available: http://www.medicines.org.uk/emc/medicine/1699/SPC/Konakion+MM+Paediatric+2+mg+0.2+ml/

eMC (2013) Summary of Product Characteristics – Voltarol Suppositories [online] Available: http://www.medicines.org.uk/emc/medicine/1344/SPC/Voltarol+Suppositories/

Fry, M., Dacey, C. (2007) Factors contributing to incidents in medicine administration. Part 1. *British Journal of Nursing* 16 (9), pp. 556–559.

Griffith, R. (2013) Nurses must report adverse drug reactions. *British Journal of Nursing* 22 (8), pp. 484–485.

Hale, T. (2012) *Medications and Mothers' Milk*, 15th edn. Amarillo: Hale Publishing.

Harkanen, M., Turunen, H., Saano, S., Velhvilainen-Julkunen, K. (2013) Medication errors: what hospital reports reveal about staff views. *Nursing Management* 19 (10), pp. 32–37.

Jones, W. (2013) *Breastfeeding and Medication*. London: Routledge.

Jordan, S. (2010) *Pharmacology for Midwives*. Basingstoke: Palgrave.

Meetoo, D. (2012) Diabetes dilemma: errors and alerts in insulin therapy *British Journal of Nursing* 21 (13) p 770

MRHA (2013) Midwives Exemptions [online] Available: http://www.mhra.gov.uk/Howweregulate/Medicines/Availabilityprescribingsellingandsupplyingofmedicines/ExemptionsfromMedicinesActrestrictions/Midwives/index.htm

MHRA (2009) Off-label or unlicensed use of medicines: prescribers' responsibilities [online] Available: http://www.mhra.gov.uk/Safetyinformation/DrugSafetyUpdate/CON087990

National Prescribing Centre (2008) *Moving towards personalising medicines management: Improving outcomes for people through safe and effective use of medicines* [online] Available: http://www.npc.nhs.uk/resources/personalising_medicines_management_web.pdf

National Patient Safety Agency (2004) *Seven Steps to patient safety. An overview guide for NHS staff* NPSA London [online] Available: http://www.nrls.npsa.nhs.uk/resources/collections/seven-steps-to-patient-safety/?entryid45=59787

NMC (2011) *NMC Circular 07/2011 Changes to midwives exemptions* http://www.nmc-uk.org/Documents/Circulars/2011Circulars/nmcCircular07-2011-Midwives-Exemptions.pdf

NMC (2010) *Standards for Medicine Management*. London: NMC.

NMC (2009) *Standards for Pre-Registration Midwifery Education*. London: NMC.

Rang, H.P., Dale, M.M., Ritter, J.M., Flower, R., Henderson, G. (2012) *Rang and Dale's Pharmacology*, 7th edn. Edinburgh: Elsevier.

Tingle, J. (2012) The scale of errors in prescribing medication in general practice. *British Journal of Nursing* 21 (10), pp. 618–619.

World Health Organization (2008) Medicines: *safety of medicines – adverse drug reactions. Factsheet 293* http://www.who.int/mediacentre/factsheets/fs293/en/ (accessed July 2013).

345

Chapter 16

Emergencies in midwifery

Liz Smith

University of Hull, Hull, UK

Brenda Waite

Diana Princess of Wales Hospital, Grimsby, UK

Learning outcomes

On completion the reader will be able to:

- describe the management of shock and the process of maternal resuscitation
- explain the predisposing factors, signs and symptoms of key obstetric emergencies
- discuss the role of the midwife in the management of key obstetric emergencies
- recognise the psychosocial care needs of the woman and family during and following emergency situations.

Introduction

Although pregnancy and childbirth are usually normal physiological events, complications and emergencies can arise. The role of the midwife in recognising and providing immediate care for obstetric emergencies is central to improving outcomes for women and their babies. This chapter aims to provide an outline of key obstetric emergencies in pregnancy and childbirth with an emphasis on the immediate care the midwife should provide to support the woman physiologically and psychologically until the interprofessional team can initiate medical and/or surgical interventions. The chapter is not intended as a definitive guide to all obstetric emergencies and will provide an overview only of those covered. Guidance for further reading and a 'finding out more' section can be found at the end of the chapter.

The chapter begins with assessment, shock and maternal resuscitation to provide an understanding of general approaches to immediate care in emergencies and then addresses the specifics of some key complications.

Fundamentals of Midwifery: A Textbook for Students, First Edition. Edited by Louise Lewis.
© 2015 John Wiley & Sons, Ltd. Published 2015 by John Wiley & Sons, Ltd.
Companion website: www.wileyfundamentalseries.com/midwifery

Assessment

The effective assessment of women is essential to the detection of deviations from the normal and in particular in determining those conditions likely to cause significant deterioration in maternal and/or fetal wellbeing. To be effective, however, assessment needs to be holistic and individualised; results of observations, screening tests and examinations need to be considered in context with baseline norms for that woman and the overall trends they demonstrate. It is vital that as much information as possible is gathered within assessment whether that is part of an antenatal examination, intrapartum observations or a postnatal examination. It is therefore important not just to focus on the physical results, but to communicate effectively with the woman to find out about how she feels and any symptoms she may be experiencing. It is also essential to use observational skills; it is sometimes easy to get carried away with checking pulse and blood pressure and not notice the fact that the woman has become pale and clammy for instance. Record keeping is also a key element of noticing trends – blood pressure may still be within normal limits but is demonstrating an overall upward trend. This is why assessment tools such as the partogram are useful in monitoring progress in labour and Modified Early Obstetric Warning Scoring Systems (MEOWS) are recommended for use in obstetrics as well as intensive and high dependency units (see Figure 16.1). It is not sufficient to record findings from assessments; midwives need to think about what the data indicates in terms of well-being and health in order that any deterioration is picked up quickly as early recognition of abnormalities and complications such as those discussed in this chapter can improve outcomes for mother and baby. Box 16.1 outlines some key indicators of effective assessment.

Shock

Shock is defined as a syndrome of impaired tissue oxygenation and perfusion due to a variety of causes (Worthley 2000). In essence this means that the cardiovascular system fails to deliver enough oxygen and nutrients to the tissues to meet metabolic needs. The effect of shock and the associated lack of oxygen will lead to metabolic acidosis, cell swelling, necrosis, organ failure and death unless both the symptoms and cause are treated.

Shock is classified into four types:

- **Hypovolaemic** – this can be haemorrhagic as in ante or postpartum haemorrhage or due to severe dehydration which can occur in association with hyperemesis or severe gastroenteritis.
- **Cardiogenic** – this can be due to ischaemia, infarction, myopathy or arrhythmias.
- **Distributive** – this includes septic, neurogenic and anaphylactic shock.
- **Obstructive** – includes shock due to pulmonary or amniotic fluid embolism.

Shock can also be divided into phases which describe its progression:

- **Stage One:** Compensated shock where the body activates mechanisms to compensate for the effects of shock and the patient demonstrates subtle signs and symptoms.
- **Stage Two:** Uncompensated shock where signs and symptoms become obvious and the patient may demonstrate reduced neurological function, oedema and respiratory distress. Medical management is essential to prevent deterioration to Stage Three.
- **Stage Three:** Irreversible shock where the patient deteriorates rapidly as damaged cells start to die.

Signs and symptoms of shock are outlined in Table 16.1.

OBSTETRIC EARLY WARNING CHART.   FOR MATERNITY USE ONLY

NAME: _____   DOB: _____

CHI: _____   WARD: _____

Contact doctor for early intervention if patient triggers one red or two yellow scores at any one time

	Date:																
	Time:																
RESP (write rate in corresp. box)	>30																>30
	21–30																21–30
	11–20																11–20
	0–10																0–10
Saturations	90–100%																90–100%
	<90%																<90%
O2 Conc.	%																%
Temp	39 38 37 36 35																39 38 37 36 35
HEART RATE	170 160 150 140 130 120 110 100 90 80 70 60 50 40																170 160 150 140 130 120 110 100 90 80 70 60 50 40
Systolic blood pressure	200 190 180 170 160 150 140 130 120 110 100 90 80 70 60 50																200 190 180 170 160 150 140 130 120 110 100 90 80 70 60 50
Diastolic blood pressure	130 120 110 100 90 80 70 60 50 40																130 120 110 100 90 80 70 60 50 40
Passed Urine	Y or N																Y or N
Lochia	Normal																Normal
	Heavy/Foul																Heavy/Foul
Proteinuria	2+																2+
	> 2+																>2+
Liquor	Clear/Pink																Clear/Pink
	Green																Green
NEURO RESPONSE (√)	Alert																Alert
	Voice																Voice
	Pain/ Unresponsive																Pain/ Unresponsive
Pain Score (no.)	2–3																2–3
	0–1																0–1
Nausea (√)	Yes (√)																Yes (√)
	No (√)																No (√)
Looks unwell	Yes (√)																Yes (√)
Looks unwell	No (√)																No (√)
Total Yellow Scores																	
Total Red Scores																	

Figure 16.1 Modified Early Obstetric Warning Scoring System chart. Source: Reproduced with permission of NHS Forth Valley.

Box 16.1   Effective clinical assessment

- Observation of general appearance noting any pallor, clamminess, lethargy or obvious discomfort.
- Ask the woman about how she feels – ask open questions to allow her to say how and what she is feeling rather than simply responding to focused closed questions.
- Vital sign recordings and other observations such as blood loss, peripheral perfusion, oedema, and urinalysis.
- Assessment should be informed by and linked to history and diagnosis but should also be thorough and holistic to avoid missing co-existing problems.
- Accurate, contemporaneous record keeping.

Table 16.1   Signs and symptoms of shock

Blood pressure	Systolic blood pressure is lower than 90 mmHg. Initially however blood pressure may rise due to compensatory mechanisms such as increased cardiac rate and contractility, vasoconstriction and water and salt conservation by the kidneys. A normal blood pressure therefore does not necessarily mean the woman is not in Stage One shock.
Pulse	Weak and rapid even at rest.
Skin	Pale, cool and clammy due to vasoconstriction and stimulation by sympathetic nervous system which causes sweating.
Mental state	Altered mental state which may result in confusion, agitation and restlessness.
Urine output	Reduced (normal urine output ranges from 0.5–2 mL/h/kg body weight).
Thirst	Occurs due to loss of extracellular fluid.
Nausea	Due to impaired gastrointestinal blood flow as a result of vasoconstriction.
Blood pH	Low due to acidosis.

Assessment of the woman should follow the recognised standard of ABCDE (see Box 16.2) and urine output. If the baby is still in utero any assessment should also address fetal wellbeing.

Management of shock

The principles of treatment and management are:

- Treat the cause (for example; haemorrhage, pulmonary embolism, sepsis).
- Maintain airway and give oxygen therapy.
- Restore cardiac output and perfusion by fluid resuscitation and drugs.
- Provide analgesia where required.

The effectiveness of the management can be assessed by the stabilisation of vital signs, increased urinary output and improved mental state. Continued assessment and evaluation is essential and should continue after the woman is apparently stabilised. It is also important that,

Box 16.2   ABCDE assessment of the critically ill patient

A = AIRWAY
- Check airway is not obstructed if patient is unconscious
- Give oxygen

B = BREATHING
- Check rate, depth and sound of breathing
- Note whether chest expansion is equal
- Record oxygen saturation if possible

C = CIRCULATION
- Observe for cyanosis (central or peripheral)
- Heart rate
- Capillary refill time

D = DISABILITY
- Conscious level

E = EXPOSURE
- Examination should be thorough whilst maintaining privacy and dignity

(Based on UK Resuscitation Council 2010)

despite the need for emergency treatment and care, basic needs such as information and support are not forgotten. As with all resuscitation situations a member of the multidisciplinary team should take responsibility for the provision of information and reassurance; it is a frightening situation for the woman and any family members present at the time and they will all need compassionate support throughout. It is also helpful for women to have clear explanations when they are sufficiently recovered to be able to discuss what happened to them. Record keeping is also a vital function and a member of the inter-professional team should be allocated to ensure that all actions and treatments are carefully and accurately recorded.

Maternal resuscitation

The incidence of cardiopulmonary arrest is rare in pregnancy and childbirth and is most strongly associated with the birth itself. Although it is a rare occurrence, Billington and Stevenson (2007) suggest that the incidence is approximately 1:30,000; the outcomes are poor, but regular updating of knowledge and skills by staff is the best method of maximising the chance of survival (Boyle and Yerby 2011; Centre for Maternal and Child Enquiries (CMACE) 2011). It is also vital to ensure that equipment is checked and maintained regularly and that all staff is fully aware of emergency telephone numbers.

The Confidential Enquiry into Maternal Deaths (CMACE 2011) identifies both direct and indirect causes of death during pregnancy, childbirth and the postnatal period and those most likely to result in a need for resuscitation are listed below.

- pulmonary embolism
- amniotic fluid embolism
- haemorrhage (antepartum and postpartum)
- pre-eclampsia and eclampsia
- septic shock
- anaesthetic causes (e.g. high spinal block, intubation difficulties)
- cardiac disease
- respiratory disease.

Basic life support

This section utilises the Resuscitation Council (UK) (2010) guidelines; however the normal physiological changes associated with pregnancy mean that adaptations to resuscitation procedures have to be made to overcome the problems presented by the altered physiology. The algorithm for basic life support is shown in Figure 16.3, to provide an overview of the process of maternal resuscitation. Early basic life support interventions are the key to the success of resuscitation, but it is important to remember that it is a 'holding' intervention to maintain the patient whilst medical personnel and the necessary equipment arrive to instigate advanced life support measures (Resuscitation Council (UK) 2010). Just as early basic life support is vital so is early access to advanced life support and it is therefore essential to note the differences in the algorithm for arrests occurring out of hospital (community).

Approach with care

Always assess the area around the woman for potential hazards as an injured rescuer is no use to her. Any obstacles should be moved out of the way and if the floor is wet a sheet or similar can be used to place over the wet area to minimise the risk of slipping. If the woman is in the birthing pool she will need to be lifted out and placed on the floor or bed (this should be done in accordance with patient handling hospital policy).

Shake and shout

Gently shake her shoulders and ask her loudly if she is alright to try and gain a response. If the baby is still in utero, wedge the right hip with a pillow or blanket to reduce pressure on the aorta and inferior vena cava.

Summon help

If she does not respond, then help should be summoned. In hospital this should be done by means of the emergency buzzer, and whoever answers should call the emergency resuscitation team (a full cardiac arrest team plus obstetric personnel should be requested and a neonatal/paediatric team if the baby is in utero). In the community setting, anyone in the vicinity that can help should be asked to summon an ambulance using 999. It is essential that the person ringing for an ambulance has specific and appropriate information to give to the emergency services.

Airway

Inspect the mouth for vomit, blood or any other obstruction. Suction can be used to clear the airway, but finger sweeps should only be used if the obstruction can be clearly seen and lifted out. Any action taken in this respect should not take a large amount of time. The airway should be opened by means of a head tilt, chin lift and jaw thrust combined (see Figure 16.2 and Box 16.3). Placing a pillow or blanket under the shoulder blades will assist with opening the airway and being able to visualise the vocal cords during advanced life support.

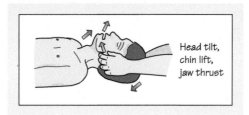

Figure 16.2 · Head tilt, chin lift, jaw thrust. Source: Blundell and Harrison 2013, Chapter 13, Station 30, p. 38. Reproduced with permission of John Wiley & Sons.

Box 16.3   Airway opening manoeuvres (Figure 16.2)

HEAD TILT – CHIN LIFT MANOEUVRE
    Place a hand on the forehead and tilt the head back gently into a neutral position with the neck slightly extended. Place the fingers (not thumb) of the other hand under the bony part of the lower jaw and lift the mandible upward and outward.

JAW THRUST MANOEUVRE
    Place two or three fingers under each side of the lower jaw at its angle and lift the jaw upward and outward.

Breathing
    Look, listen and feel for normal breathing.

- Look for chest movement but remember this may be difficult due to splinting of the diaphragm by the uterus and baby and/or enlargement of the breasts.
- Listen for breath sounds.
- Feel for air on your cheek.
- This assessment should take no longer than 10 seconds.
- NOTE: If you are alone in the woman's home or community setting this is the point at which you should summon an urgent paramedic ambulance.

Chest compressions
    Give 30 chest compressions if the woman is not breathing.

Rescue breaths
    Use a bag-valve-mask or pocket mask to provide two breaths whilst keeping the airway open (as shown in Box 16.4). Ideally oxygen should be used for the breaths but there should be no delay if it is not available. The procedure should continue with 30 compressions followed by two rescue breaths until help arrives and takes over to provide advanced life support.

Continuing resuscitation
    The airway will be secured by means of intubation or the insertion of a laryngeal mask airway. Compressions will be continued but a defibrillator will be attached to monitor any cardiac rhythm and provide shocking where appropriate. There will be a need to cannulate to gain intravenous (IV) access and provide fluid resuscitation with crystalloid or colloid boluses. Drugs such as adrenaline will be given intravenously.

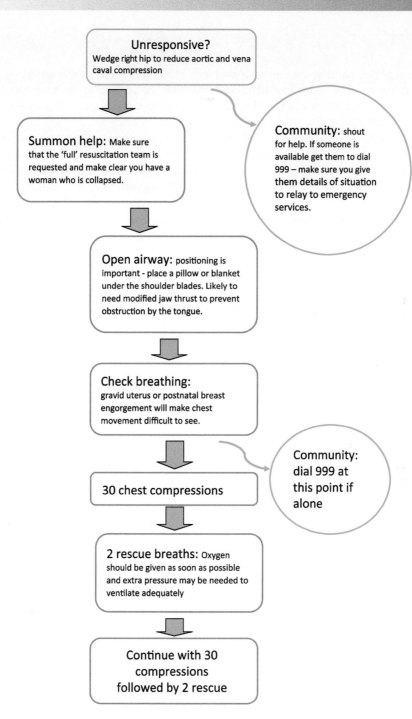

Figure 16.3 Basic life support. Source: Based on Resuscitation Council (UK) 2010.

Box 16.4   Giving chest compressions

Place the heel of one hand in the centre of woman's chest (lower half of the sternum). Place the heel of the other hand over the first hand and interlock the fingers. Make sure your hands are placed over the bony sternum not the ribs and that they are not too low (not over the abdomen or bottom end of the sternum).

Position yourself vertically above the woman and with your arms straight press down on the sternum. The pressure should aim to move the sternum down by about 5–6 cm; however this is quite hard to do if the woman has been tilted to reduce pressure on major vessels. After the compression release all pressure whilst keeping hands in contact with the chest (this allows blood to flow back into the heart).

Compression and release should take equal time and should be provided at an approximate rate of 100–120 compressions per minute (the 'Staying Alive' rhythm).

For women who are undelivered and over 20 weeks at the time of the arrest, delivery by caesarean section is urgent and is normally performed without moving the woman to the operating theatre.

All actions taken must be carefully recorded with accurate times (always use the same clock or watch to avoid inaccuracy).

Any family present will need supporting. They may wish to witness the resuscitation attempts and if so should be supported in their need to be present and provided with information about the procedures by a member of the team allocated to look after them.

Following a resuscitation event it is normal for staff to feel emotional and support should always be offered. Whilst formal support, often through midwifery supervision, is important, so is peer support. Feelings of inadequacy and questioning are common whether the resuscitation was successful or not and debrief can be helpful in resolving these (Boyle and Yerby 2011).

Antepartum haemorrhage

Antepartum haemorrhage (APH) is defined as bleeding from the genital tract from 24 weeks gestation and before the birth of the baby. APH poses significant risk to both mother and baby and is associated in particular with stillbirth and neonatal death. There are two main types of APH: placental abruption (also known as abruptio placentae) and placenta praevia. However there can also be what is known as incidental bleeding from lesions of the genital tract such as cervical polyps, vaginal infection or carcinoma of the cervix. See Box 16.5 for predisposing factors for APH.

Placental abruption

Bleeding occurs when a normally situated placenta separates, either partially or fully, from the uterine wall. The bleeding can be revealed, i.e. obvious bleeding per vaginum (P.V.), concealed where the blood remains trapped between the placenta and the uterus, or mixed where both occur. The degree of separation will determine whether it is categorised as severe, moderate or mild. The cause of separation may not be apparent, but there is an association with sudden decompression as with rupturing membranes where polyhydramnios is present, trauma (road traffic accidents, falls or a blow to the abdomen), hypertensive disease and external cephalic version.

Box 16.5   Predisposing factors for antepartum haemorrhage

- Threatened miscarriage
- Previous caesarean section (placenta praevia)
- History of miscarriage and induced abortion (placenta praevia)
- High parity (>3)
- Older age (>35 years)
- Maternal cocaine use
- Smoking
- Hypertensive disorders (placental abruption)
- Multiple pregnancy
- Domestic abuse (placental abruption)

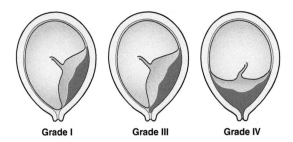

Grade I   Grade III   Grade IV

Figure 16.4   Grades of placenta praevia. Source: Cruickshank and Shetty 2009, Figure 17.1, p. 117. Reproduced with permission of Cruickshank and Shetty.

Signs and symptoms include:

- bleeding – since this can be concealed the degree of bleeding does not indicate the severity of the abruption
- shock (see earlier section)
- abdominal pain which may be associated with backache
- abdominal tenderness on gentle palpation and where bleeding may be concealed there may be increased abdominal girth and tension
- fetal distress – a history of reduced or excessive movements may be reported and the fetal heart may show signs of distress or be absent.

Placenta praevia

Placenta praevia occurs when the placenta is implanted partially or wholly within the lower uterine segment. This is classified into four types (Figure 16.4):

- **Type I** – the placenta encroaches into the lower uterine segment but does not extend to the cervical os.
- **Type II** – the edge of the placenta reaches to the internal cervical os but does not cover it.
- **Type III** – the placenta partially covers the internal cervical os.
- **Type IV** – the placenta completely covers the internal cervical os.

Management of APH

Any bleeding in pregnancy must be taken seriously and a hospital admission for assessment is necessary, however small and apparently insignificant the loss is. A history of the blood loss and the events associated with it, including any sexual intercourse, is vital, though where obvious heavy loss and shock are apparent the time taken for this may be limited. Clinical assessment of vital signs, particularly pulse and blood pressure, gentle abdominal examination and auscultation of the fetal heart should be carried out and a cardiotocograph (CTG) recording initiated. Vaginal examination should not be carried out, even with a speculum until a scan has ruled out placenta praevia. Blood tests for full blood count and clotting studies should be carried out and group and cross matching ordered if necessary. Where shock is a feature of presentation this should be treated as discussed in the previous section. The priority should be in resuscitating and stabilising the woman before delivering the baby. It should be remembered that deterioration can occur rapidly so even if the blood loss is limited on admission, observation of maternal and fetal wellbeing should be continued.

Even a relatively small blood loss can be anxiety provoking for the woman and her family and it is important that all care is thoroughly explained and an atmosphere of calm professionalism is maintained. Communication between the midwife, the woman and her family should be honest and understanding of the concerns and anxiety the situation will provoke. Inappropriate reassurance is both unprofessional and damaging to trust and confidence.

If there is a need to deliver the baby steroid injections to mature the fetal lungs will be required if the gestation is below 34 weeks, and where possible arrangements should be made for neonatal staff to meet the woman and her family. If delivery is not imminent and the woman is rhesus negative then anti-D immunoglobulin should be offered as an intramuscular (IM) injection. A clear management plan for the remaining days/weeks of pregnancy should be agreed with the woman; this may include planned caesarean section or induction depending on the nature of the APH.

Unfortunately the abruption or degree of bleeding may result in stillbirth. It is advisable if possible to deliver the baby vaginally in these circumstances and the contractions will help to control the bleeding. The support of the midwife in such circumstances is essential to the woman and her family, but peer support for the staff caring for the woman is also vital (see Chapter 17: 'Bereavement and loss' where care and support is discussed in greater depth).

Postpartum haemorrhage

Postpartum haemorrhage (PPH) can be primary or secondary. Primary PPH is generally defined as blood loss from the genital tract of 500 milliliters (mL) or more in the first 24 hours following birth (Crafter 2011). However it should be noted that for some women, e.g. those with pre-existing anaemia, a loss of less than 500 mL will constitute a PPH because the loss will be sufficient to cause symptoms of excessive blood loss. Major and minor PPH is categorised in Table 16.2. See Box 16.6 for predisposing factors for PPH.

Table 16.2   Categorisation of postpartum haemorrhage

Minor PPH		500–1000 mL
Major PPH	Moderate	1000–2000 mL
	Severe	>2000 mL

Box 16.6   Predisposing factors for postpartum haemorrhage

- Over-distension of the uterus, e.g. polyhydramnios, multiple pregnancy, macrosomic baby
- Obesity
- Raised blood pressure (more than 140/90)
- Previous caesarean section
- Previous PPH
- Clotting disorders
- Prolonged labour
- Precipitate labour
- Injudicious use of syntocinon
- Instrumental or operative delivery
- Mismanagement of the third stage

Table 16.3   Causes of postpartum haemorrhage (Anderson and Etches 2007)

	Cause	Approximate incidence
TONE	Atonic uterus – feels 'boggy' on palpation	70%
TRAUMA	Perineal, vaginal wall or cervical tears	20%
TISSUE	Retained placenta and/or membrane	10%
THROMBIN	Clotting abnormalities	1%

Secondary PPH is defined as abnormal or excessive bleeding from the genital tract from 24 hours to 12 weeks after birth (Royal College of Obstetricians and Gynecologists (RCOG) 2009).

Major obstetric haemorrhage remains a leading cause of maternal death; therefore timely recognition and intervention is vital to improve outcomes for affected women (CMACE 2011). The factors which can predispose to primary PPH are listed below; however in many cases no risk factors are identified (Mousa and Alfirevic 2009; RCOG 2009).

The causes of primary PPH are usefully identified as the 'Four Ts' a mnemonic device which assists with both recognition of cause and appropriate management (Table 16.3).

The 'Four Ts' should be systematically reviewed to establish the cause of PPH and initiate treatment (Figure 16.5). Combinations of causes can occur and therefore assessment should consider this.

As can be seen from Table 16.3, the commonest cause of PPH is an atonic uterus where the uterus fails to adequately contract following delivery of the baby. The failure to contract means that the large venous sinuses within the uterus are not ligated by the muscle fibres and blood loss can be rapid. A partially contracted uterus can, however, lead to more insidious bleeding which presents as trickling loss that can be missed if the midwife is not observant. When bleeding occurs palpation of the uterus quickly determines whether it has contracted or not; it should not feel bulky or boggy (Tone). The contracted uterus feels firm centrally located on the abdomen, below the umbilicus. If it is not contracted, it is possible to 'rub up' a contraction

358

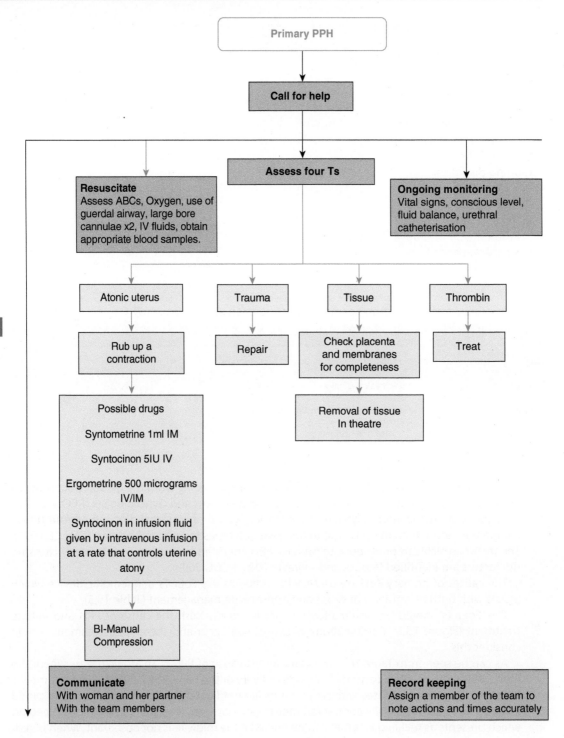

Figure 16.5   Management of postpartum haemorrhage (PPH).

abdominally by a firm circular massaging action with the palpating hand. If the placenta has not been delivered then this should be attempted once a contraction has been achieved. The placenta and membranes should be carefully checked for completeness as even a fragment of placenta or membrane can impede contraction of the uterus (Tissue). It is also useful to empty the bladder by means of a catheter as a full bladder can impede uterine contraction (and delivery of the placenta). If possible, it is helpful to put the baby to the breast as this aids uterine contraction (see Chapter 8: 'Postnatal midwifery care' and Chapter 10: 'Infant feeding', where oxytocin release in response to nipple stimulation is discussed in greater depth). In excessive uterine bleeding, any placental products remaining in the uterus need to be removed in theatre. Following an actively managed third stage of labour where Syntometrine 1 mL IM (made up of 5 international units (IU) of oxytocin and 500 micrograms of Ergometrine) is commonly used in women who do not have pre-existing hypertension or pre-eclampsia; for further bleeding caused by an atonic uterus oxytocic drugs can be given either intravenously or intramuscularly. A single dose of Ergometrine 500 micrograms IV is recommended to treat an atonic uterus; however the same contraindications apply as for the use of Syntometrine. In a hospital setting, if the woman has pre-existing hypertension or pre-clampsia, Syntocinon 5 IU can be administered by slow intravenous injection. These interventions can be followed up by adding Syntocinon to an intravenous solution and administering by continuous intravenous infusion, set at a rate to control uterine atony (Crafter 2011).

Bi-manual compression of the uterus may need to be employed where bleeding persists despite drug treatments or where an infusion cannot be commenced (e.g. home birth). Bi-manual compression involves using one hand in the vagina to push up against the uterus whilst the other hand compresses the fundus through the abdominal wall. This is an uncomfortable procedure for the woman, but can prevent excessive bleeding and provide time to gain access to alternative means of controlling the haemorrhage.

Any form of haemorrhage is a frightening occurrence for patients and their families, but PPH occurs at a time when the woman and her partner are expecting to celebrate the birth of their baby, therefore it can be particularly distressing. The blood loss can be rapid and obvious and the woman's partner in particular can find the experience to be very frightening. It is essential, therefore, that the interprofessional team behave with utmost professionalism and this is best achieved by there being a clear team leader who directs everyone in their assigned tasks and co-ordinates the care and management of the woman. It is also important that communication is maintained with the woman and her partner to keep them informed about the situation. They should be provided with the care and support they need throughout. In the drive to treat and manage the haemorrhage it is easy to forget to support the woman and her partner, but it is a very important part of the overall management and can make the difference between a situation where both are aware of a problem that is being appropriately and professionally managed and a distressingly bad experience with lasting psychological consequences.

Obstetric interventions

If the uterus fails to contract following administration of oxytocin (Syntometrine or Syntocinon) and/or Ergometrine then Carboprost (Hemabate) may be administered. Carboprost augments the contractility of the uterine muscles and 250 micrograms is administered by deep intramuscular injection and can be repeated at 15–90 minute intervals (Billington and Stevenson 2007). Misoprostol, a synthetic prostaglandin, may be given instead of Carboprost, but as this is administered per rectum and there is as yet limited research to support its use (Mousa and Alfirevic 2009), it is not in common usage.

Surgical interventions include uterine packing, the insertion of a tamponade balloon, a B-Lynch uterine compression suture or arterial embolisation. Hysterectomy is avoided if at all possible and is considered a 'last resort' intervention to save the woman's life.

The midwife's role throughout obstetric management is to continue to ensure that the woman and her partner are kept fully informed and supported, to continue to monitor vital signs and ensure that all interventions are recorded accurately.

Continuing midwifery care

Complications following PPH include anaemia, genital tract infection and disseminated intra-vascular coagulation (DIC). It is essential for midwives to remain vigilant following the stabilisation of the woman for signs and symptoms of complications. The monitoring of vital signs, fluid balance and blood profile should continue for some time following cessation of bleeding and analgesia should be administered as appropriate. A postnatal debrief is also good practice to allow the woman to discuss what happened and to have any of her queries and concerns addressed.

Pre-eclampsia and eclampsia

360

Pre-eclampsia is a disorder unique to pregnancy that has the potential to cause both fetal and maternal morbidity and mortality. It is characterised by hypertension and significant proteinuria and generally occurs after the first 20 weeks of pregnancy. Pre-eclampsia is now thought of as a syndrome (a collection of signs and symptoms that are recognised as a condition) rather than a disease that can be diagnosed by a specific test and it affects major organs and systems in a progressive and unpredictable manner (Robson 2002).

There is a tendency to put figures to hypertension (Box 16.7), for example NICE (2010) define mild hypertension as 140–149/90–99 mmHg, but the absolutely vital aspect of monitoring blood pressure is to take into account the woman's baseline recording. Therefore, if a woman's booking blood pressure was 100/60 mmHg and this was the pattern of recording for the first half of pregnancy and she then presented at 28 weeks with a BP of 120/80 mmHg she is hypertensive as both systolic and diastolic pressures have increased by 20 mmHg. Levine et al. (2000) suggest that a rise of 30 mmHg in systolic or 15 mmHg in diastolic blood pressure (on two separate occasions) should be considered as a standard for the diagnosis of pre-eclampsia. It is recommended that automated blood pressure recording systems are not relied on for assessing

Box 16.7 Hypertensive disorders in pregnancy

Gestational hypertension: new hypertension presenting after 20 weeks without significant proteinuria.
Pre-eclampsia: new hypertension presenting after 20 weeks with significant proteinuria.
Severe pre-eclampsia: is pre-eclampsia with severe hypertension and/or with symptoms, and/or biochemical and/or haematological impairment.
Eclampsia: is a convulsive condition associated with pre-eclampsia.

(NICE 2010)

Box 16.8   Investigations for pre-eclampsia screening

- 24-hour urine collection and analysis for total protein and creatinine clearance
- Full blood count
- Blood chemistry
- Liver function tests
- Coagulation profile
- Scan for fetal size, amniotic fluid volume and Doppler studies

blood pressure due to the risk of underestimation; manual recording by means of a sphygmomanometer is the method of choice (Lewis 2001). The incidence of pre-eclampsia is estimated at 2–3% with eclampsia affecting approximately 1:2000 pregnancies and although the incidence of eclampsia is falling, it remains a significant cause of maternal mortality (CMACE 2011). The exact aetiology of pre-eclampsia remains unknown, but many theories suggest that there is a placental trigger followed by a maternal systemic response (Billington and Stevenson 2007). There is thought to be a familial tendency with a 25% increase in risk if the woman's mother had pre-eclampsia and a 40% increase if her sister suffered from it. There is an increased risk associated with multiple pregnancies, and if a hydatidiform mole forms then the condition may well appear before 20 weeks.

The condition is defined by the hypertension and proteinuria that are easily monitored during pregnancy by regular blood pressure measurements and urinalysis; however it also causes oedema, coagulopathy, impaired renal function and liver dysfunction. Additionally the affects of pre-eclampsia on placental function can lead to intrauterine growth retardation and fetal hypoxia (see Box 16.8, Investigations for pre-eclampsia screening). It is essential, therefore, that the progress and effects of pre-eclampsia are fully investigated on diagnosis.

Hypertension can be managed by drug therapy and NICE (2010) recommend Labetalol as a first line treatment although Methyldopa and Nifedipine may also be used. Blood pressure should be monitored to evaluate the effectiveness of treatment. A plan of care is essential and women should be encouraged to participate in the decision making process particularly as induction of labour may be necessary.

Severe or fulminating pre-eclampsia is the worsening maternal condition that signals impending eclampsia (Holmes and Baker 2006; see Box 16.9) and it is important that midwives recognise the signs and symptoms and ensure that medical assessment and treatment is accessed urgently. The aim of care and management is to control hypertension, inhibit convulsions and prevent coma and therefore prevent fetal and maternal mortality.

Eclampsia is the occurrence of convulsions after 20 weeks gestation and up to 10 days post-delivery in association with the signs and symptoms of pre-eclampsia. Whilst many women will demonstrate developing pre-eclampsia in the days or weeks preceding an eclamptic fit, some will not experience any obvious deviation from the norm until the convulsion occurs. (See Box 16.10 for immediate care of the woman with eclampsia.) It is important that a diagnosis of eclampsia is not assumed, but that other cerebral causes of convulsions such as epilepsy are also considered. Antenatal eclampsia is associated with both maternal and neonatal mortality and morbidity; therefore once the woman is stabilised, delivery should follow as soon as possible.

Box 16.9   Signs and symptoms of fulminating pre-eclampsia

- Sharp rise in blood pressure
- Diminished urine output – increased proteinuria
- Headache – frontal persistent
- Drowsiness and confusion
- Visual disturbances
- Nausea and vomiting
- Excessive swelling, particularly of the face and neck

Box 16.10   Immediate care of the eclamptic woman

- Summon help (obstetric team and an anaesthetist or paramedic ambulance as appropriate).
- Protect the woman from injury during the fit.
- Manage Airway, Breathing and Circulation according to the principles of resuscitation.
- Monitor and record vital signs (including fetal heart if appropriate).
- Record all drug treatment accurately as given.

An eclamptic fit generally presents in distinct phases:

- *Prodromal* – where the fit is preceded by possible visual disturbances, muscular twitching, facial congestion, foaming at the mouth and deepening loss of consciousness.
- *Tonic* – generalised muscular spasm and rigidity, absent respiration and cyanosis.
- *Tonoclonic* – intermittent contraction and relaxation of all muscles (convulsive movement) associated with stertorous breathing, increased salivation and possible incontinence of urine and faeces.
- *Post-ictal state* – gradual return to consciousness, re-establishment of respiration (breathing may be deep and rapid). The woman may be lethargic or in a confused and agitated state following a fit and may not remember what has happened.

The current accepted treatment of eclampsia is magnesium sulphate which has been shown to be an effective hypotensive and anticonvulsant agent (Duley et al. 2010). The protocols for dosage may vary locally, but a loading dose given by slow intravenous injection is then followed by a slow intravenous infusion. Toxicity can occur leading to depressed respiration, drowsiness, loss of tendon reflexes, double vision and reduced urine output; therefore it is essential that the overall condition of the woman is monitored both for hypertension and associated complications and for signs of toxicity. Blood levels of magnesium will be checked during treatment. Psychological support for the woman and her family is very important as this is a time of great anxiety. Transfer to a general intensive care or high dependency unit may be necessary in some cases and midwifery care should not only be continued, but is essential in providing ongoing support and specialist care.

Box 16.11   Pre-disposing risk factors for shoulder dystocia

Pre-pregnancy or antenatal factors:
- Maternal Body Mass Index >30 kg/m^2
- Diabetes mellitus – pre-existing or gestational
- Previous shoulder dystocia
- Induction of labour
- Excessive maternal weight gain
- Macrosomia
- Post-term pregnancy

Intrapartum factors
- Prolonged first stage of labour
- Prolonged second stage
- Oxytocin augmentation
- Operative vaginal delivery

(RCOG 2012; Allen 2011)

Shoulder dystocia

Shoulder dystocia is defined as a cephalic vaginal delivery where additional obstetric manoeuvres are required to deliver the fetus after the head has delivered (RCOG 2012). It occurs when the anterior shoulder of the fetus becomes impacted on the maternal symphysis pubis or, less commonly, the posterior shoulder on the sacral promontory. Its incidence is reported with a wide variety of figures but the largest studies suggest up to 0.6 to 0.7% of vaginal births and it can be associated with significant perinatal mortality, as well as maternal morbidity in terms of perineal trauma and haemorrhage.

Although it is not possible to predict shoulder dystocia, there are a number of pre-disposing factors that put a woman at higher risk (see Box 16.11). Many occurrences however are in the absence of any risk factors. Shoulder dystocia is usually first suspected when there is some difficulty in delivering the face by extension, often extra maternal effort is required to free the chin from the perineum. There is often a noticeable retraction of the head, usually referred to as 'turtle-necking' resulting in the chin being forced up into the perineum and the cheeks puffing out. Restitution will often not occur spontaneously and gentle traction with the next contraction does not result in the birth of the body. Once recognised, it is imperative that help is summoned immediately as there is a low rate of hypoxia ischaemic injury to the baby if the head-to-body delivery time is less than five minutes (Leung et al. 2011).

It is important to remember that excessive traction to the head must *never* be applied; similarly, fundal pressure must *never* be instigated as both of these will dramatically increase the chance of brachial plexus injury, the most common injury to the neonate following a case of shoulder dystocia, although this injury can occur without such complications at delivery (Doumouchtsis and Arulkumaran 2009). It is highlighted in the RCOG (2012) Shoulder Dystocia

Guidelines, that maternal pushing should be discouraged as this may exacerbate the situation, further impacting the shoulders.

Maternal and fetal morbidity can be reduced if staff have had training in how to manage this obstetric emergency and have a clear strategy to follow (Draycott et al. 2008; Allen 2011). A widely used strategy is that prompted by the mnemonic HELPERR:

Help

Call for assistance by activating the recognised obstetric emergency drill appropriate to the setting.

Evaluate for episiotomy

Although this is a bony obstruction problem, it can be useful to perform an episiotomy if the perineum is restricting access to perform the internal manoeuvres.

Legs

Position the mother to lie flat with both thighs hyper flexed up onto the abdomen (known as McRoberts' manoeuvre; see Figure 16.6). This has a twofold effect of straightening the lumbosacral arch and flexing the fetal spine, allowing the posterior shoulder to pass over the sacral promontory and drop into the hollow of the sacrum. This can then allow the anterior shoulder to pass under the symphysis pubis and deliver.

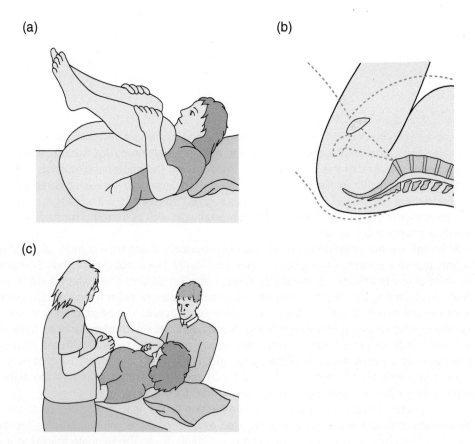

(a)

(b)

(c)

Figure 16.6   McRoberts' manoeuvre. Source: Simkin and Ancheta 2011, Figure 8.7, p. 263. Reproduced with permission of John Wiley & Sons.

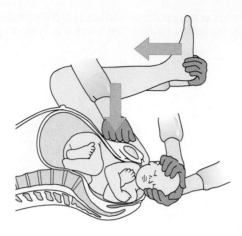

Figure 16.7 Suprapubic pressure. Source: Simkin and Ancheta 2011, Figure 8.8, p. 264. Reproduced with permission of John Wiley & Sons.

Pressure

External pressure applied over the symphysis pubis, similar to the action of cardiopulmonary resuscitation, but from behind the fetal shoulder at an angle of 45 degrees, can assist in releasing the anterior shoulder by moving it into the oblique angle (Figure 16.7).

In practice, it is often found that these two manoeuvres alone will resolve the problem and have been reported successful in up to 90% of cases (RCOG 2012). If unsuccessful then further measures must be employed.

Enter

Sometimes a more direct pressure on the fetal shoulders is necessary to reduce the distance between the shoulders and rotate the fetus into the oblique diameter. This is performed by positioning two fingers under the pubic arch, behind the anterior shoulder and pushing it forward. This may be accompanied by pressure on the front of the posterior shoulder. If this is unsuccessful a rotation can be attempted in the opposite direction with the manoeuvre termed Woods Screw.

For this manoeuvre, pressure needs to be applied behind the posterior shoulder, pushing it forward and performing a 180 degree rotation to make the anterior shoulder become the posterior one, thus releasing it and allowing delivery (see Figure 16.8).

Remove the posterior arm

This manoeuvre is technically difficult, especially if the baby's posterior arm is not flexed across its chest. The person attempting delivery is required to insert their hand in front of the baby to grasp the forearm of the posterior arm and sweep it across the chest and over the face to deliver it. If the arm does not deliver, it can be used to assist in rotation as in the Woods Screw. This manoeuvre does carry a higher risk of fracturing the humerus of the neonate.

Roll the patient

If possible, the woman may be assisted to move into the 'all-fours' position and a further attempt made to deliver the posterior shoulder (which is now uppermost).

This final manoeuvre may be attempted first in the home birth situation, where extra personnel are not available to perform the McRoberts' manoeuvre. Indeed the order of all of these may be adjusted according to the situation but *no longer than 30 seconds* should be spent on each attempt before moving onto another.

1. Apply pressure with tips of index and middle fingers to ANTERIOR shoulder to attempt to move shoulders into the oblique diameter. This is known as Rubin II manoeuvre.

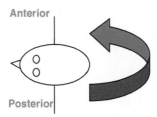

2. If no rotation occurs, use fingers of other hand to apply pressure to the anterior aspect of the POSTERIOR shoulder at the same time as applying pressure to the anterior shoulder as above. This is known as the Woodscrew manoeuvre.

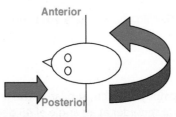

3. If there is still no rotation, remove second hand on anterior aspect of posterior shoulder and slide fingers of the first hand from the anterior shoulder to the posterior aspect of the POSTERIOR shoulder and attempt to rotate in the opposite direction. This is known as the reverse woodscrew manoeuvre.

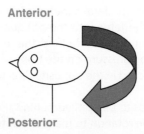

Figure 16.8   Enter manoeuvres for shoulder dystocia.

It is very important in these situations to allocate a member of the team to document the execution, timing and success of all manoeuvres employed to facilitate delivery. Documenting the position of the fetus, delivery time of the head, delivery time of the baby and head-to-body delivery interval is also an essential element of accurate record keeping.

NOTE: All enter manoeuvres should be completed within 60–90 seconds.

Thromboembolism

Thromboembolism is the term that encompasses the two pathological conditions of deep vein thrombosis (DVT) and pulmonary embolism (PE). Deep vein thrombosis is the formation of a blood clot (thrombus) in one of the deep veins, usually in the leg, resulting in partial or complete obstruction of the blood flow (National Institute for Health and Care Excellence (NICE) 2009). Pulmonary embolism is caused by a thrombus that has become dislodged and travelled back through the venous return and on to the vessels in the lung where it obstructs the pulmonary arterial system.

Due to the effect of the physiological changes of pregnancy, the pregnant woman has a five times greater risk of developing these conditions (Springel 2013), especially if she develops some of the complications of pregnancy or has an operative delivery. Although these events can occur throughout the pregnancy, studies show that the highest incidence is during the first trimester and in the postpartum period where the risk has been estimated to be up to 20 times higher than in a non-pregnant woman of the same age (Greer 2012). As these conditions have serious implications and prompt treatment is necessary, it is important for the midwife to understand when a woman may be at even greater risk from her medical history and require referral for consideration of thromboprophylaxis, as well as recognise the signs and symptoms of both conditions. (See Box 16.12 for the risk factors associated with venous thromboembolism.)

Women in the high-risk group are recommended to have thromboprophylaxis through the pregnancy; those in the intermediate group should be considered for antenatal thromboprophylaxis; and those in the lower risk group should be advised regarding mobilisation and the avoidance of dehydration. This risk assessment should be undertaken at booking with the midwife, at any point during the pregnancy where the risk may be affected and in the postnatal period (see Chapter 8: 'Postnatal midwifery care' where thromboembolism is also discussed).

367

Box 16.12   Risk factors for venous thromboembolism (RCOG 2009)

HIGH RISK
Known thrombophilia
Previous recurrent VTE

INTERMEDIATE RISK
Previous history of VTE
Family history of VTE
Maternal disease: cardiac disease, systemic lupus erythematosus (SLE), Inflammatory bowel disease

OTHER FACTORS: 3 factors or more = INTERMEDIATE RISK; less than 3 = LOWER RISK
Obesity
Anaemia
Gross varicose veins
Smoking
Systemic infection
Dehydration
Immobility
Pre-eclampsia
Multiple pregnancy
Age >35

Signs and symptoms of a thromboembolism

Although a DVT does not always cause symptoms, the most common presentation is pain and/ or swelling in the lower leg; however many pregnant women have lower leg oedema making a clinical diagnosis difficult. Springel (2013) suggests a mid-calf circumference measurement of greater than 2 cm difference between the limbs may have more significance for DVT, especially if the problem is experienced in the left leg as the incidence of left DVT is higher in pregnancy.

Similarly, many of the signs and symptoms of a PE are non-specific such as shortness of breath, cough and chest pain. Although these may be contributed to other causes, any suspicion of VTE must be treated whilst investigations are carried out to confirm or rule out the diagnosis (RCOG 2007).

Management of a thromboembolism

Treatment for pregnant women with a DVT or PE is usually a twice daily regime of low molecular weight heparin (LMWH) such as Clexane or Fragmin, but the use of graduated compression stockings and leg elevation are also recommended (Greer 2012).

In the case of sudden collapse of a pregnant woman, a massive PE should be suspected which is a life-threatening condition. Immediate resuscitative measures should be commenced as documented in the section on shock and basic life support. In the hospital setting an emergency call must be initiated. An urgent peri-mortem caesarean section may be required if the collapse occurs antenatally or during labour. In a community setting initial resuscitative measures should be undertaken after ensuring a 999 call is initiated first if alone.

Key points

- Recognition and response to emergencies by midwives can make a significant difference to the outcome for women and their families.
- Support for women, their families and midwives is essential following an emergency.
- Regular updates and skills drills will support midwives in managing emergency situations.

Conclusion

This chapter has introduced the topic of emergencies in midwifery. The early detection of complications and deviations from the normal in pregnancy and childbirth are a vital part of midwifery care. Midwives can provide interventions in emergency situations that can enhance the outcomes for the mother and baby and work with the interprofessional team to provide obstetric and medical management. Whilst the assessment, detection and first-line treatment of emergencies is absolutely vital so is the psychological support midwives can provide for the woman and her family. Communication is central to this support; it is essential that midwives have the knowledge and skill to offer information and explanations as emergencies are anxiety provoking and frightening situations. Record keeping in relation to the interventions given and the timing of these is also key to ensuring that safe, effective care is provided throughout.

End of chapter activities
Crossword

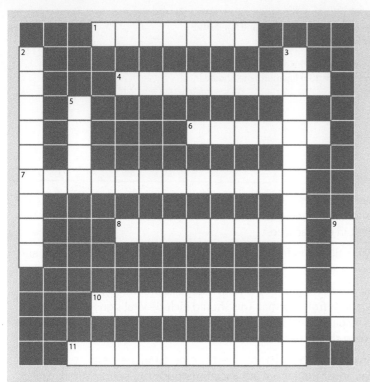

Across

1. Low molecular weight drug used in the treatment of thromboembolism.
4. Placental separation in the antenatal period.
6. Tissue damage cause of PPH.
7. One of the major symptoms of pre-eclampsia.
8. The blood pressure reading that is below 90 mmHg in shock.
10. Type of shock associated with pulmonary embolism.
11. Eclampsia is characterised by this.

Down

2. The 'B' in ABC assessment in basic life support stands for this.
3. Essential element of MDT working.
5. Essential element of all emergencies.
9. The second 'E' in the HELPERR mnemonic.

Find out more

Below is a list of things you can find out about to enhance your knowledge of the issues and topics covered in this chapter. Make notes using the chapter content, the references and further reading identified, local policies and guidelines and discussions with colleagues.

What are the normal ranges for pulse, blood pressure and respiratory rate in pregnancy?	
What is the mechanism of shock?	
Check the resuscitation equipment for adults in your clinical area and familiarise yourself with the equipment and emergency drugs.	
Find out what the local guidelines and policies are for the management of pre-eclampsia, ante-partum haemorrhage, post-partum haemorrhage, shoulder dystocia and thromboembolism.	

Glossary of terms

Advanced life support   Involves measures such as endotracheal intubation, intravenous cannulation and fluid resuscitation and drug therapy which in addition to basic life support measures are aimed at resuscitating a patient in cardiac arrest.

Antepartum haemorrhage (APH)   Bleeding from the genital tract from 24 weeks gestation and before the birth of the baby.

Assessment   Thorough physical assessment relevant to the stage in pregnancy, labour or post-natal period to diagnose any deviations from normal. This should include vital signs such as pulse, temperature, blood pressure and respiratory rate and a thorough history. A written record of each assessment is essential for informing the next one.

Basic life support   Combination of rescue breaths and chest compressions necessary to maintain some circulation following cardiac arrest until more advanced methods can be instituted.

Deep vein thrombosis   Formation of a blood clot (thrombus) in one of the deep veins, usually in the leg, resulting in partial or complete obstruction of the blood flow.

Eclampsia   A convulsive condition associated with pre-eclampsia.

Gestational hypertension   New hypertension presenting after 20 weeks without significant proteinuria.

Hypovolaemia   Low circulating volume due to fluid loss commonly caused by haemorrhage.

Placental abruption   Normally sited placenta separates either partially or wholly from the uterine wall causing haemorrhage and fetal distress. This may also be known as *abruptio placenta*.

Placenta praevia   The placenta is sited in the lower segment of the uterus. Type IV placenta praevia will be situated over the internal cervical os.

Postpartum haemorrhage (PPH)   Defined as blood loss from the genital tract of 500 mL or more following birth however less than 500 mL in a compromised patient (e.g. a woman with anaemia) can constitute a PPH if it causes symptoms of hypovolaemia.

Pre-eclampsia   New hypertension presenting after 20 weeks with significant proteinuria.

Pulmonary embolism   Obstruction of the pulmonary arterial system by a thrombus that has become dislodged and travelled back through the venous return and on to the vessels in the lung.

Severe pre-eclampsia   Pre-eclampsia with severe hypertension and/or with symptoms, and/or biochemical and/or haematological impairment.

Shock   A syndrome of impaired tissue oxygenation and perfusion due to a variety of causes and means that the cardiovascular system fails to deliver enough oxygen and nutrients to the tissues to meet metabolic needs. The effect of shock and the associated lack of oxygen will lead to metabolic acidosis, cell swelling, necrosis, organ failure and death unless both the symptoms and cause are treated.

Shoulder dystocia   cephalic vaginal delivery where additional obstetric manoeuvres are required to deliver the fetus after the head has delivered.

Thromboembolism   The term that encompasses the two pathological conditions of deep vein thrombosis (DVT) and pulmonary embolism (PE).

References

Allen, R.H.A. (2011) Shoulder Dystocia. *Medscape* [online] Available: http://emedicine.medscape.com/article/1602970-overview#showall. [10 June 2013]

Anderson, J.M., Etches, D. (2007) Prevention and management of postpartum haemorrhage *American Family Physician* 75, pp. 875–882.

Billington, M., Stevenson, M. (eds) (2007) *Critical Care in Childbearing for Midwives*. Oxford: Blackwell Publishing.

Blundell, A., Harrison, R. (2013). *OSCEs at a Glance*, 2nd edn. Oxford: John Wiley & Sons Ltd.

Boyle, M., Yerby, M. (2011) Maternal and neonatal resuscitation. In: Boyle, M. (ed.) (2011) *Emergencies Around Childbirth*, 2nd edn. London: Radcliffe Publishing.

Centre for Maternal and Child Enquiries (CMACE) (2011) Saving Mothers' Lives: reviewing maternal deaths to make motherhood safer: 2006–2008. The Eighth Report on Confidential Enquiries into Maternal Deaths in the United Kingdom. *BJOG*, 118 (Suppl. 1), pp. 1–203.

Crafter, H. (2011) Intrapartum and primary postpartum haemorrhage. In: Boyle, M. (ed.) *Emergencies Around Childbirth*, 2nd edn. London: Radcliffe Publishing.

Cruickshank, M., Shetty, A. (2009). *Obstetrics and Gynaecology: Clinical Cases Uncovered*. Oxford: Wiley-Blackwell.

Draycott, T.J, Crofts, J.S., Ash, J.P., Wilson, L.V., Yard, E., Sibanda, T., Whitelaw, A.. (2008) Improving neonatal outcome through practical shoulder dystocia training. *Obstetrics and Gynaecology* 112 (1), pp. 14–20.

Doumouchtsis, S.K., Arulkumaran, S. (2009) Are all brachial plexus injuries caused by shoulder dystocia? *Obstetrical and Gynaecological Survey* [online] Vol.54 (9). Available: http://journals.lww.com/obgynsurvey/Abstract/2009/09000/Are_All_Brachial_Plexus_Injuries_Caused_by.22.aspx [10 June 2013]

Duley, L., Gülmezoglu, A.M., Henderson-Smart, D.J., Chou, D. (2010) Magnesium sulphate and other anti-convulsants for women with pre-eclampsia. *Cochrane Database of Systematic Reviews*.

Holmes, D., Baker, P.N. (eds) (2006) *Midwifery by Ten Teachers*. London: Hodder Arnold.

Greer, I.A. (2012) *Thrombosis in pregnancy: updates in diagnosis and management*. ASH education book [online] Vol. 2012(1) Available: http://asheducationbook.hematologylibrary.org/content/2012/1/203.full [11 June 2013]

Leung, T.Y., Stuart, O., Sahota, D.S., Suen, S.S., Lau, T.K., Lao, T.T. (2011) Head-to-body delivery interval and risk of fetal acidosis and hypoxic ischaemic encephalopathy in shoulder dystocia. *BJOG* 118 (4), pp. 474–479.

Levine, R., Elwell, M., Hauth, J., Curet, L., Catalano, P., Morris, C. (2000) Should the definition of preeclampsia include a rise in diastolic blood pressure >/=15mmHg to a level <90mmHg in association with proteinuria? *American Journal of Obstetrics and Gynecology* 183, pp. 787–792.

Lewis, G. (ed) (2001) *Why mothers die 1997–1999: the fifth report of the confidential enquiries into maternal deaths in the United Kingdom*. London: RCOG Press.

Mousa, H.A., Alfirevic, Z. (2009) Treatment for postpartum haemorrhage. *Cochrane Collaboration Intervention Review*. Chichester: John Wiley.

National Institute for Health and Clinical Excellence (2009) *Deep vein thrombosis*. London: NICE.

National Institute for Health and Clinical Excellence (2010) *The management of hypertensive disorders during pregnancy (CG107)*. London: NICE.

Robson, S. (2002) Pre-eclampsia and eclampsia. In: Maclean, A., Neilson, J. (eds) (2002) *Maternal morbidity and mortality*. London: RCOG Press.

Royal College of Obstetricians and Gynaecologists (RCOG) (2007) *The acute management of thrombosis and embolism during pregnancy and the puerperium. Green-top Guideline No. 37b*. London: RCOG.

Royal College of Obstetricians and Gynaecologists (RCOG) (2009) *Prevention and management of postpartum haemorrhage Green-top Guideline No 52*. London: RCOG.

Royal College of Obstetricians and Gynaecologists (RCOG) (2009) *Reducing the risk of thrombosis and embolism in pregnancy and the puerperium Green-top Guideline No. 37a*. London: RCOG.

Royal College of Obstetricians and Gynaecologists (RCOG) (2012) *Shoulder Dystocia Green-top Guideline No.42*, 2nd edn. London: RCOG.

Simkin, P., Ancheta, R. (2011). *The Labor Progress Handbook: Early Interventions to Prevent and Treat Dystocia*, 3rd edn. Ames, IA: John Wiley & Sons, Inc.

Springel, E.H. (2013) Thromboembolism in pregnancy. *Medscape* [online] Available: http://emedicine.medscape.com/article/2056380-overview. [12 June 2013]

UK Resuscitation Council (2005) *Systematic approach to the acutely ill patient*. London: UKRC.

UK Resuscitation Council (2010) *Adult Resuscitation Guidelines*. London: UKRC.

Worthley, L.I. (2000) Shock: a review of pathophysiology and management. *Critical Care Resuscitation* 2 (1), pp. 55–65.

Chapter 17

Bereavement and loss

Liz Smith
University of Hull, Hull, UK

Brenda Waite
Diana Princess of Wales Hospital, Grimsby, UK

Learning outcomes

By the end of this chapter the reader will be able to:

- discuss the theories relating to bereavement and loss
- utilise theories of bereavement and loss to inform care
- recognise that bereavement practices may be influenced by culture and religion
- understand the value of support for women, their families and colleagues.

Introduction

Whilst pregnancy and childbirth are generally associated with the joy and happiness of a new baby there are unfortunately some pregnancies which do not end happily and midwives need to draw on all their skill to support the parents and their family through their loss. It is important to remember, however, that loss is not just associated with miscarriage, stillbirth and neonatal death; it is also associated with premature birth, unexpected illness and abnormality irrespective of the ultimate outcome. In order to provide sensitive care to women and their families, midwives need to have an understanding of the theories of grief whilst remembering that these are theories not facts and that everyone is different. This chapter will therefore discuss the main theories of grief in the context of midwifery and consider some of the situations where midwives can make a difference to the experience of loss for women and their families.

Terminology

In order to enhance understanding of theory and of care needs it is necessary to use terminology appropriately. The terms associated with loss are often used interchangeably but in truth have differing meanings.

Fundamentals of Midwifery: A Textbook for Students, First Edition. Edited by Louise Lewis.
© 2015 John Wiley & Sons, Ltd. Published 2015 by John Wiley & Sons, Ltd.
Companion website: www.wileyfundamentalseries.com/midwifery

Grief – is a natural and personal response to loss and is multidimensional involving emotional, physical, behavioural, cognitive, social and spiritual aspects (Greenstreet 2004; Buglass 2010).

Mourning – is the active and outward expression of grief and contributes to its resolution.

Bereavement – is the state of having experienced a loss and is often associated with the period of time following the loss. It is this association with time that often leads people to have erroneous beliefs about how long someone should grieve for.

Stroebe et al. (1993) summarise the links between the terms by suggesting that bereavement is a state of loss that triggers a grief reaction that is associated with behaviours that are known as mourning. Responses to loss are affected by culture and religion as well as personality and circumstances (Buglass 2010) and it is important therefore to treat everyone as an individual and every situation as unique.

Theories

The theories associated with responses to loss can assist midwives in understanding the process of grief, but it should be remembered that a theory is not an absolute fact; those experiencing bereavement will not necessarily follow one single theory and behaviour cannot necessarily be predicted. Theories do provide a guide and an explanation of some of the behaviours acted out by individuals.

Possibly the best known theory of grief in healthcare comes from Kübler-Ross (1969). Her work is commonly used by healthcare professionals and is based on clinical impressions gained when working as a psychiatrist with dying patients (Buglass 2010). Kübler-Ross (1969) identified five stages of grief that are moved through and these are:

* denial
* anger
* bargaining
* depression
* acceptance.

There is an assumption that people move through the stages in order having completed one stage before going on to the next; however this is not so and the theory is criticised as being too linear and rigid. If it is taken more as a cycle that people move through in both directions at times, it is perhaps more helpful but it has to be accepted that some people never really reach acceptance. The loss of a baby, particularly by miscarriage or stillbirth, is something that some parents and their family do not fully accept and events or stressors can send them back through the stages almost from the beginning. Anecdotal evidence does suggest, however, that what happens following the loss can impact on the process of grief. Those who experienced perinatal loss in the past suffered from the lack of mementoes and limited emotional care, and this ultimately affected their ability to come to acceptance.

Bowlby (1973) based his four stage model on his influential theory of attachment. Unlike Kübler-Ross his stages of grief are overlapping and flexible. They are:

* shock
* yearning and protest
* despair
* recovery.

There are clear similarities to Kübler-Ross' stages with 'yearning and protest' having some link with the two stages of denial and anger, but the language does perhaps better fit with perinatal loss. Parents and families are frequently very shocked at their loss which they have very little if any time to prepare for (with the exception of some neonatal deaths and planned termination for major abnormality). The idea of yearning and protest has resonance with the loss of a baby as does despair. Recovery seems to be a better description of how many view their progress and is more suggestive of 'getting on with life' despite the loss. Parkes (1998) presented a theory which is very similar to Bowlby with four stages which are:

* shock or numbness
* yearning and pining
* disorganisation and despair
* recovery.

Again Parkes (1998) emphasised that the stages are not linear and could be experienced several times. A trigger for returning to earlier stages could be an anniversary (Parkes 1998) and this can be important when the date of birth is also the date of death as the anniversary is particularly poignant. A trigger for some women can also be a new pregnancy when the joy is mixed with anxiety and sadness for the baby they lost.

Worden (1982, 1996) developed a non-linear and dynamic model which involves the bereaved person working to accept the loss and the pain and adjusting to the loss by 'relocation of the deceased person in one's life' (1996, p.15). Again there are similarities to other models and an emphasis on recovery not being reliant on forgetting the person who has died, but rather coming to terms with their loss. It is important not to suggest that life will be the same as it was before the bereavement as this is not possible. Work by Rando (1985, 1986) on parental grief suggests that although the physical relationship may have been lost, the emotional bond is not. Worden (1982) suggested that part of the process of grief was adjusting to changes in role, identity and status associated with the loss of their loved one. Perinatal loss is associated with a significant change in role and identity, as parents and family expected to have a new baby to relate to so their expected role as mother, father, grandparent etc is no longer relevant in the context of the deceased baby. Rubin and Malkinson (1993) support this and suggest that parenthood can enhance a person's sense of identity and perinatal loss therefore involves a loss of self in relation to social roles.

Dual-process models of coping with bereavement such as that of Stroebe (1998) suggest that people have to cope with both loss and restoration-oriented factors and they will oscillate between the two. Whilst loss-oriented processes link with the stages of grief expressed by other theorists, restoration-oriented processes are related to coping with everyday life and building new roles and relationships. Dual process models have been criticised for placing too much emphasis on coping (Buglass 2010), but they do recognise that both expressing and controlling feelings are part of grief. Parents and families can sometimes feel guilty about coping and being able to control their feelings and it is important that they are reassured that this is 'normal'.

The value of the theories of grief is not in expecting everyone to behave according to any one theory, but to help the midwife understand the possible stages women and their families may go through and to therefore understand that their behaviour is part of the process. It is also helpful when reassuring grieving individuals that they are not 'going mad' or behaving abnormally as they sometimes believe. Staged models (see Figure 17.1) for the most part help us understand that the process can move backwards as well as forwards through their grieving and the dual-process theory highlights that the process is not just about loss it is also about coping and adjusting to life without the baby and their expected future.

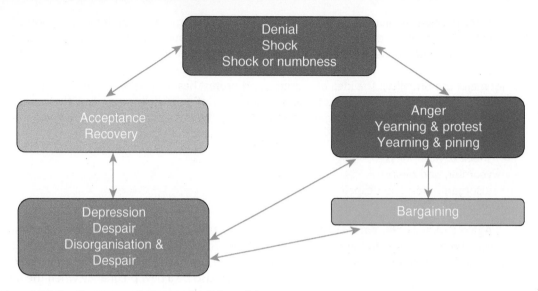

Figure 17.1   Summary of stages of grief models.

Communication

Communication underpins effective midwifery care whatever the situation, but communicating in relation to breaking bad news and caring for bereaved women and their families is particularly challenging for many midwives. Walter (2010) suggests that practitioners need to be aware of their own assumptions about grief and loss and Schott and Henley (1996) state that there is a need for healthcare practitioners to understand their own style of communication before they can adapt to meet the needs of different people and situations. Walter's (2010) suggestion is important as it reminds practitioners that their own assumptions can limit sensitivity to the needs of women and their families and can therefore lead to poor communication and care. Kohner and Henley (2009) highlight how, for example, professionals can wish to protect parents from the distress of their experience which ultimately results in poor communication. This desire to protect is based on assumption and a paternalistic approach to care that does not empower women and their families. However this does not mean that communication and care should not be sensitive and sympathetic to the distress women and their families will inevitably experience, but it is important that midwives provide communication that best meets the needs of those in their care.

Box 17.1 highlights the basic principles of good communication and these apply when breaking bad news and caring for those who are grieving as much as they do in any other circumstance. It is important that it is not assumed that first names should be used because someone is distressed for example, and even where this may be acceptable it is wise to check what name the person wishes to be known by (some people do not use their first name, may prefer or dislike shortened versions of their name and some cultures order their names differently). The use of jargon and colloquial language is also detrimental to understanding and can lead to frustration on the part of women and their families as they struggle to comprehend what they are being told. Assessing what is being understood by questioning and allowing a chance for concerns or queries to be expressed ensures that the process of communication is as effective as it can be given the circumstances. Inclusive communication is important as fathers and

Box 17.1   Basic principles of good communication

- Good manners – respect and courtesy, introduce yourself and find out how others wish to be addressed.
- Communicating to meet clients' needs – avoid jargon and colloquial language, assess knowledge and understanding.
- Encourage questions and expression of concerns or worries.
- Be non-judgmental and inclusive.
- REMEMBER TO LISTEN AS WELL AS TALK.

grandparents can feel excluded and feel that the focus of both communication and care is on the woman when they also need to understand and be cared for, to enable them to care for each other. An understanding of the theory of grief and loss can help midwives deal with the responses women and their families may make to their bereavement and thereby enhance the non-judgmental approach.

Research by Nordlund et al. (2012) highlights the need to show respect to the baby within communication. Describing the baby as 'the miscarriage', 'the fetus' or 'it' was perceived as being very hurtful and offensive. The research also demonstrated that the respondents felt that a lack of respect for their circumstances was shown by professionals who talked about irrelevant topics and who were too upbeat. Another interesting comment from a respondent highlighted how she felt upset that some professionals were seen by her to be hugging and supporting one another in a way they had not provided support to her. This latter finding highlights the problem of whether it is appropriate and professional to show emotion in relation to their loss. The comment would imply that it is acceptable to cry with the woman and her family when that emotion is about their experience, but professional behaviour would be to keep personal feelings for later as much as possible. The research also demonstrates that non-verbal communication is also important to women and their families. Respondents reported lack of eye contact from professionals which they found distressing. See Box 17.2 for principles of sensitive communication.

As with all aspects of care communication in relation to bad news and care following bereavement needs to take into account cultural need and language barriers. Interpreters and taped/written information should be utilised to minimise language barriers so that no-one is denied access to the information and support they are entitled to.

Culture and religion

There is much information available within healthcare about cultural and religious beliefs relating to grief and mourning rituals and whilst this information is undoubtedly useful it is also very generalised. Walter (2010) makes the important point that although individuals are shaped by their culture they are not 'determined by it' and similarly religion and culture interact with one another. There may be a tension between what the individual wants and what their culture requires them to do and if healthcare professionals merely use the cultural information available to shape their communication and the choices offered they may not be fully meeting the individuals' needs at best and at worst they may be contributing to the tension experienced. The

377

Box 17.2   Principles of sensitive communication

- Privacy – most Maternity Units have a Family Room for caring for bereaved families, but where this is not available there must be privacy and no interruptions.
- Avoid assumptions – allow the woman and her family to take control as much as possible in relation to the amount, pace and language of the information provided.
- Provide choices where possible.
- Allow time and do not be uncomfortable with silence whilst the woman and her family are absorbing information or dealing with their emotions.
- Be honest and truthful.
- Co-ordinate information giving so that women and their families are not overwhelmed.
- Recognise when someone does not wish to talk.

Box 17.3   Issues to consider in relation to cultural and religious preferences

- Etiquette in respect of talking about death – the use of appropriate language about death and the deceased.
- Cultural/religious rituals – in relation to handling the body (who is allowed, how the body should be prepared and dressed) and whether burial or cremation is required.
- What ceremonies or rituals are required during the period of mourning.
- How grief is expressed – is public wailing/crying expected or is grief expressed quietly and in private.
- Gender roles in mourning.

most essential element of meeting cultural and religious need, therefore, is to communicate effectively and not be afraid to ask what the woman and her family want. It is also important to recognise that the theories discussed earlier in this chapter are all Western, and do not therefore necessarily apply to everyone (Walter 2010). As Mander (2006) suggests, stereotype-based assumptions about preferences of bereaved parents have to be avoided. Box 17.3 offers some guidance as to issues that midwives may wish to gently ask about to determine cultural or religious preferences. It may be difficult to ask questions about preferences and rituals when women and their families are distressed, however, it is better to ask than to cause further distress and offence by making assumptions.

Care around the time of death

Privacy may be required for prayer and some families may want a religious leader or chaplain to be present. Christians may want their baby to be baptised.

Some cultures have customs that require the extended family to gather at the bedside and wherever possible this should be accommodated.

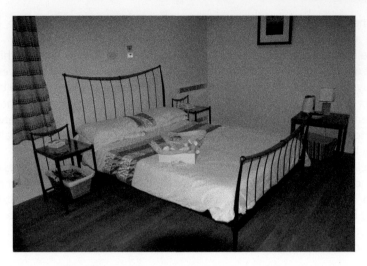

Figure 17.2   A private comfortable environment on a labour ward for parents who have experienced loss. Source: Women and Children's Hospital Hull and East Yorkshire NHS Trust, reproduced with permission of Janet Cairns, Head of Midwifery.

The provision of privacy should not leave parents and families feel unsupported; they need to know how to contact a midwife when they need to so the call bell system should be fully explained to ensure they do not feel isolated and fearful (SANDS 1995). Labour wards may have rooms specifically for the care of women and families following loss as shown in Figure 17.2.

Care following loss

It is important to remember that this is a situation where what is generally accepted as good practice does not meet everyone's needs. This may be for cultural or religious reasons, but it may just be that it is not how the individual wants to be cared for. It is also important to remember that the woman and her family may not know what they want or what their culture or religion expects of them in respect of the loss of their baby, so they will need time to make decisions and to consult with others.

Some parents may not wish to see or hold their baby after death at all, whilst others may want the baby to be washed before they hold her/him as their cultural beliefs are that the fluids associated with birth are unclean. There may be rituals associated with the preparation of the body and who performs these. Where staff are asked to prepare the body it is important to ask about clothing and positioning. Some Orthodox religions (e.g. Orthodox Jews, some Muslims and Hindus) may require healthcare staff to wear gloves when handling the body. Care should be taken in relation to jewellery and the placing of flowers with the body may not be acceptable to some parents.

Naming the baby may be important for some parents regardless of how early in the pregnancy the loss occurs, whilst for others it may not be appropriate. When names are given it is good practice to use them in discussions with parents.

Photographs of the baby are generally welcomed by parents; however some may have strong objections to this practice. It is important to sensitively ascertain why parents do not want photographs as some do regret not having them later. Offering to take photographs and keeping them with the notes may be appropriate for those who are unsure, but not for those who have an objection to it.

Some religions and cultures do not permit post mortem examination, so this is a subject that should be approached with extreme sensitivity and honesty about the answers such an examination may provide. It is the need for answers that create a tension between beliefs and wishes for parents at times, so understanding this can enhance communication. Where there is a legal requirement for a post mortem this can cause considerable distress for parents who did not want this to happen. It is important for communication between professionals to minimise the impact on both the parents and the body of the baby where possible.

Some religions require cremation whilst others require burial, though these rulings may differ between adults and children. For example for Hindu and Sikh adults are cremated, but children are buried. Funerals and ceremonies relating to death vary between both cultures and religions. There may be rules relating to women that are difficult to understand for Western midwives, as women generally may worship separately within the religion and in some cultures women are seen as unclean following birth.

Midwifery care

Whilst there are some general principles to be applied to all situations of grief and loss within maternity care as discussed above, there are also some aspects of care that present particular challenges or need specific considerations. The following section will consider these challenges and specific needs.

Stillbirth

A stillbirth is legally defined as a baby born after the 24th week of pregnancy that has not breathed or shown any sign of life (Stillbirth Definition Act 1992). Stillbirths can occur at any stage during the last 16 weeks of pregnancy and there is not always any warning that there is anything wrong with the fetus or the woman. Sometimes however women identify that they are aware that the baby is not moving as much or at all and then it is vital that they are admitted for fetal monitoring and if a heartbeat is not detected an ultrasound scan should be done to confirm the diagnosis of stillbirth. Sensitive and empathetic care is absolutely vital during both the monitoring and scan and following the diagnosis. There may be a temptation to be overly reassuring whilst seeking the fetal heart but this can damage the trust between midwife and woman and can cause confusion when the diagnosis is finally confirmed. A professional approach keeps the woman informed of what is happening and why, whilst demonstrating an understanding of the anxiety and even panic she will be experiencing. Reassurance that everything is being done for her by calm, competent staff is what she needs at this very difficult time.

Whilst it is necessary to get the baby delivered before the complications set in, the woman and her family require time to absorb the bad news and understand what will happen next. Women will want to know why their baby died and whether they could have done anything to prevent it. They are often overwhelmed with guilt even though they will have done nothing wrong. It can be difficult to address their concerns because even following the post mortem results it is not always possible to say why the baby died. Even when there is evidence of a cause, the full results of the post mortem and any other tests such as microbiology take time. A follow-up appointment will be necessary at around 6 weeks following the birth to discuss findings and answer any questions.

Emotional support and honest professional information giving is crucial for the woman and her family. Holding the baby and the taking of mementoes such as hand and foot prints will all be helpful. The midwife who delivered the baby can sign and issue the stillbirth certificate which will be necessary for the registration of the death. Funeral arrangements can be made by the hospital or can be done privately by the family. Families may want to dress the baby in a special outfit or wish to have a cuddly toy to go in the coffin which is no problem at all where the baby will be buried, but some materials are not always suitable for cremation and advice should be sought about this.

Neonatal death

A neonatal death is defined as one that occurs within a month of birth and can be due to prematurity, congenital abnormality, infection or asphyxia associated with labour and delivery. Care is necessarily split between the paediatric team with responsibility for the baby and the midwives looking after the woman. It is essential, therefore, that communication is inclusive and co-ordinated between the teams. Whilst the practicalities of mementoes (see Box 17.4) and funeral arrangements may be managed by the neonatal staff, midwives still have a role in providing support and information giving in much the same way as they have when a stillbirth occurs. The neonatal team may only have limited involvement if death occurred as a result of a failed resuscitation at birth, and where there may be confusion as to who is responsible for what, it is vital that midwives ensure this is addressed to make sure nothing is missed or replicated unnecessarily.

Miscarriage

Traditionally women suffering early pregnancy loss requiring hospital care were admitted to gynaecology wards. However realisation that this was not a satisfactory situation for either the woman or the nursing staff on such wards has meant that increasingly cases are cared for by midwives in Early Pregnancy Units or where these are not available on Maternity Units. A miscarriage is defined as a spontaneous loss of a pregnancy before 20 weeks; however most occur before 14 weeks. Miscarriage is sometimes known as a spontaneous abortion in medical circles which can cause great distress to women as the term abortion is more commonly associated with planned termination of pregnancy and not with the unplanned and distressing loss of a wanted baby. However, early a miscarriage occurs for many women and their families, it is the loss of a baby not a pregnancy and this is an important issue when caring for them. It can be easy to dismiss the loss as less important because it occurs before the baby starts to move or even before a scan picture is available, but with pregnancy testing being readily available many women have known since the first month that they are pregnant and have made plans for their baby.

Box 17.4   Mementoes of the baby

- Photographs (and video footage for some neonatal death in NICU).
- Hand and/or foot print cards.
- Lock of hair.

REMEMBER CONSENT IS NECESSARY BEFORE MAKING THESE MEMENTOES

Cot cards and name bracelets can also be given (name bracelets will have to be replaced as per policy for transfer to the mortuary).

Figure 17.3 is an illustration of a memory box.

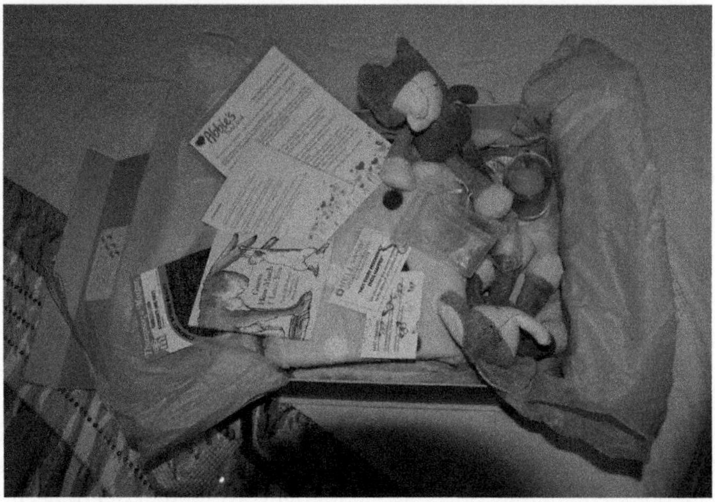

Figure 17.3   Abbie's Fund box with permission from Abbiesfund. Access the websites for more information about the charity [available online] www.abbiesfund.co.uk; www.facebook.com/abbiesfund. Source: abbiesfund.co.uk. Reproduced with permission of Katy Cowell.

Termination for fetal abnormality

Caring for women undergoing termination for fetal abnormality is particularly challenging. Because diagnosis is not made until quite late in the pregnancy most women have to endure a labour and delivery which can be quite difficult. From a grieving perspective the women and their families are not only struggling with the loss of their baby, but also their expectations of that baby. The presence of an abnormality creates guilt and anxiety as many women and their partners wonder if it was something they had done or not done that caused it. They also worry about any future pregnancies being affected in a similar way. The decision to terminate a fetus with abnormality is not an easy one and it is very important that care is non-judgmental. It is also essential that the family are allowed to make their own choices about seeing the baby. Some abnormalities can be quite frightening, but there is a danger that an overly protective approach by midwifery staff causes more harm than good as what is imagined can be worse than reality. It can be important for some families to see the baby and the abnormality to confirm their decision. Preparing the women and her family effectively can minimise the distress as can a supportive approach that gives them space to make the decision to see the baby and to spend time with him/her. Families experiencing this situation may have questions about the condition affecting their baby, so access to the paediatric team following delivery may be necessary and most will need follow up for advice regarding future pregnancies and/or genetic counselling.

Maternal death

Maternal death is fortunately rare in the United Kingdom. The national report on maternal death (Centre for Maternal and Child Enquiries (CMACE) 2011) which is published every three years identified several factors such as: obesity, social exclusion, domestic abuse and substance misuse. These are challenges that are increasingly evident in midwifery practice. An important factor in reducing maternal death is early identification of those at risk and the advocacy of a known midwife. Any maternal death is subject to formal enquiry (in order to compile a national report as noted above) and midwives will be asked to complete documentation relating to this, as will obstetricians and any other relevant healthcare professionals. This is so that any lessons that can be learnt from each individual maternal death can lead to any appropriate changes in practice.

The woman's partner and family will need emotional and practical support. They may be trying to deal with the loss of both mother and baby or to cope with the care of a baby in the absence of his/her mother. Grief may affect their behaviour and there may be disagreements about who should be doing what which will need tact and diplomacy from the midwives. There may also be legal issues to be addressed where the parents of the baby were not married.

Peer support for midwives

Midwives providing care in any situation where life is lost will be affected by their own feelings of loss and grief. This will not be as intense as the family's emotions, but will nonetheless affect their overall wellbeing. Peer support is essential in helping midwives deal with their feelings. The need for confidentiality means that unless they can talk to a colleague things can get 'bottled up'. The role of the Supervisor of Midwives is central to support following difficult situations and midwives should always access their Supervisor of Midwives for this. However, the support of close colleagues can make a significant difference. It is very easy to forget the needs of our colleagues when everyone is busy, but some will feel isolated and perhaps even feel that their peers are blaming them if people do not make an effort to speak to them. Just asking if they are alright or if they need to talk can make all the difference.

Support groups

There are a number of support groups available for parents and families who have lost a baby. SANDS the Stillbirth and Neonatal Death Society provide a helpline, an information service; publications and have local groups run by bereaved parents throughout the UK. SANDS also provide support and information for healthcare professionals.

The Miscarriage Association support women and families who have experienced miscarriage, ectopic or molar (hydatidiform mole) pregnancies. As with SANDS they provide information and have a helpline. The association also provides information for professionals.

There are also organisations that provide support in relation to specific conditions such as Anencephaly Support Group and general bereavement support organisations such as Cruse Bereavement Care who provide support for all those experiencing bereavement. There are also faith-based organisations.

Most organisations have websites and can therefore be found by a quick internet search, including many details for the three major organisations relevant to bereavement within maternity care, but remember that each woman and family member may have individual needs and there may be a group or organisation that will be better placed to meet that need, so it is important to talk to them about what they expect from bereavement support. Support groups may help, but access to formal counselling services should still be made available.

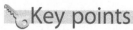
Key points

- Theories of loss and grief are useful in understanding reactions and providing effective care.
- Care needs to be respectful and sensitive to individual needs not prescriptive.
- Working with other agencies and voluntary organisations can enhance care.

Conclusion

Fortunately midwives do not have to deal with loss and grief too often, but this can make it even more challenging to care for and support women and their families when a baby dies. It is important therefore that the theories of grief are understood and that midwives know how and where to access information about cultural and religious issues relating to death and grief and also about support groups (see Box 17.5) both locally and nationally. This chapter has summarised some of the key issues and highlighted some of the circumstances that may be encountered in relation to modern midwifery practice. Good communication skills and a caring approach to the women and their families are central to good practice in this area, and gaining knowledge in respect of theory and services can only serve to enhance the care and support provided.

Box 17.5   Contact details for support groups

SANDS
28, Portland Place
London W1B 1LY
Tel: 020 7436 7940
Helpline: 020 7436 5881
Website: http://www.uk-sands.org/

The Miscarriage Association
17, Wentworth Terrace
Wakefield WF1 3QW
Tel: 01924 200795
Helpline: 01924 200799
Website: http://www.miscarriageassociation.org.uk/

Cruse Bereavement Care
PO Box 800
Richmond
Surrey TW9 1RG
Tel: 020 89399530
Helpline: 0844 4779400
Website: http://www.cruse.org.uk/

Glossary of terms

Bereavement   Is the state of having experienced a loss and is often associated with the period of time following the loss.

Grief   Is a natural and personal response to loss and are multidimensional involving emotional, physical, behavioural, cognitive, social and spiritual aspects.

Maternal death   Death during or within a year of pregnancy.

Mementoes   Keepsakes for parents such as foot and hand prints, photographs.

Miscarriage   A spontaneous loss of a pregnancy before 20 weeks.

Mourning   The active and outward expression of grief and contributes to its resolution.

Neonatal death   One that occurs within a month of birth.

Stillbirth   is legally defined as a baby born after the 24th week of pregnancy that has not breathed or shown any sign of life.

Theories   Theoretical ideas about how people grieve.

> *We were parents*
> *You played hide and seek*
> *through our dreams for years*
> *before you arrived.*
>
> *Then, once we'd tigged you*
> *– that squirm of blur*
> *inside that pulsing screen –*
>
> *we lay at night trying*
> *not to giggle; straining*
> *to hear your heartbeat.*
>
> *You made us laugh a lot,*
> *and disagree, and talk till 3am*
> *of names, and whose nose you'd get.*
>
> *And then you, who had lived*
> *with us such a blink of time,*
> *left.*
>
> *And we are left, holding*
> *onto nothing but naming books,*
> *and our lurching world.*
>
> *For you braced your whole*
> *13 cm self, and threw our*
> *planet off its axis.*

Reproduced with permission of poet and playwright, Char March, www.charmarch.co.uk

End of chapter activities

Find out more

The following activities will help you apply the content of this chapter to your place of work and enhance your knowledge of bereavement and loss.

1. Read the local policies and guidelines relevant to the loss of a baby (at any stage of pregnancy and in the neonatal period). Ask colleagues about mementoes and other care practices within maternity and neonatal services.

2. Find out about local support groups and the information available in your place of work about these groups. Do you need more information? Is there a need for more information about faith-based groups relevant to your client groups?

3. Try and gain more information about the religious practices you are most likely to have to facilitate (e.g. if you have a high number of Muslim women accessing care try and find out what is required for the major groups within the Islamic faith). A genuine wish to improve services should be received well by religious leaders and groups, but you will need to ensure your approach is professional and tactful.

4. Read more about theories of bereavement and loss using the references and further reading lists for this chapter and any other relevant material you may find.

References

Bowlby, J. (1973) *Attachment and Loss: Separation, Anxiety and Anger Vol II*. London: Hogarth Press.

Buglass, E. (2010) Grief and bereavement theories. *Nursing Standard* 24 (41), pp. 44–47.

Centre for Maternal and Child Enquiries (2011) Saving Mothers' Lives. *BJOG* 118, pp. 1–203.

Greenstreet, W. (2004) Why nurses need to understand the principles of bereavement theory. *British Journal of Nursing* 13 (10), pp. 590–593.

Kohner, N., Henley, A. (2009) *When a Baby Dies: The Experience of Late Miscarriage, Stillbirth and Neonatal Death* (revised edn). London: Routledge.

Kübler-Ross, E. (1969) *On Death and Dying*. New York: Macmillan.

Mander, R. (2006) *Loss and Bereavement in Childbearing*. Abingdon: Routledge.

Nordlund, E. Borjesson, A. Cacciatore, J. Pappas, C. Randers, I., Radestad, I. (2012) When a baby dies: Motherhood, psychosocial care and negative affect. *British Journal of Midwifery* 20 (11), pp. 780–784.

Parkes, C.M. (1998) Bereavement in adult life. *British Medical Journal* 316 (7134), pp. 856–859.

Rando, T.A. (1985) Bereaved parents: particular difficulties, unique factors and treatment issues. *Social Work* 30 (1), pp. 19–23.

Rando, T.A. (1986) *Parental Loss of a Child*. Champaign, IL: Research Press Company.

Rubin, S.S., Malkinson, R. (1993) The death of a child is forever: The life course impact of child loss. In: Stroebe, M.S., Stroebe, W., Hansson, R.O. (1993) *Handbook of Bereavement: Theory, Research and Intervention*. New York: Cambridge University Press, pp. 285–299.

Schott, J., Henley, A. (1996) *Culture, Religion and Childbearing in a Multiracial Society*. Oxford: Butterworth Heinemann.

Stillbirth Definition Act (1992) available on: http://www.legislation.gov.uk/ukpga/1992/29/pdfs/ukpga _19920029_en.pdf

Stillbirth and Neonatal Death Charity (SANDS) (1995).

Stroebe, M.S. (1998) New directions in bereavement research: exploration of gender differences. *Palliative Medicine* 12 (1), pp. 5–12.

Stroebe, M.S., Stroebe, W., Hansson, R.O. (1993) *Handbook of Bereavement: Theory, Research and Intervention*. Cambridge: Cambridge University Press.

Walter, T. (2010) Grief and culture: a checklist. *Bereavement Care* 29 (2), pp. 5–9.

Worden, J.W. (1982) *Grief Counselling and Grief Therapy: A Handbook for the Mental Health Practitioner*. New York: Springer.

Worden, J.W. (1996) *Children and Grief: When a Parent Dies*. New York: Guilford Press.

Chapter 1 To be a Midwife

Crossword solution grid:

Across
- 5. CLINICAL REASONING
- 8. HIGH QUALITY
- 9. PARTNERSHIP
- 10. RESPONSIBLE
- 13. RESPECT
- 15. PROBLEM SOLVE
- 16. SOCIALISATION
- 18. COMPASSION

Down
- 1. RESILIENCE
- 2. SUPERVISOR OF MIDWIVES
- 3. CARING
- 4. RECORD KEEPING
- 5. COMMUNICATION
- 6. ONE HUNDRED
- 7. DIRECTED
- 11. PEOPLE
- 12. SKILL
- 14. NMC
- 17. TITLE / LEARN

Fundamentals of Midwifery: A Textbook for Students, First Edition. Edited by Louise Lewis.
© 2015 John Wiley & Sons, Ltd. Published 2015 by John Wiley & Sons, Ltd.
Companion website: www.wileyfundamentalseries.com/midwifery

Chapter 2 Teamworking

```
                    ¹H                              ²O
                     U                               P
      ³P             M        ⁴C                      T
   ⁵W O M A N        I     ⁶C O U R A G E             I
      W             L        L                       M
      ⁷E F F E C T I V E L E ⁸A D E R ⁹S H I P
      R             T        A       C       B       S
                    Y        B       C       A       M
                             O       O       R
              ¹⁰H A N D O V E R       U
                             A       N
      ¹¹M A N A G E M E N T   T      ¹²R
                             I       A   O
                             O    ¹³B U L L Y I N G
      ¹⁴T A K E A C T I O N   I       E
                             L       M
                      ¹⁵S    I       O
              ¹⁶M O T I V A T E D
                      X       Y       E
                             L
```

Chapter 3

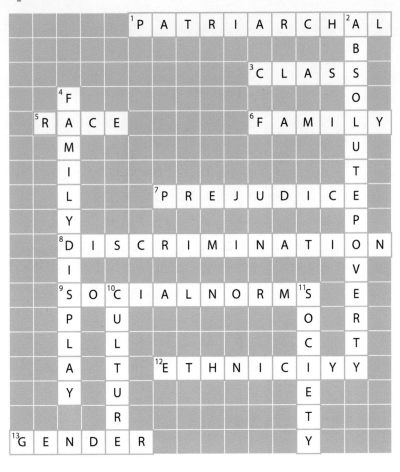

Chapter 4

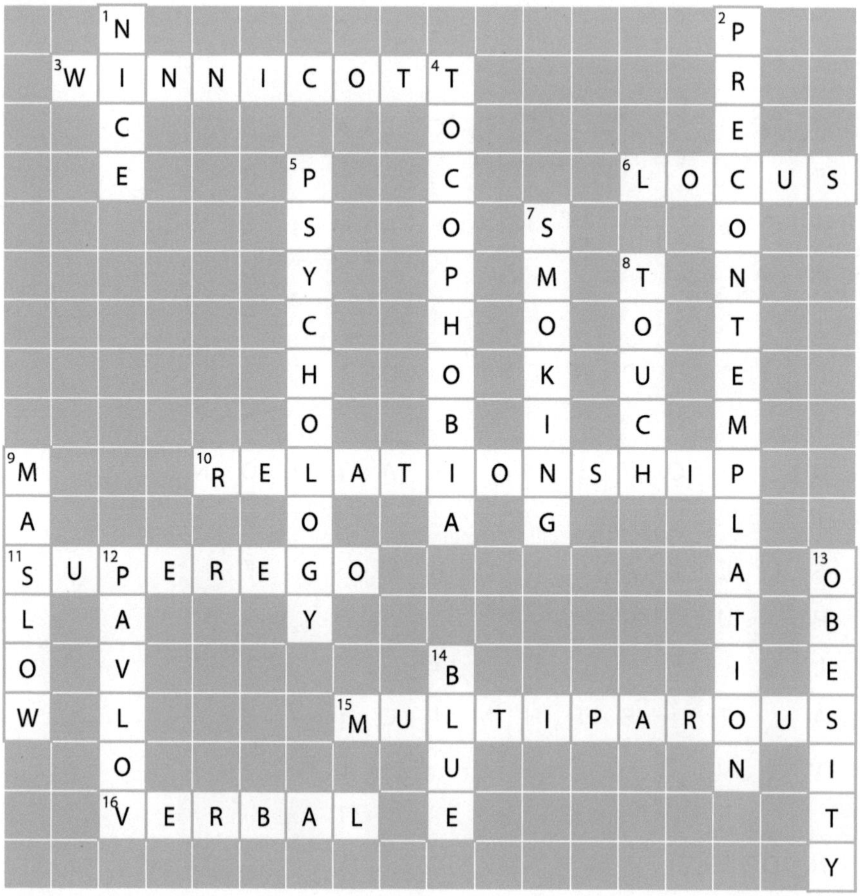
1 NICE
2 PRECONTEMPLATION
3 WINNICOTT
4 TOCOPHOBIA
5 PSYCHOLOGY
6 LOCUS
7 SMOKING
8 TOUCH
9 MASLOW
10 RELATIONSHIP
11 SUPEREGO
12 PAVLOV
13 OBESITY
14 BLUE
15 MULTIPAROUS
16 VERBAL

Chapter 5

				¹B	L	E	N	D	²E	D		³C
									X			O
		⁴P	⁵R	E	P	A	R	A	T	I	O	N
			O					E				F
			U	⁶T		⁷A		N				I
⁸S			T	R		D		D				N
U			I	A		V		E				E
R			N	D		A		D				M
R			E	I		N						E
O				T		C						N
G		⁹A	D	O	L	E	S	C	E	N	T	
A				N		D						
T				A								
¹⁰F	E	R	T	I	L	I	T	Y				

Chapter 6

Across

7. TOXOPLASMOSIS
9. MIDWIFERYLED
12. MONITOR
13. NULLIPAROUS
14. TRIMESTER

Down

1. CERVIX
2. GUIDELINE
3. ENGAGEMENT
4. ANTENATAL
5. MATERNITY
6. CONSTIPATION
8. PHLEBOTOMIST
10. WHOOLEY
11. ABNORMAL

Chapter 7

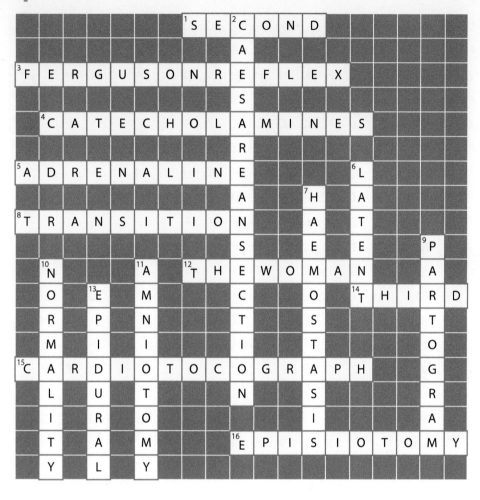

Crossword solution:

1 Across: SECOND
2 Down: CAESARSEAN
3 Across: FERGUSONREFLEX
4 Across: CATECHOLAMINES
5 Across: ADRENALINE
6 Down: LATEE
7 Down: HATE
8 Across: TRANSITION
9 Down: PATOGRAGRA
10 Down: NORMALITY
11 Down: AMNIOTOMY
12 Across: THEWOMAN
13 Down: EPIDURAL
14 Across: THIRD
15 Across: CARDIOTOCOGRAPH
16 Across: EPISIOTOMY

Chapter 8

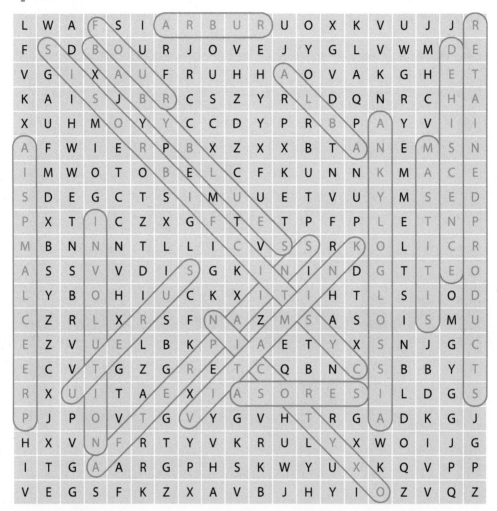

1. Physiological process of the uterus returning to be a pelvic organ: involution
2. Often detected within the antenatal period but may occur postnatally: pre eclampsia
3. May manifest with a pyrexia, inflammation and painful breasts: mastitis
4. The hormone secreted by the posterior pituitary gland at the initiation of the baby sucking at the breast: oxytocin
5. Three words used to describe the stages and colour of lochia: rubra, serosa, alba
6. May be detected from newborn bloodspot screening: cystic fibrosis
7. May present clinically as; a tender uterus on abdominal palpation, excessive and or offensive lochia and or pyrexia retained products
8. Mother feeling emotional and tearful around the third day postnatally, referred to as baby blues
9. Returns to a pelvic organ after approximately 10-14 days uterus
10. Name used to describe the breakdown and separation of caesarean section wound site dehiscence

11. Postpartum contractions, often stronger in multiparous women afterpains
12. Recommended for newborns as a prophylaxis treatment after birth to prevent haemorrhagic disease vitamin K
13. Alternative name for tongue tie Ankyloglossia
14. Number of blood spots required on the specimen sample for completion of newborn screening four

Chapter 9

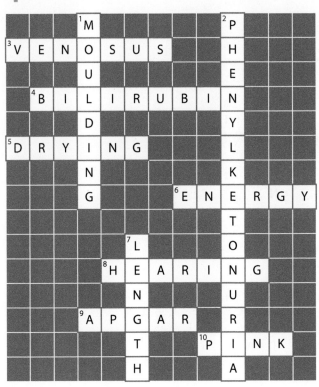

Chapter 10

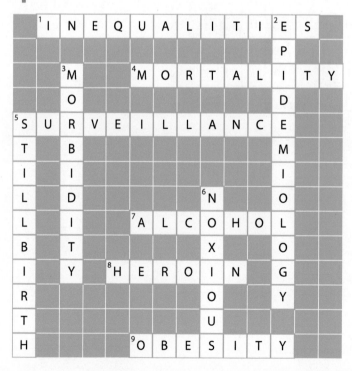

Crossword solution (Chapter 10):

Across:
2. OXYTOCIN
3. PROGESTERONE
7. LACTIFEROUS
8. LACTOCYTES
9. FULL

Down:
1. MYPEPIA
2. ENDED
4. ENDED
5. PROLACTIN
6. STRESS
7. LOBES
8. LIA

Chapter 11

Crossword solution (Chapter 11):

Across:
1. INEQUALITIES
4. MORTALITY
5. SURVEILLANCE
7. ALCOHOL
8. HEROIN
9. OBESITY

Down:
1. STILLBIRTH
2. EPIDEMIC
3. MORBIDITY
6. NOXIOUS

Chapter 12

¹C	O	²M	P	L	I	A	N	C	E	
		E								
		N					³S	I	X	
⁴V	A	S	E	⁵C	T	O	M	Y		
		T		O						
		R		I		⁶B	⁷F			
		U		L		A	E			
		A				R	M			
		T				R	I	⁸W		
		I				I	D	E		
⁹P	R	O	G	E	S	T	E	R	O	N	E
		N			R		M	K		

Chapter 13

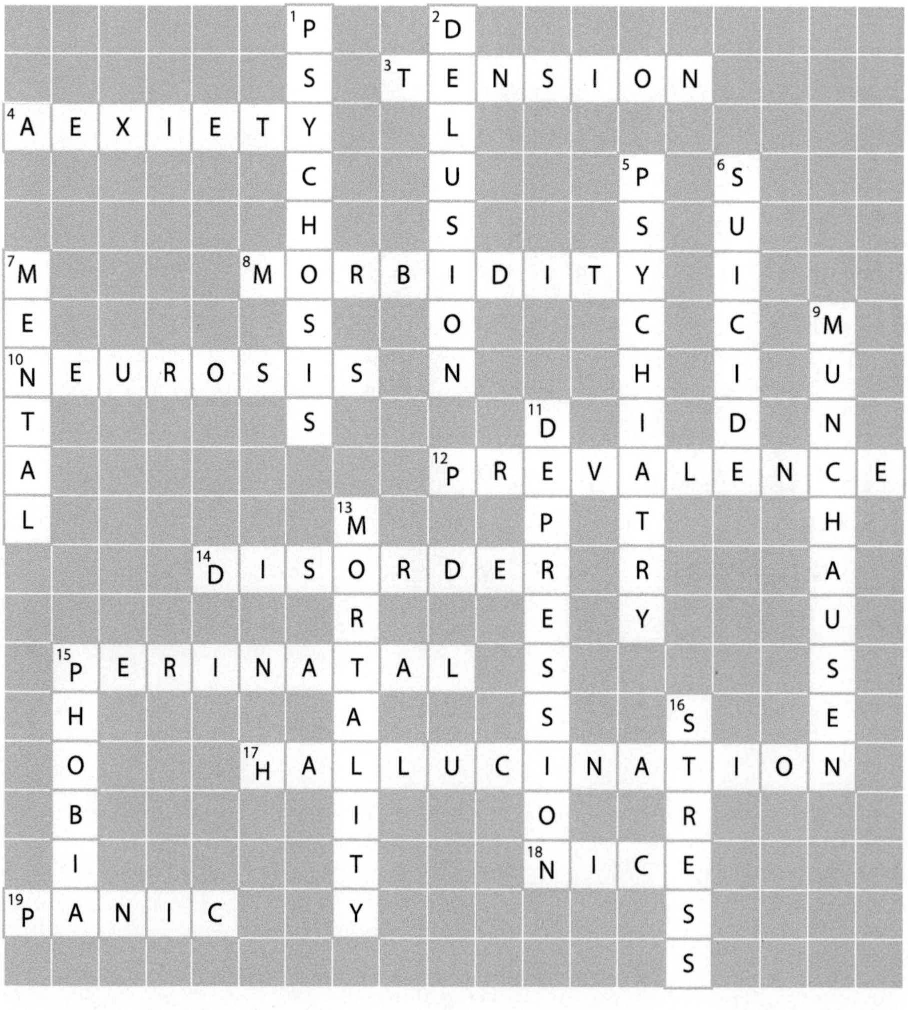

The crossword grid answers are:

Across:
- 3. TENSION
- 4. AEXIETY
- 8. MORBIDITY
- 10. NEUROSIS
- 12. PREVALENCE
- 14. DISORDER
- 15. PERINATAL
- 17. HALLUCINATION
- 18. NICE
- 19. PANIC

Down:
- 1. PSYCHIATRY
- 2. DELUSION
- 5. PSYCHIC
- 6. SUICIDE
- 7. MENTAL
- 9. MUNCHAUSES
- 11. DEPRESSRY
- 13. MORBIDITY
- 16. STRESSS

Chapter 14

Answers																			
E	+	+	+	+	+	+	+	+	+	+	+	+	+	+	+	+	R	+	+
H	R	+	Y	+	+	+	+	+	+	+	+	+	+	+	+	Y	E	+	+
R	C	U	+	D	+	+	+	+	+	+	+	+	+	+	H	S	G	+	+
C	E	R	T	H	O	M	E	O	P	A	T	H	Y	P	A	A	U	M	+
+	O	L	A	C	+	B	+	+	+	+	+	+	O	F	N	+	L	A	+
+	+	N	A	E	N	+	+	+	+	+	+	S	E	E	C	+	A	C	+
+	+	+	T	X	S	U	+	+	+	+	O	T	C	M	+	+	T	+	+
E	+	+	+	R	A	E	P	+	+	L	Y	D	N	+	+	+	I	+	+
N	+	+	Y	O	T	R	U	I	+	O	+	+	+	+	+	+	O	+	+
E	+	+	+	G	G	L	I	H	C	T	H	E	R	A	P	Y	N	+	+
R	+	+	+	O	N	+	P	O	E	A	E	C	N	E	D	I	V	E	L
G	+	+	+	L	I	+	+	S	N	+	+	+	+	+	+	+	+	A	+
Y	+	+	+	O	L	+	+	+	+	+	+	+	+	+	+	+	T	+	+
+	+	+	+	X	A	+	+	+	+	+	+	+	+	+	+	S	+	+	+
+	+	+	+	E	E	+	+	+	+	+	+	+	+	+	Y	+	+	+	+
+	+	+	+	L	H	+	+	+	+	+	+	+	R	+	+	+	+	+	+
+	+	+	+	F	+	+	E	C	I	O	H	C	C	+	+	+	+	+	+
Y	P	A	R	E	H	T	O	N	P	Y	H	+	+	+	+	+	+	+	+
+	+	+	+	R	+	+	+	+	+	+	+	+	+	+	+	+	+	+	+
+	+	+	+	+	+	+	+	+	+	+	+	+	+	+	+	+	+	+	+

(Over, Down, Direction)
ACUPUNCTURE (11, 11, NW)
ANECDOTES (17, 4, SW)
BODY (7, 5, NW)
CAM (19, 6, N)
CHOICE (13, 17, W)
CONTROL (1, 4, SE)
CRYSTAL (14, 17, NE)
ENERGY (1, 8, S)
EVIDENCE (19, 11, W)
HEALING (6, 16, N)

HOMEOPATHY (5, 4, E)
HYPNOTHERAPY (12, 18, W)
NMC (14, 8, NE)
PHILOSOPHY (8, 11, NE)
REFLEXOLOGY (5, 19, N)
REGULATION (18, 1, S)
RELAXATION (1, 3, SE)
RESEARCH (8, 9, NW)
SAFETY
THERAPY (11, 10, E)

Chapter 15

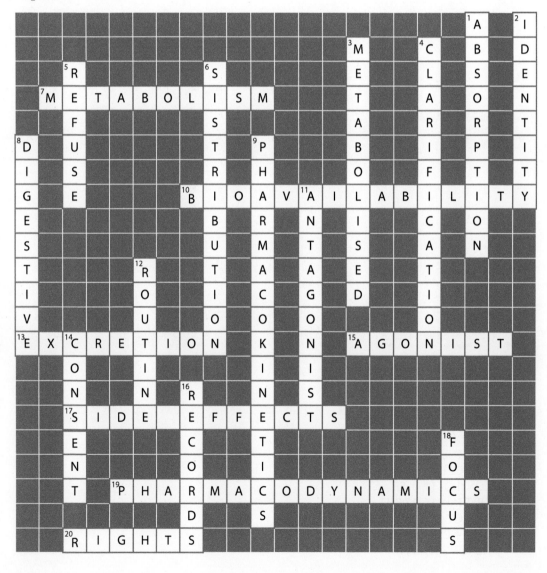

Chapter 16

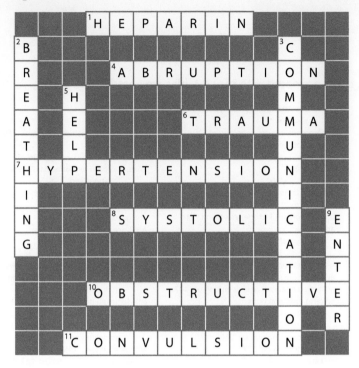

Index

Note: Figures are noted with f; boxes are noted with b; and tables are noted with t.

Fundamentals of Midwifery: A Textbook for Students, First Edition. Edited by Louise Lewis.
© 2015 John Wiley & Sons, Ltd. Published 2015 by John Wiley & Sons, Ltd.
Companion website: www.wileyfundamentalseries.com/midwifery